Common Enemies

Common Enemies

Disease Campaigns in America

RACHEL KAHN BEST

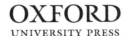

OXFORD
UNIVERSITY PRESS

OXFORD
UNIVERSITY PRESS

Oxford University Press is a department of the University of Oxford. It furthers
the University's objective of excellence in research, scholarship, and education
by publishing worldwide. Oxford is a registered trade mark of Oxford University
Press in the UK and certain other countries.

Published in the United States of America by Oxford University Press
198 Madison Avenue, New York, NY 10016, United States of America.

Library of Congress Cataloging-in-Publication Data
Names: Best, Rachel Kahn, 1982– author.
Title: Common enemies : disease campaigns in America / Rachel Kahn Best.
Description: New York, NY : Oxford University Press, [2019] |
Includes bibliographical references.
Identifiers: LCCN 2018059881 | ISBN 9780190918415 (pbk. : alk. paper) |
ISBN 9780190918408 (hardcover : alk. paper) | ISBN 9780190918422 (Universal PDF) |
ISBN 9780190918439 (electronic publication)
Subjects: LCSH: Medical policy—United States. |
Health services accessibility—United States. | Social medicine—United States. |
Social movements—United States.
Classification: LCC RA418.3.U6 B47 2019 |
DDC 362.10973—dc23
LC record available at https://lccn.loc.gov/2018059881

1 3 5 7 9 8 6 4 2

Paperback printed by Sheridan Books, Inc., United States of America
Hardback printed by Bridgeport National Bindery, Inc., United States of America

Contents

Acknowledgments

This project began as my dissertation in the sociology department at UC Berkeley, guided by four insightful and generous dissertation committee members. Mike Hout was always ready with perceptive comments on graphs and tables and advice on how to write prose that people might actually want to read. Each meeting with him yielded new ways to express quantitative data clearly. Meanwhile, some of the best ideas in this book were incubated in Ann Swidler's office. Ann is an uncommonly generous thinker. Each time I met with her, she would imagine the best possible argument I could make with my data and then forever remember it as my argument. Laurie Edelman was a sounding board, strategist, and collaborator, helping me navigate the process of research design and publication. Ann Keller contributed her expert understanding of patients' activism and provided insightful, detailed comments on my drafts. Other Berkeley faculty generously provided advice and comments, including Claude Fischer, Neil Fligstein, Marion Fourcade, Calvin Morrill, and Margaret Weir. I benefited from an incredible community of sociology graduate students, including many who read drafts of dissertation chapters. Special thanks go to Hana Brown, Sarah Garrett, Alex Janus, Daniel Laurison, Laura Mangels, and Sarah Quinn. At Berkeley, I also benefited from feedback from the Inequality Workshop; the Research Group on Multilevel Modeling; the Center for Culture, Organizations, and Politics; and the Empirical Legal Studies Workshop. A fantastic team of Berkeley undergraduates helped me collect data on congressional hearings: Caitlin Green, Sophie Harrison-Wong, Katherine Hood, David Lee, Willie Jo Marquez, Greg Mooney, Kate Sousa, and Shanna Zhu. When I traveled to NIH headquarters, Michael Boyle of the NIH Office of Budget and David Cantor and Barbara Harkins of the Office of NIH History provided invaluable assistance with data collection.

After completing my PhD, I collected additional data for the book as a Robert Wood Johnson Foundation Scholar in Health Policy Research at the University of Michigan. During my fellowship, Chris Bail, Rick Hall, Daniel Lee, Helen Levy, and Edward Norton were especially generous with their time and feedback. The administrative support of Gail Pieknik and Theresa Ramirez facilitated the project immensely. Nate Carroll, Anup Das, David Jones, Nelson Saldana, Mrinalini Tavag, Jay Thaker, and Qing Zheng provided incomparable research assistance. Staff at the Schlesinger Library at the Radcliffe Institute for Advanced Study helped me navigate the archives.

Drawing on data from my dissertation and postdoctoral research, I wrote the book while a faculty member in the Department of Sociology at the University of Michigan. My Michigan colleagues have been impossibly generous, reading drafts of my work and providing sage advice. Thanks are due to Barbara Anderson, Renee Anspach, Elizabeth A. Armstrong, Jennifer Barber, Deirdre Bloome, Sarah Burgard, Rob Jansen, Jaeeun Kim, Greta Krippner, Sandra Levitsky, Roi Livne, Alexandra Murphy, Jason Owen-Smith, Pam Smock, and Kiyoteru Tsutsui. Scholars from other campuses, including Elizabeth M. Armstrong, Phil Brown, Paul Burstein, Steve Epstein, Emily Marshall, Isaac Martin, Stefan Timmermans, and Edward Walker, also provided comments and advice. I owe an especially large debt to Barbara Anderson, Renee Anspach, Elizabeth A. Armstrong, Elizabeth M. Armstrong, Jessica Garrick, Sandra Levitsky, Roi Livne, Jason Owen-Smith, and Edward Walker for reading the full manuscript. I received fantastic research assistance from Jessica Garrick, Dana Kornberg, and Johanna Masse. Librarians Hailey Mooney and Justin Joque provided important advice and assistance.

I also received generous and insightful feedback from anonymous reviewers at the *American Sociological Review*; the *Journal of Health Politics, Policy, and Law*; and Oxford University Press. Both journals provided permission to reuse portions of the articles I published there.[1] My editor, James Cook, has been a thoughtful and calming influence, helping shepherd the manuscript through the publication process. I received excellent feedback at several seminars, workshops, and conferences, including talks at the University of Arizona, Duke University, the University of Michigan, and the annual meetings of the American Sociological Association and the Robert Wood Johnson Foundation Scholars in Health Policy Research. Research funds were provided by the Office of NIH History; the UC Berkeley Science, Technology and Society Center; Berkeley Law's Empirical Legal Studies fellowship; the Robert Wood Johnson Foundation; and the University of Michigan.

[1] Best, "Disease Politics and Medical Research Funding"; Best, "Disease Campaigns and the Decline of Treatment Advocacy."

I am also grateful for my friends and family. Nick and Yen Azzaro, Todd and Tanya Berenz, Erin Bonar, Zlato Buchs Fagundes, Kate Duchowny, and Grace and Edward Kim spent a Thanksgiving dinner helping me brainstorm titles for this book. My grandfather, Alfred Kahn, an economist, encouraged me to do research that would make the world better and not just be an "exercise in econometrics." My mother, Hannah Kahn, a choreographer, showed me how to turn creativity into daily labor, sometimes exhilarating and often tedious, and how to manage the anxiety associated with letting people see your completed work. My father, Arthur Best, a law professor, inspired a commitment to logical thinking and a fascination with empirical patterns and always combined productivity with humor and self-deprecation. My husband, Holice Kil, has shared laughter and non-sociological conversation and has worked with me to build an egalitarian marriage, a goal that required wrestling with more biological, logistical, and cultural constraints than I ever expected. Our children, Fred and Edie, have provided a welcome break from research and writing. I apologize to them for this book's disappointing lack of superheroes, animals, and illustrations.

I have been incredibly lucky to work at institutions that gave me the time and freedom I needed to complete this project. As a graduate student at Berkeley, I received funding and support to spend several years conducting independent and unpredictable dissertation research. My postdoctoral fellowship from the Robert Wood Johnson Foundation gave me two years with few external obligations, time that let me rethink my dissertation project, expand its scope, and double the amount of data. As an assistant professor at the University of Michigan, I twice received time off teaching and a delay in my tenure clock after giving birth to a baby. This time allowed me to figure out how to be a parent, teacher, and writer simultaneously. The university also provided generous start-up research funds that let me complete this project without seeking grant funding. The staff at Gretchen's House Childcare Center, particularly Paula Steffen and Banu Bostanci, provided expertise, warmth, and love that let me be in my office from 9 to 5 without worrying about my children. These luxuries are increasingly rare as PhD programs reduce time to degree, the postdoctoral fellowship I received has been discontinued, many faculty members teach more courses and receive less internal research funding, and excellent childcare is rare and expensive. Having received so many advantages, I feel a great responsibility for this book to really be something special. If it falls short, the fault is all mine.

Abbreviations

ACS	American Cancer Society
ACT UP	AIDS Coalition to Unleash Power
ADA	American Diabetes Association
ADHD	attention deficit hyperactivity disorder
AHA	American Heart Association
AIDS	acquired immune deficiency syndrome
BCA	Budget Control Act of 2011
BEA	Budget Enforcement Act of 1990
BRDPI	Biomedical Research and Development Price Index
CDC	Centers for Disease Control and Prevention
CF	cystic fibrosis
CGD	Taft Corporate Giving Directory
COPD	chronic obstructive pulmonary disease
CP	cerebral palsy
CPI-U-RS	Current Population Index research series using current methods
DALYs	disability-adjusted life years
DOD	Department of Defense
DOD-CDMRP	Department of Defense Congressionally Directed Medical Research Program
FDA	Food and Drug Administration
FY	fiscal year
GRH	Gramm-Rudman-Hollings Balanced Budget and Emergency Deficit Control Act of 1985
HHS	Health and Human Services
HIV	human immunodeficiency virus
ICD	International Classification of Diseases
IOM	Institute of Medicine
IRS	Internal Revenue Service
MDA	Muscular Dystrophy Association
NBCC	National Breast Cancer Coalition
NCCS	National Center for Charitable Statistics
NCI	National Cancer Institute

NHC	National Health Council
NIAID	National Institute of Allergy and Infectious Diseases
NIH	National Institutes of Health
NMSS	National Multiple Sclerosis Society
NTA	National Tuberculosis Association
NTEE	National Taxonomy of Exempt Entities
OMB	Office of Management and Budget
PHS	Public Health Service
PSA	prostate-specific antigen
RCDC	Research, Condition, and Disease Classification system
RPG	research project grant
UCP	United Cerebral Palsy
WFA	Women's Field Army
WHO	World Health Association

Common Enemies

Introduction

Diseases in American Public Life

In the mid-twentieth century, fewer than 1% of Americans identified health as the most important problem facing the country.[1] But if their answers to public opinion polls suggested a lack of interest in health, their actions showed something different. Three quarters of urban Americans donated to a campaign against tuberculosis, ushering in an era of mass philanthropy.[2] Millions of mothers knocked on doors collecting dimes to fight polio, welcomed by porch lights signaling that a majority of households were waiting to donate.[3] They raised more than any charity in history except the Red Cross.[4] Millions more volunteered to fight cancer and heart disease.[5]

By 2010, disease campaigns still eclipsed collective responses to seemingly more important problems. Only 1% of Americans chose disease as "the most important problem facing the world in the future," while 14% focused on global warming and threats to the environment.[6] Yet three times as many participated in the Race for the Cure than joined the largest march against climate change.[7] Breast cancer patients and their friends and families filled the streets of dozens of cities, raising hundreds of millions of dollars a year to fight breast cancer.[8] Like the mid-century marching mothers, twenty-first-century Americans felt comfortable asking their friends and neighbors to help fight disease. Millions emptied buckets of ice water on their heads and asked their Facebook friends for donations to

---

[1] McCombs and Zhu, "Capacity, Diversity, and Volatility," 511.
[2] Carter, *Gentle Legions*, 19; Marts, *Generosity of Americans*, 127; Sills, *Volunteers*, 176–78, 182; Zunz, *Philanthropy in America*.
[3] Sills, *Volunteers*, 160.
[4] Oshinsky, *Polio*, 69.
[5] American Association of Fund-Raising Counsel, "Giving USA," 9.
[6] Yeager et al., "Measuring Americans' Issue Priorities," 129.
[7] Dastagir, "Climate-Change March"; Munguia, "How Many People"; Susan G. Komen Breast Cancer Foundation, "Race for the Cure."
[8] Sulik, *Pink Ribbon Blues*; Susan G. Komen for the Cure, *2010–2011 Annual Report*.

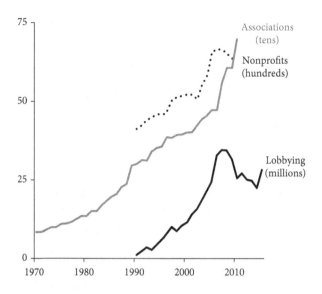

Figure I.1   Growth of disease advocacy, 1970–2015

Number of disease-related voluntary associations (tens); number of disease-related nonprofits with budgets over $25,000 in constant 1987 dollars (hundreds); total lobbying expenditures by disease organizations (millions).

fight amyotrophic lateral sclerosis.[9] Disease awareness ribbons decorated an ever-expanding array of consumer products.[10] Hundreds of national voluntary associations and thousands of nonprofits targeted diseases, and disease advocates lined up to lobby Congress (see Figure I.1).

Disease philanthropy and activism have spurred medical advances, from the polio vaccine to treatments for HIV/AIDS. In academia, fully two-thirds of research and development funding now goes to the life sciences.[11] In the public sector, the political appeal of fighting disease has led the United States to fund more biomedical research than any other country in the world.[12] Exposed to a dizzying array of awareness campaigns, Americans feel less healthy and seek screening and treatment for more and more conditions.[13]

---

[9] ALS Association, "ALS Ice Bucket Challenge"; ALS Association, "What We Do"; Serres, "Two Years Later"; Steel, "Ice Bucket Challenge."

[10] Charity Walks Blog, "Charity Walk Events"; craftsnscraps.com, "Awareness Ribbon Colors."

[11] Stephan, *How Economics Shapes Science*, 237.

[12] Murphy and Topel, "Introduction," 2.

[13] Brownlee, *Overtreated*, 199; Welch, Schwartz, and Woloshin, *Overdiagnosed*, 8–9, 89, 198.

Why are diseases the problems Americans come together to address? Why do some diseases attract more attention than others? And how has fighting one disease at a time changed how we distribute charitable dollars and which health policies we pursue? Answering these questions requires tracing the records left by thousands of organizations targeting hundreds of diseases. Drawing on the first comprehensive data on a century of disease campaigns, this book reveals why disease campaigns became so central to American public life, why certain diseases rose to prominence, and how fighting one disease at a time changes how we distribute resources, conceptualize problems, and promote health.

The common enemies we can agree to fight may not be the greatest threats to our collective well-being. Disease campaigns tend to concentrate resources on a few favored diseases, systematically neglect stigmatized conditions, and prioritize uncontroversial goals. Yet the same forces that limit the potential of individual disease campaigns to improve our health also stimulate the vast outpouring of resources. Disease campaigns are limited and lopsided but also big-hearted and bounteous, and they do more good than harm.

Shifting the Focus to Disease Campaigns

Because of the limited ways we study agendas and advocacy, scholars still don't know why disease campaigns became so prominent or how they have changed charity and public policy. To answer these questions, researchers must look beyond contentious politics and explore the creation of consensus. And they must zoom out from individual organizations to understand fields of interacting organizations and movements.

From Conflict to Consensus

Researchers have studied individual disease campaigns, but their theoretical interests have led them to focus on the most contentious ones. Ironically, *because* health movements have been so generative for answering questions about medicalization, biomedicine, and expertise, we've "sampled" them in a way that doesn't let our knowledge accumulate to an accurate understanding of the whole field. Scholars interested in how conditions come to be understood as medical have focused on movements targeting contested illnesses, from Gulf War–related illness to fibromyalgia.[14] Scholars focused on challenges to the rising power of corporations in biomedicine focus on relatively radical disease campaigns and those that identify environmental effects on health.[15] Scholars focused on changing relations between experts and laypeople seek out movements that redefine expertise and broaden lay participation in science and medicine.[16] These studies have disproportionately focused on the most contentious and political disease campaigns. We've paid much less attention to bigger, more bureaucratic organizations that target established diseases and defer to scientific expertise.

This disproportionate focus on the most contentious disease campaigns reflects a broader bias in work on social movements and agenda setting. Scholars tend to assume that real politics involves conflict, and so they study contentious issues and clashing values.[17] For instance, one influential article argued that "any social movement of potential political significance will generate opposition."[18] Some define their object of study as "contentious politics."[19] Studies of agenda setting define an issue as "a conflict between two or more identifiable groups" and the agenda as "a general set of political controversies."[20] Scholars describe social problems as involving

[14] Armstrong, *Conceiving Risk, Bearing Responsibility*; Barker, *The Fibromyalgia Story*; Barrett, "Illness Movements"; Brown, *Toxic Exposures*; Brown et al., "Gulf of Difference"; Brown et al., "Embodied Health Movements"; Brown et al., "Health Politics of Asthma"; Brown, Morello-Frosch, and Zavestoski, *Contested Illnesses*; Cable, Shriver, and Mix, "Risk Society and Contested Illness"; Conrad and Potter, "From Hyperactive Children"; Dumit, "Illnesses You Have to Fight to Get"; Kempner, *Not Tonight*; Klawiter, *Biopolitics of Breast Cancer*; Kroll-Smith and Floyd, *Bodies in Protest*; McCormick, *No Family History*; Saguy and Riley, "Weighing Both Sides"; Taylor, *Rock-a-by Baby*; Zavestoski et al., "Science, Policy, Activism, and War."

[15] Brown, *Toxic Exposures*; Brown et al., "Health Politics of Asthma"; Clarke et al., "Biomedicalization," 184; Hess, "Beyond Scientific Controversies"; McCormick, *No Family History*; Murphy, *Sick Building Syndrome*.

[16] Anglin, "Working from the Inside Out"; Bell, *DES Daughters*; Bix, "Disease Chasing Money and Power"; Brown et al., "Embodied Health Movements"; Brown et al., "Gulf of Difference"; Callon and Rabeharisoa, "Growing Engagement"; Epstein, *Impure Science*; Hess, "Medical Modernisation"; Hogg, *Patients, Power & Politics*; Murphy, *Sick Building Syndrome*; Panofsky, "Generating Sociability"; Rabeharisoa, "Experience, Knowledge and Empowerment"; Rabeharisoa and Callon, "Involvement of Patients' Associations"; Taylor, *Rock-a-by Baby*; Wehling, Viehover, and Koenen, *Public Shaping*.

[17] Armstrong, *Forging Gay Identities*, 6, 12; Downey, "Elaborating Consensus," 337; Lowi, "American Business," 681; McCarthy and Wolfson, "Consensus Movements," 273; Nelson, *Making an Issue of Child Abuse*, 29; Polletta, "Mobilization Forum," 475.

[18] Meyer and Staggenborg, "Movements, Countermovements," 1630. Some movements are rarely studied because they "are so unambitious in their aims or moderate in their tactics as to be boring" to researchers. Polletta, "Mobilization Forum," 476.

[19] McAdam, Tarrow, and Tilly, *Dynamics of Contention*.

[20] Cobb and Elder, *Participation in American Politics*, 82, 14; see also Nelson, *Making an Issue of Child Abuse*, 27.

"the values and interests of various groups which are frequently in direct or indirect opposition to each other."[21] And so when researchers collect data on which issues are targeted by social movements, they often track which issues people *protest* about, revealing the prominence of civil rights, human rights, women's rights, the environment, education, and peace.[22] But these may not be the same issues for which people raise money from their neighbors, companies advertise their support, and politicians compete to claim credit for addressing.

Studies of public agenda setting take a seemingly more neutral approach, asking people to identify the "most important problem facing this country today." The most common answers include crime, the economy, the environment, and international relations.[23] But when people actually volunteer, donate, and march, they focus on a very different set of problems than they mention in surveys. Few people would rank breast cancer as the most important problem facing our nation. But for many, a "race for the cure" might be their only participation in a public event to target a problem. Volunteers often avoid activities that seem "political" or controversial, focusing instead on problems that feel "close to home" and "do-able," selecting uncontroversial goals like supporting schools and opposing drugs.[24] To understand why some issues attract more attention than others, we need to complement data on opinions and protests with data on organizations and finances, tracking where people actually put their time and money.

Uncontroversial campaigns are sometimes called "consensus movements" or "valence issues," supported by large majorities and attracting little or no organized opposition.[25] Theorists suggest that consensus campaigns tend to be short-lived and subnational since as movements grow in scope and geography, they will almost invariably challenge existing interests and attract controversy.[26] But there is reason to believe that they may actually persist,

---

[21] Haines, "Depoliticization of Social Problems," 120.

[22] Bearman and Everett, "Structure of Social Protest"; Jung, King, and Soule, "Issue Bricolage."

[23] Jennings and Wlezien, "Distinguishing Between Most Important Problems"; McCombs and Zhu, "Capacity, Diversity, and Volatility"; Yeager et al., "Measuring Americans' Issue Priorities."

[24] Of course, there are things about schools and drugs that could arouse debate, but volunteers tend to define them in ways that maximize consensus—for instance, arguing that a campaign is "for the children," a frame that makes the solutions seem "obvious to anyone with common sense." Eliasoph, *Avoiding Politics*, 23, 2, 44, 61, 246.

[25] Baumgartner and Jones, *Agendas and Instability*, 150–51; Campbell et al., *Elections and the Political Order*, 170–74; Downey, "Elaborating Consensus"; Lofland, "Consensus Movements"; Lofland, *Polite Protesters*; McCarthy and Wolfson, "Consensus Movements," 273–74; Nelson, *Making an Issue of Child Abuse*, 27.

[26] McCarthy and Wolfson, "Consensus Movements," 275.

grow, and attract resources. Social movements may be most successful when they imply "that justice and the common good can be addressed at the level of national consensus."[27] Consensus movements can co-opt various groups, from friendship circles to churches to voluntary associations, attracting large numbers of volunteers.[28] Corporate money flows to "safe" issues.[29] Government agencies join in the pursuit of uncontroversial goals, and Congress finds it easier to distribute resources.[30] Disease campaigns have multiplied over the course of a century, changing how we fund medical research and promote public health. To observe these effects, we can't ignore consensus campaigns.

From Organizations to Fields

Despite a rich tradition of studying individual disease movements, we lack a comprehensive overview of disease campaigns. Most studies focus on a single organization or disease movement; a handful study several diseases but not the entire field.[31] These studies have yielded an important understanding of the roots of individual campaigns and the effects of particular movements.[32] But to understand disease advocacy in the aggregate—to document its historical prominence, explain its appeal, and trace its overall effects—we need data on diverse fields of organizations targeting multiple diseases over decades. These data depart from traditional methods of studying advocacy and agendas in two ways.

To understand disease campaigns, we first need to cast a wide net, accepting fuzzy boundaries between various types of advocacy.

---

[27] Bellah et al., *Habits of the Heart*, 200–203.

[28] Eliasoph, *Avoiding Politics*, 2, 44, 61, 246; McCarthy and Wolfson, "Consensus Movements," 284–85.

[29] Lofland, *Polite Protesters*, 69.

[30] Hayes, *Lobbyists and Legislators*, 32, 97; McCarthy and Wolfson, "Consensus Movements," 289.

[31] For reviews, see Brown et al., "Embodied Health Movements"; Epstein, "Patient Groups and Health Movements"; Epstein, "Politics of Health Mobilization"; Hess et al., "Science, Technology, and Social Movements"; Landzelius, "Patient Organization Movements"; Rabeharisoa, "Experience, Knowledge and Empowerment." A few researchers have conducted surveys of patients' organizations, but these cross-sectional data cannot accurately track changes in the field of disease campaigns over time. Baggott, Allsop, and Jones, *Speaking for Patients and Carers*; Keller and Packel, "Going for the Cure"; Wood, *Patient Power?*

[32] Case studies have identified disease movements that attracted research funding, changed how research is conducted, and transformed patients' experiences. For reviews, see Epstein, "Patient Groups and Health Movements"; Epstein, "Politics of Health Mobilization"; Hess et al., "Science, Technology, and Social Movements"; Rabeharisoa, "Experience, Knowledge and Empowerment."

Traditionally, scholars thought of social movements and interest groups as separate phenomena, defining social movements as marginalized groups adopting disruptive tactics and interest groups as political insiders using institutionalized tactics. But it's not easy to draw such a clean line in practice, both because these variables are continua, not dichotomies, and because individual organizations may adopt different strategies at different times.[33] I use the term "advocacy organizations" to refer to both interest groups and social movement organizations.[34] I use "disease campaigns" to refer to an even broader constellation of actors and organizations, including nonprofits and self-help groups that are not consciously political.[35] Since the boundaries between advocacy organizations and policymakers can also be fuzzy,[36] these campaigns can also include government actors and policies.

Second, studies of advocacy organizations rarely collect data across numerous issues and over time.[37] But understanding the effects of disease campaigns requires zooming out to study multiple organizations and movements, rather than narrowing our attention to individual advocacy organizations or single diseases. Existing studies also tend to focus on issues targeted by active movements or movements that achieved policy successes—sampling on the dependent variable in a way that makes it difficult to tell whether advocacy matters.[38] Looking across dozens of diseases,

---

[33] Andrews and Edwards, "Advocacy Organizations"; Burstein, "Interest Organizations"; Burstein, "Social Movements and Public Policy"; Gamson, *Strategy of Social Protest*, 138; McAdam, Tarrow, and Tilly, *Dynamics of Contention*; Polletta, "Mobilization Forum"; Tarrow, "Foreword."

[34] Andrews and Edwards, "Advocacy Organizations." Other scholars have adopted the terms "state-oriented challengers," "publics," and "interest organizations." Amenta and Caren, "Legislative, Organizational, and Beneficiary Consequences"; May, "Reconsidering Policy Design"; Burstein, "Interest Organizations."

[35] Polletta argues that "the lines separating movement groups from, say, interest groups, charities, terrorist organizations, unions, nongovernmental organizations, and self-help groups often reflect the idiosyncrasies of how subfields have developed rather than anything intrinsic to the phenomena themselves." Polletta, "Mobilization Forum," 475.

[36] Armstrong and Bernstein, "Culture, Power, and Institutions"; Epstein, *Inclusion*; Goldstone, *States, Parties, and Social Movements*; Santoro and McGuire, "Social Movement Insiders"; Skrentny, *Minority Rights Revolution*; Wolfson, *Big Tobacco*.

[37] Baumgartner and Leech, *Basic Interests*; Giugni, "How Social Movements Matter," xxiv; Heaney and Rojas, "Hybrid Activism," 1053; Larson and Soule, "Sector-Level Dynamics," 293; McAdam and Scott, "Organizations and Movements," 9; Minkoff, *Organizing for Equality*, 5. Scholars are aware of this problem, and increasing numbers have begun looking across multiple issues and over time. Baumgartner and Leech, *Basic Interests*; Bearman and Everett, "Structure of Social Protest"; Clemens, *The People's Lobby*; Gamson, *Strategy of Social Protest*; Giugni, *Social Protest and Policy Change*; Hojnacki et al., "Studying Organizational Advocacy," 390; Soule and King, "Competition and Resource Partitioning."

[38] Burstein, "Interest Organizations," 54; Leech, "Lobbying and Influence," 540; Olzak, "Analysis of Events," 121; for notable exceptions, see Biggs and Andrews, "Protest Campaigns and Movement Success"; Gamson, *Strategy of Social Protest*; King, Bentele, and Soule, "Protest and Policymaking."

including those not targeted by advocacy, allows for more conclusive tests of whether advocacy organizations secure benefits for their constituents—for example, did the National Breast Cancer Coalition convince the government to fund more breast cancer research?[39]

In addition to documenting the effects of individual advocacy organizations, field-level data can reveal how their outcomes interact. Do organizations or movements compete in a zero-sum game, fighting for space on a finite political agenda?[40] Or do they create opportunities for each other, operating synergistically?[41] For example, when breast cancer research funding increases, is the money being taken away from other diseases?

Finally, studying fields can reveal advocacy's aggregate effects, above and beyond the benefits achieved by any one campaign. In the policy arena, campaigns may introduce new ideas and understandings that shape policymaking.[42] For instance, did disease campaigns change the criteria that policymakers and scientists used to decide how to fund medical research? These aggregate effects only become visible with data on the field of disease campaigns over time.

Finding the Right Data

This book draws on multiple types of quantitative and qualitative data to provide the first comprehensive look at disease campaigns in America. Moving beyond studies of individual organizations or single diseases, I collected data on the entire field of disease campaigns over decades. Rather than relying on the recollections of living people, I sought out the traces that organizations leave in records and documents. Rather than building a narrow definition of advocacy into the sampling strategy, I compiled data on nonprofits, voluntary associations, congressional witnesses, and lobbyists. To answer questions about why some diseases have more advocacy than

---

[39] Amenta and Young, "Making an Impact"; Burstein, Einwohner, and Hollander, "Success of Political Movements"; Gamson, *Strategy of Social Protest.*

[40] Hilgartner and Bosk, "Rise and Fall of Social Problems"; Kingdon, *Agendas, Alternatives, and Public Policies*; McCombs, *Setting the Agenda*; Zhu, "Issue Competition."

[41] Hilgartner and Bosk, "Rise and Fall of Social Problems"; Kingdon, *Agendas, Alternatives, and Public Policies*; Skrentny, "Policy-Elite Perceptions"; Skrentny, *Minority Rights Revolution.*

[42] Armstrong and Bernstein, "Culture, Power, and Institutions"; Best, "Disease Politics and Medical Research Funding"; Campbell, "Ideas, Politics, and Public Policy"; Guetzkow, "Beyond Deservingness"; Rochefort and Cobb, "Agenda Access"; Stone, "Causal Stories."

others and whether advocacy shapes the research funding a disease receives, I created a quantitative data set with information on 92 diseases from 1960 to 2015. To understand which goals disease advocacy organizations pursue, I created a second data set with information on 1,744 unique disease advocacy organizations from 1960 to 2014. I also draw on qualitative data and secondary sources that date back to the beginning of the twentieth century. The data provide new insights into how fields of campaigns develop and how they change politics, policy, and society.

The *Encyclopedia of Associations* sheds light on over half a century of advocacy.[43] Since the 1950s, its publishers have tried to identify all national voluntary associations and asked them to describe their main goals and activities. Reading through the annual volumes, identifying disease-related organizations, and analyzing the content of their listings, I tracked how many associations targeted each disease in each year, how they described their goals, and how their agendas changed over time.

Congressional hearings reveal advocates' public efforts to influence policy. For decades, the House committee overseeing appropriations for labor, health and human services, and education[44] held hearings that reserved significant time for testimony from "interested individuals" with relatively low barriers to entry.[45] The hearing transcripts create an accessible record of which organized interests sought to influence health and social welfare policies and the goals they pursued. I classified all the witnesses who testified at these hearings, revealing increases over time in the prominence of disease advocates. And I analyzed the content of their testimony, tracking changes in what disease advocates asked for and how they justified their claims.

I also collected financial data about disease advocacy organizations. Each year, most nonprofits with budgets exceeding a modest threshold must file Internal Revenue Service forms that become publicly available. These filings reveal a wide range of disease charities and provide financial information on

---

[43] The *Encyclopedia* is ideal for studying large national organizations across long time periods but has less complete coverage of smaller, local, radical, and unstable organizations. Andrews et al., "Sampling Social Movement Organizations"; Martin, Baumgartner, and McCarthy, "Measuring Association Populations"; Minkoff, "Macro-Organizational Analysis"; Bevan et al., "Understanding Selection Bias"; Johnson and Frickel, "Ecological Threat," 321–22; Walker, McCarthy, and Baumgartner, "Replacing Members with Managers?"

[44] Prior to 1980, the committee oversaw labor, health, education, and welfare.

[45] Stolberg, "Patients Lobby."

their budgets and lobbying expenditures. The Senate Lobbying Disclosure Act Database provides further records of disease-related lobbying. Other records reveal corporate sponsorship of disease advocacy. While corporate funding often leaves no written trace, I was able to track grants to disease organizations reported in the *Taft Corporate Giving Directory*, which compiles information on programs that account for a majority of all corporate charitable donations.[46] I also collected data on grants that the pharmaceutical company Eli Lilly made to disease organizations, based on the company's disclosures.

I also tracked public policy responses to disease. Historical data on medical research funding from the National Institutes of Health (NIH) and the Department of Defense let me document how much research funding various diseases received over time. I also compiled data on health laws passed by Congress. These data yield information on disease campaigns in the policy realm and provide a chance to trace disease advocacy's effects on research budgets.

I collected additional information about diseases that might help explain why some receive more attention than others. Data on the mortality and disability attributed to different diseases allow me to see whether these measures of severity line up with the amount of advocacy and funding diseases receive and whether the relationship between health burden and political attention changes over time. To trace the relationship between advocacy and various types of stigma, I identified preventable diseases, mental illnesses, and infectious conditions.

I complement these quantitative data with several types of qualitative data. I drew on two archives related to breast cancer advocacy. I conducted a small number of interviews with various participants in disease politics. I also relied on a wide range of primary and secondary sources, including studies of philanthropy, charity, and social work conducted at various points in the twentieth century and news coverage of disease politics and NIH policymaking. The Appendix provides detailed descriptions of all data sources. This mix of quantitative and qualitative data reveals why disease campaigns dominate and how they change the ways we distribute resources and promote health.

---

[46] Taft Group, *Corporate Giving Directory*, 1995, vii; Taft Group, *Corporate Giving Directory*, 2005, xiii.

Unbalanced Benevolence

This book argues that disease campaigns became the battles Americans can agree to fight for three reasons: the perception of health as a universal and/or deserving goal, the appeal of narrowly targeted campaigns, and the strategic avoidance of controversy. These three sources of disease campaigns' appeal encourage campaigners to neglect stigmatized conditions, cluster around a few diseases, and prioritize uncontroversial goals.

Universal or Valorized Beneficiaries

Problems that are imagined to affect everyone and policies that distribute benefits universally arouse less controversy than those that affect subsets of the population.[47] These features of our political culture create consensus around health issues. We all have bodies, and we all see ourselves as potentially sick. The risks of death and disease are perceived as more widely shared than, for example, the risk of poverty.[48] Although almost all causes of death and disability affect the poor at greater rates than the rich,[49] not all diseases are preventable; and in the long term, neither are physical decline and death. And so the need for health is not seen as political in the way that the need for money is. One influential economist argues that people would choose contemporary medical care over all other developments in the past century.[50] Whether this is true or not probably depends on the race, gender, and sexual orientation of the person you ask. But clearly, for many people, efforts to improve health are especially valuable. Americans view health as a preeminent goal and a virtue, prizing it over other social goods. Health is imbued with moral significance, becoming almost sacred.[51]

The perception of health as a universally shared and uniquely important goal means that disease campaigns can fairly easily be portrayed as

---

[47] Lowi, "American Business"; Skocpol, *Boomerang*, 167. Issues with universal beneficiaries may *not* attract the most advocacy since interest groups have less incentive to form when a policy's benefits are widely dispersed. Wilson, *The Politics of Regulation*.

[48] Heimer, "Social Structure, Psychology, and the Estimation of Risk," 501; Rehm, Hacker, and Schlesinger, "Insecure Alliances."

[49] Link and Phelan, "Social Conditions"; Phelan et al., "'Fundamental Causes.'"

[50] Larry Summers, quoted in Smith, *Epic Measures*, 70.

[51] Clarke et al., "Biomedicalization"; Conrad, "Medicalization and Social Control," 223; Metzl and Kirkland, *Against Health*.

universally beneficial. This book argues that in the early twentieth century campaigns against tuberculosis, polio, cancer, and heart disease built consensus by arguing that everyone stood to benefit from their activities. It was no accident that these were infectious diseases and widespread chronic conditions; it made sense for everyone to feel at risk. Nancy Tomes attributes some of their appeal to the need for "a seemingly neutral ground for building consensus" in a nation "riven by gender, racial, ethnic, and class differences."[52]

While these early disease campaigns made universal claims, arguing that they would protect everyone from infectious diseases and widespread chronic conditions, many contemporary disease campaigns see patients[53] with particular diseases as their constituents. When problems affect a defined subgroup of the population, policies tend to distribute benefits to groups perceived as deserving and blameless and to punish or ignore stigmatized groups.[54] Therefore, the new disease campaigners work to make the case that their patients are deserving of public help. This is harder to do with diseases that are stigmatized— those whose patients are scorned, excluded, stereotyped, and discriminated against.[55] And so contemporary disease campaigns disproportionately target rarer but unstigmatized chronic conditions, revealing how conceptions of worthiness shape advocacy and policy.[56]

In extreme cases, stigma can motivate powerful activism. The stigmatization of gay men and AIDS patients in the 1980s inspired a triumphant social movement. But without a comparable combination of extreme neglect, immediate emergency, and threat of repression, the lower levels of stigma attached to preventable, infectious, and mental illnesses tend to inhibit mobilization. When publicly identifying oneself as a patient invites judgment and discrimination, patients are less likely to mobilize.[57] When

[52] Tomes, *Gospel of Germs*, 19.

[53] Scholars struggle over which terms to use for people experiencing a disease, recognizing that "patients" may imply passivity, "consumers" may imply commercialization, and people "living with" a disease excludes those who have died. Baggott, Allsop, and Jones, *Speaking for Patients and Carers*, 4–5; Tomes, "Patients or Health-Care Consumers?" I use the term "patients" due to its colloquial familiarity.

[54] Gilens, *Why Americans Hate Welfare*; Lieberman, *Boundaries of Contagion*; Schneider and Ingram, "Social Construction of Target Populations"; Skrentny, "Policy-Elite Perceptions"; Skrentny, *Ironies of Affirmative Action*; Skrentny, *Minority Rights Revolution*; Steensland, "Cultural Categories."

[55] Pescosolido and Martin, "The Stigma Complex," 91.

[56] Steensland, "Cultural Categories"; Schneider and Ingram, "Social Construction of Target Populations."

[57] Beard, "Advocating Voice"; Carpenter, "Is Health Politics Different?," 290; Kedrowski and Sarow, *Cancer Activism*; Siplon, *AIDS and the Policy Struggle*.

they do, their claims are met with less attention and sympathy than those of patients with unstigmatized diseases.[58] Focusing on universal beneficiaries or valorized groups helps build consensus and attract resources to address problems but creates imbalances in the types of problems that are addressed.

Narrow Causes

While broad *impact*—affecting large segments of the population—helps problems attract attention, broad *focus*—targeting large, unspecific goals—does not. Another source of disease campaigns' appeal is the fact that they target one disease at a time. Organizations, from for-profit firms to social movement organizations, benefit from finding a specialized niche.[59] Organizations that are overly general or that attempt to span multiple categories are less likely to attract funding, survive, and achieve their goals.[60] In the policy realm, it's often easier to pass public policies that target narrow

[58] Cultural contexts mean that claims on behalf of some problems and people are more resonant than others, creating a more favorable "discursive opportunity structure" for some advocates than others. Best, *Threatened Children*, 17, 176–77; Ferree, "Resonance and Radicalism," 309; McCammon et al., "Movement Framing"; Skrentny, "Policy-Elite Perceptions," 1797.

[59] Baumgartner and Jones, *Agendas and Instability*; Browne, "Organized Interests"; Gamson, *Strategy of Social Protest*, 41–49; Gray and Lowery, "Demography of Interest Organization Communities"; Heinz et al., *The Hollow Core*; Hsu, Hannan, and Koçak, "Multiple Category Memberships"; Levitsky, "Niche Activism"; McCarthy and Zald, "Resource Mobilization and Social Movements," 1234; Olzak, "Effect of Category Spanning"; Walker and Stepick, "Valuing the Cause"; Zald and McCarthy, "Social Movement Industries," 15; Zuckerman, "Categorical Imperative."

[60] Baumgartner and Jones, *Agendas and Instability*; Browne, "Organized Interests"; Brulle and Jenkins, "Foundations and the Environmental Movement," 160; Gamson, *Strategy of Social Protest*, 41–49; Gray and Lowery, *Population Ecology of Interest Representation*; Heinz et al., *The Hollow Core*; Hsu, Hannan, and Koçak, "Multiple Category Memberships"; Olzak, "Effect of Category Spanning"; Walker and Stepick, "Valuing the Cause," 24; Zuckerman, "Categorical Imperative." In an apparent contradiction, Heaney and Rojas argue that social movement organizations that "hybridize" multiple categories have an advantage in mobilization. Heaney and Rojas, "Hybrid Activism." But Heaney and Rojas's hybrid organizations operate at the *intersection* of categories, becoming more narrowly targeted (e.g., a feminist anti-war organization). In contrast, the generalists and category-spanners described by previous researchers operate at the *union* of categories, broadening their focus (e.g., MoveOn.org, which Heaney and Rojas call "nonantiwar focused"). By showing that narrower organizations fare better than generalists, Heaney and Rojas actually provide further support for the organizational advantages of specialization. Similarly, Wang and colleagues argue that "boundary spanning," broadly defined, can either facilitate or hamper movements' effectiveness. But when they narrow their focus to one type of boundary spanning—the attempt to cover a broad range of "issues, identities, and tactical repertoires"—they concur with previous researchers' findings about the negative effects of broad organizational identities. Wang, Piazza, and Soule, "Boundary-Spanning in Social Movements," 179.

problems than broad ones.[61] While specialized campaigns are more ef-fective, they have limitations. When we target a few specific causes, there are always other important problems that attract less attention. Narrowly specialized advocacy organizations may be disinclined to pursue broader goals.[62] Narrowly targeted policies and specialized bureaucracies may have trouble implementing ideas that cross organizational categories.[63]

This book shows that Americans donate much more to targeted campaigns against particular diseases than to broader efforts to improve public health. In the case of diseases, there are a few big "winners" (tu-berculosis, then polio, then AIDS and breast cancer) and other diseases that are neglected by comparison. Compared to multi-disease campaigns, campaigns against single diseases tend to focus on goals that fit well with disease categories, like targeted research and awareness campaigns. They are less likely to pursue goals that cross disease categories, including basic research, environmental protection, and access to medical treatment.

Avoiding Controversy

Some issues seem predestined to arouse conflict in a given society at a given time; for instance, in the contemporary United States, it would be difficult to organize a consensus campaign about abortion.[64] But consensus does not only result from the characteristics of the problem. Advocates can also nurture consensus when they decide which solutions to pursue. Goals that challenge existing interests, require structural change, and are laid out in specific terms tend to arouse more controversy than vaguely stated goals and those that focus on changing individuals' behaviors.[65] Facing pressure to

[61] Christensen and Lægreid, "Whole-of-Government"; Exworthy and Hunter, "Challenge of Joined-Up Government"; Nelson, *Making an Issue of Child Abuse*, 125, 135.

[62] Collins, *Black Feminist Thought*; Duggan, *Twilight of Equality?*, xviii, 67–68; Fung, "Associations and Democracy"; Gamson, "Hiroshima"; Gitlin, *Twilight of Common Dreams*; Gitlin, "From Universality to Difference"; Hobsbawm, "Identity Politics and the Left"; hooks, *Talking Back*; Minkoff, Aisenbrey, and Agnone, "Organizational Diversity," 525; Piore, *Beyond Individualism*; Rorty, *Achieving Our Country*; Turner, "Intersex Identities"; Waters, "Succession in the Stratification System"; Weakliem, "Race versus Class?"

[63] Christensen and Lægreid, "Whole-of-Government," 1060; Exworthy and Hunter, "Challenge of Joined-Up Government"; Gordon, *Dead on Arrival*, 234; Nelson, *Making an Issue of Child Abuse*, 125, 135; Smith, "Institutional Filters," 88–90; Weir, "Ideas and the Politics of Bounded Innovation."

[64] Meyer and Staggenborg, "Movements, Countermovements," 1641.

[65] Meyer and Staggenborg, 1640; Baumgartner and Jones, *Agendas and Instability*, 151; Gusfield, "Ownership of Social Problems," 435–39; Lofland, *Polite Protesters*, 2; Lowi, "American Business"; McCarthy and Wolfson, "Consensus Movements," 277.

attract members and donors and achieve visible successes, many advocates adjust their goals to match political opportunities and avoid arousing opposition.[66] Some minimize conflict by selecting uncontroversial goals and framing their activities as nonthreatening and apolitical.[67] When activists and policymakers sidestep conflict, they're more likely to win policy gains and public support; but these short-term gains may come with a cost: the failure to pursue larger changes and represent more diverse interests.[68]

Disease advocacy organizations vary widely in the extent to which they strategically pursue consensus. Some organizations are militant and oppositional, challenging powerful interests and demanding social change.[69] But this book identifies broader forces that push many organizations to embrace consensus goals, a process that helps explain how disease campaigns have remained so popular over the decades. Corporate influence can discourage disease advocacy organizations from focusing on environmental hazards and encourage them to launch awareness campaigns and lobby for publicly funded research.[70] Meanwhile, the pursuit of policy victories pushes disease advocates to prioritize medical research over treatment access. Underemphasizing treatment access limits the extent to which mainstream disease advocacy challenges the profound inequalities in access to healthcare in the United States.

Inefficient but Indomitable

Disease campaigns distribute resources in a way that no one would have designed. They funnel vast sums of money and attention to a few particular

[66] Diani, "Linking Mobilization Frames"; Einwohner, "Practices, Opportunity"; Ferree, "Resonance and Radicalism"; Gould, *Moving Politics*, 3; Jenkins, "Nonprofit Organizations and Political Advocacy," 319; Kingdon, *Agendas, Alternatives, and Public Policies*, 38; Klandermans, "Social Construction of Protest," 78–86; McAdam, *Political Process*; McCarthy and Zald, "Resource Mobilization and Social Movements," 1228–29; Meyer, "Protest and Political Opportunities," 127–28; Meyer and Staggenborg, "Movements, Countermovements," 1651; Tarrow, *Power in Movement*.

[67] Baumgartner and Jones, *Agendas and Instability*, 151; Lofland, *Polite Protesters*, 2, 67; McCarthy and Wolfson, "Consensus Movements," 277; Meyer and Staggenborg, "Movements, Countermovements," 1640.

[68] Einwohner, "Practices, Opportunity"; Ferree, "Resonance and Radicalism," 306–7, 339–40; Jenkins, "Nonprofit Organizations and Political Advocacy"; Kingdon, *Agendas, Alternatives, and Public Policies*; Lofland, *Polite Protesters*, 52, 74.

[69] Epstein, "Patient Groups and Health Movements," 512–13.

[70] Batt, "A Community Fractured"; Jones, "In Whose Interest?"; Rothman et al., "Health Advocacy Organizations."

diseases, neglecting others. With the exception of AIDS, the favored diseases tend to exclude stigmatized conditions. And they focus predominantly on awareness campaigns and research funding, paying much less attention to preventing disease and ensuring access to healthcare. It's easy to imagine more efficient ways to promote our collective well-being.

But arguing that the distribution of funding is *inefficient* is different from arguing that these campaigns are *harmful*. The key question is whether the money and attention devoted to disease campaigns are being taken away from other, more important goals. Do disease campaigns crowd out responses to other problems? If we weren't fighting diseases, would we be devoting more attention to broader health campaigns, fighting poverty, and pursuing social justice? Do diseases siphon resources from each other? If we weren't fighting breast cancer, would we be devoting more attention to chronic obstructive pulmonary disease? And do goals displace each other? If we weren't busy raising awareness, would we be removing carcinogens from the environment?

Some theorists argue that narrow campaigns and consensus politics harm society by displacing broader campaigns and contention. Critics of identity politics argue that movements representing narrowly defined groups fail to challenge broader systems of domination and exclusion.[71] Lofland maintains that consensus campaigns waste resources, using up "energy and talent that might otherwise be available for more openly oppositional politics" and tricking people into thinking they've made a difference.[72] Piven and Cloward argue that when poor people's movements have turned away from disruptive protest, they "blunted or curbed the disruptive force which lower-class people were sometimes able to mobilize."[73] Eliasoph suggests that by focusing on individual solutions to social problems, consensus campaigns can make people overlook the need for structural change in ways that benefit powerful people and institutions, making "problems

---

[71] Gamson, "Hiroshima"; Gitlin, *Twilight of Common Dreams*; Gitlin, "From Universality to Difference"; Hobsbawm, "Identity Politics and the Left"; Piore, *Beyond Individualism*; Turner, "Intersex Identities"; Rorty, *Achieving Our Country*; Waters, "Succession in the Stratification System"; Weakliem, "Race versus Class?"; Collins, *Black Feminist Thought*; hooks, *Talking Back*.

[72] Lofland, *Polite Protesters*, 74; see also pages 52, 71–73; Cloward and Piven, "Disruption and Organization," 596; Davis, *Secret History*, 211; Lofland, "Consensus Movements," 186; McCormick, *No Family History*, 43; Piven and Cloward, *Poor People's Movements*, xxi–xxii.

[73] Piven and Cloward, *Poor People's Movements*, xxi–xxii.

like poverty seem natural, not matters of dispute, not human creations that humans could fix."[74]

These critiques imply that if there were fewer consensus campaigns and less specialized advocacy, more people would participate in contentious politics and more organizations would challenge powerful interests and promote structural change. But we could also imagine consensus and contentious politics operating independently: maybe the people collecting dimes for polio would *not* otherwise have been marching for civil rights. There might even be positive spillovers between consensus and contentious campaigns. Specialized campaigns can sometimes help achieve broader goals.[75] Downey argues that consensus politics can change the political environment in ways that favor later contentious activism.[76] In a study of the civil rights movement, Haines found that the emergence of radical black activism caused more funding to flow to moderate civil rights organizations—money that would not otherwise have funded any civil rights organization.[77] Could the same be true in the other direction, with moderate campaigns benefiting radical activism?

By collecting data on the entire field of disease advocacy over decades, I show that rather than rearranging an existing pot of charitable resources, disease campaigns increase the size of the pot. Throughout a century of disease campaigns, reformers have tried to launch more "rational" campaigns for general public health. But they've never been able to work up the same excitement as the single-disease campaigns. In assuming that charity, advocacy, and policymaking can be rationally planned and equally divided, these efforts ignore the role of disease campaigns in attracting the money in the first place. You can't just switch from breast cancer to hepatitis or from disease campaigns to public health promotion and expect the same outpouring of charitable and public resources. If there were no disease campaigns, the money wouldn't be going to promote health or to fight poverty—the disease campaigners might just stay home and keep their money. In fact, rather than taking money away from other problems, disease

---

[74] Eliasoph, *Making Volunteers*, 117; see also pages 17, 93; Eliasoph, *Avoiding Politics*, 251; Lofland, *Polite Protesters*, 76.

[75] Bickford, "Anti-Anti-Identity Politics"; Bernstein, "Identity Politics"; Polletta, "Strategy and Identity"; Armstrong, *Forging Gay Identities*.

[76] Downey, "Elaborating Consensus."

[77] Haines, "Black Radicalization."

campaigns may have benefited other causes by institutionalizing mass philanthropy and creating a culture of giving.

Similarly, disease campaigns do not compete with each other for attention and resources in a zero-sum game. I find that disease lobbying is most
successful when budget surpluses help the medical research budget grow.
So rather than being taken from other diseases, the research funding given
to mobilized diseases tends to be "new money." In fact, gains spill over as
disease campaigns inspire spending on medical research and the funding
eventually spreads across conditions. If there were no breast cancer movement securing public funding for medical research, the money wouldn't
otherwise be going to study other diseases—the NIH budget would just be
smaller.

A field-level perspective also reveals that while many disease campaigns
fail to promote the policies that would most improve our health, they do
not crowd out campaigns for those policies. Some scholars suggest that
narrowly targeted health activism, including disease campaigns, may explain the lack of a movement for universal healthcare in the United States.[78]
Individual organizations that target diseases *are* less likely to emphasize
treatment access and shared environmental hazards than broader health organizations. But narrow goals and the pursuit of consensus help the entire
disease advocacy field grow, including more radical disease organizations
that challenge corporate interests and inequality. A mainstream campaign
encouraging mammograms does not cancel out the environmental breast
cancer movement's anti-corporate agenda—in fact, the former may help the
latter gain visibility and influence. While individual disease organizations
face pressures to choose narrower goals, the existence of disease campaigns
actually leads to more attention to broader goals as well.

This finding speaks to the potential of social movements to produce social
change, despite pressures to deradicalize. Scholars describe various forces
that make social movement organizations overly bureaucratic, insufficiently
challenging of political institutions and inequality, and insensitive to their
beneficiaries' real needs.[79] Within individual organizations, co-optation,

---

[78] Gordon, *Dead on Arrival*; Heath, Rapp, and Taussig, "Genetic Citizenship"; King, *Pink Ribbons, Inc.*, 120; Levitsky and Banaszak-Holl, "Introduction," 3. Others note that while constituency-based social movements often lobby for narrowly targeted health policies to benefit particular groups, they have also sometimes turned to demands for universal access to healthcare. Epstein, "Politics of Health Mobilization," 246; Hoffman, "Health Care Reform," 76, 79; Hoffman, *Health Care for Some*.

[79] Clemens, "Organizational Repertoires and Institutional Change"; Ferree, "Resonance and Radicalism"; Jenkins, "Radical Transformation of Organizational Goals"; Michels, *Political Parties*;

bureaucratization, and the need to ensure organizational survival may create pressure to abandon radical goals. But at the field level, there's little reason to think that these choices crowd out more radical organizations. In fact, the proliferation of individual organizations with conservative or limited goals can help the whole field grow in ways that actually help organizations with more radical goals. Recognizing the insidious pressures on individual disease campaigns does not imply that these campaigns do more harm than good overall.

Plan of the Book

This book argues that disease campaigns build their appeal by targeting universal or valorized beneficiaries, narrowing their focus, and pursuing consensus solutions. In consequence, they focus attention on some diseases and neglect others, and they prioritize uncontroversial goals, limiting their potential to improve our health. But while they distribute resources inefficiently, they are not engaged in a zero-sum competition, either with each other or with other goals.

These patterns become clear across long historical periods. Chapter 1 reveals the centrality of disease campaigns in American philanthropy and public policy in the early and mid-twentieth century. Combining the appeal of narrow causes and universal beneficiaries, philanthropists and doctors launched enormous campaigns against tuberculosis, polio, cancer, and heart disease. They created a new form of mass philanthropy in which millions of Americans volunteered and donated to solve social problems. This form spread from one disease to another and dominated American charitable giving and voluntarism for half a century. Federal investments in health at the Centers for Disease Control and the NIH also grew up around disease categories. These campaigns' outsize successes reveal the appeal of narrowly targeted campaigns, along with one of their downsides: they create a highly skewed distribution of public health dollars. But we shouldn't assume that specialized campaigns are hoarding resources that would otherwise be distributed more equitably across problems; attempts to distribute money on

---

Piven and Cloward, *Poor People's Movements*; Staggenborg, "Consequences of Professionalization"; Zald and Ash, "Social Movement Organizations."

the basis of public health needs never matched the appeal of single-disease campaigns.

Chapter 2 explains how in the second half of the twentieth century disease advocacy evolved from universal campaigns to patients' constituencies. Changes in the experience of health and illness and the nationwide expansion of political advocacy laid the groundwork for patient-led campaigns. Then, AIDS and breast cancer activists constructed a new type of disease advocacy on the foundations of the gay rights and women's health movements. Unlike the earlier disease crusades, these movements were led by patients banding together to fight diseases that affected them personally, and they blazed a trail for patients suffering from other diseases. The earlier disease crusades had used universal goals to achieve consensus and attract mass participation; patients' organizations needed to create a new kind of consensus politics. As patients' activism became increasingly legitimate, disease nonprofits proliferated, patients took over congressional hearings, and disease walks and ribbons became an inescapable feature of American public life.

The shift to disease patients' constituencies created new inequalities among diseases. Chapter 3 shows that the amount of death and disability a disease causes and the ability of disease campaigners to attract corporate donations tell us surprisingly little about how much advocacy will target a disease. In explaining why some diseases attract more attention than others, ideas and culture matter more than objective conditions. Since not all patients are equally willing or able to mobilize and not all patients are viewed as equally deserving of help, constituency-based activism tends to disadvantage stigmatized diseases in favor of those that create valorized identities. Diseases marked by various types of stigma—preventable, contagious, and mental illnesses—are targeted by much less advocacy than other diseases. The advocates who do target these conditions have more difficulty convincing policymakers and the public that their patients deserve public help.

Disease campaigns create a demand for ways to decide which diseases are most important. Chapter 4 explains that since the 1960s, advocates have introduced various criteria to highlight their diseases' impacts, from mortality to health spending. These competing claims encouraged policymakers to seek formal ways to rank and compare diseases, creating pressure to standardize the NIH budget across disease categories. The NIH pushed back and sought to preserve scientists' control over priority setting, worrying that the pursuit of narrow, disease-specific goals would funnel resources away from basic science and untargeted research. But while the *proportion* of the NIH budget targeting these goals declined slightly, the overall amounts increased dramatically, suggesting that specialized campaigns do not draw resources away from broader goals. The push for disease data did change how the government distributes money, bringing the funding distribution more in line with mortality rates. This chapter introduces a broader way of conceptualizing the effects of advocacy, beyond securing funding or passing favorable laws. Advocacy also changes how policymakers define issues and judge policies, with concrete effects on funding distributions. These aggregate changes only become visible with field-level data.

As disease campaigns multiplied in the 1980s and 1990s, critics worried that they would compete with each other for federal funding, stalling the growth of the medical research budget. Chapter 5 shows that even though diseases with the most organized patients secured huge funding increases, disease lobbying rarely became a zero-sum game. Instead, disease campaigns were most successful when the NIH budget was growing. When medical research competed with other federal spending priorities, the search for cures won out over more redistributive and politically controversial programs. Combining insights about advocacy and budget politics reveals that advocacy's effectiveness varies over time, as does the extent to which related problems compete with each other. Specialized claims do not invariably compete, nor do they necessarily doom broader goals.

Why did research become such a prominent goal in the first place? Chapter 6 asks how a disease focus shapes the types of goals advocacy organizations pursue and the types of laws Congress passes. Prevention and treatment access policies often cut across disease categories, making them less attractive goals for disease advocates than research and awareness. Corporate influence pushes organizations to prioritize awareness over prevention, and the pursuit of policy victories favors medical research over the divisive politics of access to healthcare. These pressures create a health policy portfolio that subsidizes corporate interests, underemphasizes collective risks, fails to challenge inequalities, and may actually make us less healthy by encouraging overtreatment. Yet while only a small *proportion* of organizations focus on prevention and treatment access, the phenomenal growth of disease advocacy means that large *numbers* of organizations continue to pursue the latter goals. Narrow goals outnumber broader goals but do not displace them.

Dread diseases are our common enemies, the fears everyone shares, the battles we can fight without generating opposition. To achieve this universal appeal, disease campaigns tend to neglect stigmatized diseases, target narrow categories, and avoid controversial goals. Focused on the wars we can agree to fight, we bypass other important battles. But disease campaigns cannot be blamed for our collective neglect of other important problems. Big-hearted, benevolent, and sometimes misguided, disease campaigns are a lopsided bonanza, an imperfect but indomitable blessing.

1

Charitable Crusades

Campaigns against tuberculosis, polio, cancer, and heart disease launched the mass philanthropy that underpins the American nonprofit sector. Single-disease campaigns also fostered new federal investments in public health and medical research. This chapter draws on records and secondary sources to explain disease campaigns' central role in twentieth-century public life. These early disease campaigns, which I call the "charitable crusades," created a new model for organizing. They targeted one disease at a time, a narrow focus that was more compelling than broader efforts to improve public health. They described themselves as serving the public at large (not just current patients); these universal claims implied that everyone stood to benefit from fighting infectious diseases and ameliorating common chronic conditions. Rather than disinterested charity, they were seen as insurance policies in which people pooled resources to mitigate the risk of illness. Building consensus, they mobilized mass participation by donors and volunteers. This model spread from one disease to another as campaigners shared resources and expertise and the public became accustomed to an annual calendar of appeals for donations.

Narrowly targeted campaigns do a good job of attracting mass interest. But they have a downside: they tend to distribute resources unevenly. As disease campaigns dominated philanthropy and structured health policy, critics warned that they were creating windfalls for some diseases and neglecting others. Policymakers and scientists raised concerns that organizing public policy around disease categories was preventing the development of a broader health agenda and stifling public investments in basic biomedical research. But for both philanthropy and public policy, attempts to spread the money around failed time and time again because nothing could match the appeal of a disease campaign. Specialized campaigns may not distribute funds rationally, but they attract new resources to solve problems and are preferable to the alternative: donors keeping the money in their wallets and voters feeling less supportive of public expenditures.

Conceptualizing Diseases and Campaigns

The first disease campaigns grew from fertile ground. By the early twentieth century, changes in health and medicine made diseases seem like discrete entities and solvable problems, and social changes prepared Americans to come together to solve them. Before the late nineteenth century, it would not have made sense to launch a public campaign against a particular disease since diseases were not generally thought of as discrete entities. Almost every experience of illness was thought to have multiple interacting causes and to follow an unpredictable trajectory. A few epidemic diseases were beginning to be understood to be contagious early in the nineteenth century, but even in these cases, physicians and the public believed that the illness resulted from interactions between a tainted environment and individual vulnerabilities. Diagnoses relied primarily on patients' narrative accounts of their symptoms, and personalized treatments focused on reducing individuals' vulnerability.[1]

Between 1860 and 1900, scientific developments encouraged people to think of diseases as ideal types, generally following a similar course and sharing underlying causes. Researchers developed the germ theory of disease and discovered the organisms responsible for tuberculosis, cholera, typhoid, and diphtheria. Physicians increasingly made diagnoses on the basis of clinical tests and observations, rather than patients' narrative accounts. This seemingly objective physical information encouraged physicians to think of diseases as having a shared course, development, and prognosis across individual patients' experiences. The emergence of health insurance, life insurance, epidemiology, and public health increased the demand for statistics based on disease classifications.[2] This differentiation and classification of diseases was a necessary prerequisite to launching public campaigns against diseases—you can't mobilize around a category you can't conceptualize.[3] Meanwhile, increasing faith in science, respect for physicians, and optimism about medical advances made numerous diseases seem like

---

[1] Rosenberg, *Our Present Complaint*; Starr, *Social Transformation of American Medicine*; Warner, *Therapeutic Perspective*.

[2] Anspach, "Sociology of Medical Discourse"; Reiser, *Medicine and the Reign of Technology*; Rosenberg, *Our Present Complaint*, 3, 18–23; Starr, *Social Transformation of American Medicine*, 81, 135–46; Warner, *Therapeutic Perspective*, 248–49; Tomes, *Gospel of Germs*.

[3] Taylor and Zald, "Collective Action in the Health Sector," 309.

problems that could be solved.[4] The growing belief that medical advances could conquer disease provided a powerful incentive for disease campaigns.

Another prerequisite for disease campaigns was the emergence of public campaigns against social problems. Before the late nineteenth century, most charitable efforts were made by individual do-gooders helping individual needy people. But the turn of the century saw the rise of large-scale philanthropy that sought to improve society as a whole. Progressive reformers sought to use scientific methods and bureaucratic organizations to address the causes of problems, rather than simply softening their effects.[5]

Meanwhile, more Americans were in a position to donate time and money. As disposable incomes rose, more middle- and working-class Americans could give away money.[6] Middle- and upper-class white women, pushed out of the paid labor force after industrialization, had more time for voluntary activities.[7] A flood of voluntary associations emerged in the late nineteenth century, many promoting mutual benefit by spreading risks and pooling resources.[8] Optimistic about curing diseases and ready to join together to solve problems, Americans were primed for disease campaigns.

Tuberculosis and the Invention of Mass Philanthropy

As early twentieth-century philanthropists turned their energy from helping needy individuals to solving social problems, their first mass campaign targeted a disease. The National Tuberculosis Association (NTA), founded in 1904 as the National Society for the Study and Prevention of Tuberculosis, is often remembered as the first national organization founded

[4] Mukherjee, *Emperor of All Maladies*, 22; Starr, *Social Transformation of American Medicine*, 129–38.

[5] Depending on which change they focus on—the move from individual givers to bureaucratic organizations; the shift from individual beneficiaries to social problems; the emergence of scientific management, modern fundraising, and mass participation—historians date the emergence of modern philanthropy in different decades. But there is widespread agreement that a major change had occurred by the early twentieth century. Friedman, "Philanthropy in America"; Gross, "Giving in America"; Hall, "Historical Overview"; Haveman, Rao, and Paruchuri, "The Winds of Change"; O'Neill, *Third America*, 115–16; Robbins, "Nonprofit Sector"; Rodgers, "In Search of Progressivism," 115–17; Sealander, "Curing Evils"; Wiebe, *Search for Order*; Wolfe, "Giving Philanthropy a New History"; Zunz, *Philanthropy in America*, 8–10, 30, 40.

[6] Zunz, *Philanthropy in America*, 2.

[7] McCarthy, "Women and Political Culture," 182, 192. American women also had more access to higher education than women in other countries, creating a pool of highly educated women with time to spare. Skocpol, *Protecting Soldiers and Mothers*, 340–42, 348.

[8] Clemens, *The People's Lobby*, 35; Hall, "Historical Overview," 36–39; Robbins, "Nonprofit Sector."

to fight a specific disease, or the first mass health education campaign.[9] But the NTA wasn't just the start of disease campaigns in America—it was the first time Americans came together in large numbers to raise money to fight a single problem.[10]

Focusing on a single disease was a strategic choice designed to attract the most charitable dollars. When some early members suggested that the Tuberculosis Association broaden its mission to public health in general, an official argued that "one cannot go to a community to talk generalities and get a response."[11] As tuberculosis mortality declined, there were decades of discussions about broadening the organization's focus, but the NTA did not become the American Lung Association until 1973.[12]

This narrow focus was paired with the claim that everyone would benefit from the campaign. While charitable approaches to tuberculosis had provided financial assistance to individual patients and their families,[13] the NTA conceptualized charity differently, as a "safety net against broader threats" and "a form of public thrift."[14] Tuberculosis was the leading cause of death in the United States, responsible for one in ten deaths.[15] As New York City's health commissioner explained, the campaign against tuberculosis wasn't about helping the destitute but about "making life safer and health more secure for all of us."[16] A 1922 official history of the Tuberculosis Association emphasized that everyone stood to benefit:

> Let every one who is able to help bear in mind that tuberculosis is a disease of all people, rich and poor, the educated and uneducated; that it is not confined to climates or races, but that it is universal; and that every one should be interested in combating it.[17]

---

[9] Carter, *Gentle Legions*; Cavins, *National Health Agencies*, 81; Lichtenstiger, "Philosophy and Significance," 4; Shryock, *National Tuberculosis Association*, 57; Teller, *Tuberculosis Movement*, 27; Tomes, *Gospel of Germs*, 114, 123; Zunz, *Philanthropy in America*, 47.

[10] Zunz, *Philanthropy in America*, 51. Earlier large fundraising campaigns had been humanitarian responses to disasters and the Civil War, not responses to ongoing problems. Hall, "Historical Overview," 39; McCarthy, "Women and Political Culture," 190–92; Zunz, *Philanthropy in America*, 44.

[11] Livingston Farrand, 1911, quoted in Teller, *Tuberculosis Movement*, 53.

[12] Gunn and Platt, *Voluntary Health Agencies*, 225; Shryock, *National Tuberculosis Association*, 241–45, 284–85; Teller, *Tuberculosis Movement*, 53.

[13] Cavins, *National Health Agencies*, 75.

[14] Zunz, *Philanthropy in America*, 46, 49.

[15] Shryock, *National Tuberculosis Association*, 62–63.

[16] *New York Times*, "Mayor."

[17] Knopf, *History of the National Tuberculosis Association*, 53–54.

This universal focus meant that the organization focused less on advocating for the afflicted than on protecting the public at large. Patients weren't in charge; association members often lacked personal experience with the disease.[18] In the early twentieth century, the NTA focused attention on quarantining infected people in hospitals, a practice that patients viewed with suspicion and fear of "the 'black bottle' rumored used to dispose of the dying."[19] Quarantining protected *potential* patients from *current* patients, who "were depicted as simultaneously victim and menace."[20]

If everyone was a beneficiary of the campaign, perhaps everyone should be a donor. Tuberculosis campaigners pioneered a new funding strategy, relying on millions of small donations and volunteers. Selling penny stamps called Christmas Seals, the NTA raised tens of millions a year in today's dollars.[21] In 1921, an impoverished young boy told the *San Francisco Chronicle*, "I don't always have a nickel sometimes to pay for my lunch at school . . . but I'm going to save some pennies all right to buy some of them Christmas seals with."[22] From 1924 to 1948, the NTA took in 60% more than was donated to all the museums and orchestras in the country.[23] Mass donations were made possible by mass volunteerism. By the start of the twentieth century, women's organizations were enormous, networked, and powerful.[24] While male philanthropists tended to donate money, women were more likely to volunteer their time.[25] The NTA started a tradition of enlisting them to raise money from their friends and neighbors.[26] Some years, NTA's adult volunteers numbered half a million,[27] and three million

---

[18] One exception was Dr. Lawrence Flick, a founder of the NTA, who had recovered from the disease. Flick, *Beloved Crusader*.

[19] Teller, *Tuberculosis Movement*, 91; see also Rothman, *Living in the Shadow of Death*, 180–94, 227; Shryock, *National Tuberculosis Association*, 153.

[20] Tomes, *Gospel of Germs*, 131. The focus on universal risks had both positive and negative effects for socially disadvantaged people. Arguing that protecting everyone from infection required improving the health of the poor, tuberculosis campaigners pushed for beneficial public health efforts including regulation of tenements. But the campaign also fostered the impression that "poor, uneducated, foreign-born, or nonwhite" patients might be irresponsibly spreading the disease due to poor hygiene, reinforcing stereotypes about minorities and immigrants. Tomes, 128–32.

[21] Carter, *Gentle Legions*, 77–79; Cavins, *National Health Agencies*, 84; Knopf, *History of the National Tuberculosis Association*, 55–62; Kurtz, *Social Work Year Book 1939*, 448; Oshinsky, *Polio*, 50; Shryock, *National Tuberculosis Association*, 128–32; Zunz, *Philanthropy in America*, 47–48.

[22] *San Francisco Chronicle*, "Tuberculosis Association Saves Lives."

[23] Jenkins, *Philanthropy in America*, 173.

[24] Clemens, "Organizational Repertoires and Institutional Change," 760; McCarthy, "Women and Political Culture," 193; Skocpol, *Protecting Soldiers and Mothers*, 319, 329.

[25] McCarthy, "Women and Political Culture," 192.

[26] Carter, *Gentle Legions*, 67; Zunz, *Philanthropy in America*, 71.

[27] Gunn and Platt, *Voluntary Health Agencies*, 260.

children signed on as tuberculosis "crusaders"—raising money from their neighbors and promising to maintain good hygiene.[28] In 1945, one researcher marveled that "more persons have participated in one year in this far-reaching humanitarian program for the control of a single disease than ever took part in any like philanthropic project conceived by man."[29]

The mass campaign against tuberculosis helped institutionalize a new idea: that all Americans should be giving to charity, with charitable contributions "part of the regular family budget" even for the working class.[30] The share of urban Americans making philanthropic donations jumped from 3% to 35% in the first two decades of the twentieth century. Increasingly, mass appeals replaced small local associations as the primary way Americans worked to pool resources and share risks.[31]

The NTA's model—targeting a single disease, framing the entire population as beneficiaries, and mobilizing mass participation—spread quickly. Charities that had previously assisted individual blind and deaf people adopted a public health focus, encouraging the use of silver nitrate to prevent blindness in infants, educating the public, and conducting research.[32] Campaigns against sexually transmitted diseases promised to benefit everyone, not just current patients.[33] Planning a national organization to fight mental illness, Clifford Beers sought advice from NTA officials and wrote that his organization could "do in its own field what the National Society for the Prevention and Cure of Tuberculosis has done, and is doing, in its sphere of activity."[34] These early disease organizations demonstrate the emergence of a new model for fighting disease.

Polio as a Generic Charitable Cause

Tuberculosis campaigners had invented the disease crusade, creating a model for a mass campaign to fight a single disease. A few decades later, widespread feelings of fear and vulnerability made polio another ideal target

---

[28] Zunz, *Philanthropy in America*, 49.

[29] Cavins, *National Health Agencies*, 85.

[30] Zunz, *Philanthropy in America*, 51; see also pp. 45, 51, 73–74.

[31] Zunz, 2, 74.

[32] Cavins, *National Health Agencies*, 141, 144, 155, 203; Gunn and Platt, *Voluntary Health Agencies*, 23.

[33] Cavins, *National Health Agencies*, 173, 180–83; Gunn and Platt, *Voluntary Health Agencies*, 20.

[34] Clifford Beers, 1908, quoted in Cavins, *National Health Agencies*, 96.

for a universal campaign. The disease struck communities without warning, often targeting children. Many people believed that wealthier children were more at risk, inspiring middle- and upper-class donors and volunteers.[35]

In the 1930s, Franklin Delano Roosevelt founded the National Foundation for Infantile Paralysis, also known simply as the National Foundation.[36] Like the Christmas Seals, its most successful campaign encouraged every American to make a small contribution. The "March of Dimes" featured millions of women collecting donations door to door. A researcher who accompanied one of these "marching mothers" through a working-class neighborhood reported that "perhaps three quarters of the houses had the porch light on," signaling their willingness to donate.[37] The campaign raised enormous amounts of money—when the 1945 March of Dimes brought in the equivalent of $250 million in today's dollars, it surpassed every charity in history except the Red Cross.[38] Between 1951 and 1955, it raised the modern-day equivalent of $2 billion. By some accounts, two-thirds of Americans had donated by 1954, and seven million had volunteered.[39] The size and success of the polio campaign helped shape mid-century philanthropy, ushering in a "golden age of mass fundraising" in the 1950s.[40] As philanthropy grew, a disease campaign was still leading the way.

Like the tuberculosis movement, the campaign against polio was a public crusade to eliminate a public health threat, not a push by polio patients to promote their interests. In a mid-century study of National Foundation volunteers, sociologist David Sills argued that disease associations are "unlike automobile clubs or veterans' groups" in that they "cannot obtain new members from any clearly-defined segment of the population."[41] This statement only made sense because no one considered polio patients, survivors, and family members to be the natural membership base for a polio organization. Only 18% of the volunteers for the National Foundation had any personal experience with polio, and many of those had only encountered the disease through their work in the medical profession.[42] Basil O'Connor

---

[35] Davis, *Passage Through Crisis*, 4–5.
[36] Oshinsky, *Polio*, 53.
[37] Sills, *Volunteers*, 160.
[38] Oshinsky, *Polio*, 69.
[39] Oshinsky, 89, 188.
[40] Zunz, *Philanthropy in America*, 70, 176; see also Oshinsky, *Polio*, 5; Putnam, *Bowling Alone*.
[41] Sills, *Volunteers*, 80.
[42] Sills, 86–91, 193.

had already served as the architect of the March of Dimes when, by coincidence, his daughter was diagnosed; he wrote that in all his years with the foundation he had "never dreamed . . . of polio hitting [his family]."[43]

Reflecting the fact that their motivations were not specific to polio, 70% of volunteers belonged to at least three other public interest organizations. They spoke about these organizations relatively interchangeably, saying "if someone had asked me to do something definite for the Red Cross, I probably would have done that" and "I'm always tied up in some outside activity."[44] Some participated to raise their social status and advance their careers. Volunteers told Sills that "we all felt that we'd like our names associated with sponsoring this drive" and that "all of us want to be identified with something as fine as this." They viewed polio as a shared risk, calling the campaign "the cheapest paid-up insurance policy you can get—only a dime."[45] Their efforts amplified the tuberculosis movement's model for a mass disease campaign.

Chronic Campaigns

As infectious diseases, tuberculosis and polio were sensible targets for mass campaigns. Containing the diseases lessened everyone's risk, and subsidizing patients' treatments could be viewed as social insurance. In contrast, two other dominant mid-century disease campaigns targeted widespread chronic illnesses. While not infectious, these diseases were so common that everyone could feel at risk. Like the tuberculosis and polio campaigns, the crusades against cancer and heart disease were mass philanthropic responses to broadly shared threats.

The American Society for the Control of Cancer, later called the American Cancer Society (ACS), was founded in 1913. Reflecting spillovers across disease campaigns, its early meetings were attended by tuberculosis movement leaders.[46] The ACS also followed the tuberculosis and polio model by relying on large numbers of female volunteers. In the 1930s, the society mobilized a 100,000-strong "Women's Field Army" (WFA) to

---

[43] Oshinsky, *Polio*, 153; see also p. 46.
[44] Sills, *Volunteers*, 88; see also pp. 30, 60.
[45] Sills, 106, 94, 92, 99, 170, 171.
[46] Cavins, *National Health Agencies*, 119.

distribute educational materials, get people to their doctors' offices, help poor patients, sew bandages, and raise money.[47] The WFA gave women a rare outlet for political activity and the opportunity to participate in "a safe and vital battle." But some of their activities, including helping women to avoid unwanted pregnancies and calling for public funding for healthcare, proved too political for the ACS leadership. The ACS dissolved the WFA in the 1940s.[48] The next form of mass participation was willfully apolitical, focused more exclusively on fundraising. In the 1940s, philanthropists led by Mary Lasker launched the Annual Cancer Crusade, which sent hundreds of thousands of volunteers door to door to ask for donations. The campaign raised $4 million in its first year, $50 million in today's dollars, with returns increasing over the decades.[49] By the 1980s, the ACS had 2.5 million volunteers, comprising over 2% of all the volunteers in the United States.[50]

Like polio volunteers, ACS members were active across many causes and often had no particular personal connection to cancer. When asked why he was recruited for a leadership position, an ACS vice president explained, "I was a joiner, headed the Red Cross drive, active on the zoo board and the Junior Chamber of Commerce, the local hospital board."[51] One mid-century researcher described a typical volunteer for the ACS as a woman who "tried cancer as one might try window-box gardening or canasta. She might have looked into polio or heart disease or muscular dystrophy, but the Cancer Society was conveniently located, and a friend of hers had died of cancer not long before."[52] Accurate or not, this somewhat dismissive description reveals the public perception that ACS members were philanthropists helping a cause, not cancer patients pursuing their interests.

The American Heart Association (AHA) also drew resources and expertise from earlier campaigns. The NTA directly sponsored the AHA, providing a majority of its budget in the 1920s and 1930s.[53] In the late 1940s, Mary Lasker drew on her experience with the cancer campaign and convinced the AHA to start mass fundraising. A television campaign in the late 1940s successfully attracted donations and raised the association's public

[47] Breslow, *History of Cancer Control*, 783; Carter, *Gentle Legions*, 152–53; Ross, *Crusade*, 31.
[48] Davis, *Secret History*, 112–29.
[49] Ross, *Crusade*, 193.
[50] Ross, xv.
[51] Lane Adams, quoted in Ross, 41.
[52] Carter, *Gentle Legions*, 14–15.
[53] Carter, 175; Shryock, *National Tuberculosis Association*, 242.

profile. By 1960, the association had 1.5 million volunteers.[54] Other health organizations also turned to lay control and professional fundraising. The American Diabetes Association (ADA) was founded as a professional association for physicians, in 1940. After decades of debates, the ADA admitted lay members and expanded fundraising in 1970.[55] Similarly, physicians founded several organizations to fight epilepsy, later partnering with medical researchers and philanthropists.[56]

Concerns About Disease Dominance

Disease campaigns dominated mid-century American philanthropy. Paired with the Red Cross and the National Society for Crippled Children and Adults, the campaigns against tuberculosis, polio, cancer, and heart disease were called the "Big Six" in philanthropic circles because of their impressive scale and success. When combined with the Red Cross and Community Chest campaigns, these four disease organizations accounted for fully a third of non-religious and educational philanthropy in America.[57] Huge numbers of urban Americans reported that they had donated money to fight tuberculosis (77%), polio (70%), heart disease (45%), and cancer (43%).[58] A contemporary observer called disease campaigns "the largest social movement in the United States," noting that with the exception of the civil rights movement, "health voluntarism stands virtually alone nowadays as a means whereby millions of Americans assemble for direct action against an array of national problems."[59] When Arnaud Marts mapped American charity in the 1960s, he counted over 70,000 organizations affiliated with 40 disease associations. By comparison, there were only 45,000 Parent Teacher Associations and 7,500 public libraries.[60] In the 1970s, the ACS, the AHA, the National Foundation, and the American Lung Association (descended from the NTA) were still the largest health philanthropies, each raising over $40 million per year (over $200 million in today's dollars).[61] Among the

[54] Carter, *Gentle Legions*, 174–78; Cavins, *National Health Agencies*, 163–64.
[55] American Diabetes Association, *Journey & and the Dream*, 98, 141.
[56] American Epilepsy Society, "History of AES"; Cavins, *National Health Agencies*.
[57] Sills, *Volunteers*, 176–78.
[58] Sills, 182.
[59] Carter, *Gentle Legions*, 19.
[60] Marts, *Generosity of Americans*, 127. The 70,000 organizations include, for example, each of the Tuberculosis Association's 2,000 state and local associations.
[61] American Association of Fund-Raising Counsel, "Giving USA," 42.

22 largest national health philanthropies, 90% targeted a single malady.[62] The ACS, the National Foundation, and the AHA each reported over two million volunteers per year, second only to the United Way and UNICEF.[63] Disease campaigns had swept the country.

The unprecedented scale and success of disease campaigns raised concerns. In every decade, critics worried that a few favored diseases were receiving too much money at the expense of other pressing public health priorities. In 1919, the president of the Rockefeller Foundation argued that "the health of a community is, after all, not a group of special interests. . . . To exalt one of them, to get it out of focus, and to urge it at the expense of other essential factors, is unscientific, wasteful and misleading."[64] In 1936, a prominent public health professor argued that the proliferation of disease campaigns spawned "dissipation of effort of the professional worker, and confusion in the mind of the public."[65] In the 1940s, public health leaders expressed "dismay" at the "spectacular returns" of the polio campaign, given the disease's relatively low prevalence.[66] Regarding polio and tuberculosis, critics asked,

> Can the whole private health movement be well served when two voluntary health movements, fighting two diseases, obtain from the public $26,000,000 in one year, while very many other public health dangers of greater individual or collective importance must be combatted by all the other voluntary health movements with only a small fraction of this amount?[67]

These critics worried about asymmetrical funding successes; others worried that fragmentation would eventually doom even the most successful campaigns. In the 1930s, Louis Dublin, a board member of the American Social Hygiene Association, argued that voluntary health associations would inevitably cannibalize each other since they "all draw on the same small number of persons who have a social conscience."[68]

---

[62] Blendon, "Changing Role of Private Philanthropy in Health Affairs," 653.

[63] American Association of Fund-Raising Counsel, "Giving USA," 9.

[64] George Vincent, 1919, quoted in Gunn and Platt, *Voluntary Health Agencies*, 184; see also Shryock, *National Tuberculosis Association*, 184–85.

[65] Hiscock, "Opportunities of Voluntary Health Agencies," 53.

[66] Gunn and Platt, *Voluntary Health Agencies*, 214–15.

[67] Gunn and Platt, 216.

[68] Dublin, "Social Hygiene Movement," 67.

Whether they worried about the lopsided funding distribution or the self-defeating effects of multiple appeals to the same donors, the critics agreed that a single public health fundraising campaign would be preferable. Surely public health experts could distribute the funds more rationally. Dublin predicted that if all the health associations joined forces for fundraising, "the American public would not only be aroused but won over . . . I am convinced that the plan will succeed ultimately. . . . It has the virtue of simplicity and rationality and, therefore, nothing will ultimately stop its realization."[69] To early twentieth-century public health advocates, a unified campaign seemed destined to succeed. People could donate to a single pool of funds, which would be rationally distributed by experts to the areas of greatest need. What could go wrong?

In 1913, officials from the major health associations met to discuss ways to coordinate and streamline their activities.[70] The National Public Health Congress, founded in 1914, sought to unite the major disease campaigns.[71] In 1921, 14 voluntary health associations formed the National Health Council (NHC), hoping to replace the "competitive and confusing duplication of appeals for funds" with "a substantial pooling of the separate appeals for the safeguarding of the health of the people."[72] However, while many smaller health agencies favored collaboration, three of the four dominant disease associations stated that there would be *no* advantages to unification, and none fully supported the plan.[73] The NHC's own board and staff were reluctant "to give up their special activities and participate constructively in joint programs."[74] The NHC survives to this day, but it never fulfilled its goals of replacing single-disease campaigns and rationalizing the distribution of health charitable dollars. In 2014, it took in less than one-fiftieth as much as the March of Dimes.

While the NHC sought to combine all voluntary health drives, federated giving went even further, seeking to combine all philanthropy. During World War I, fundraisers worried that donors and volunteers were becoming fatigued by repeated drives and concluded that "financial

---

[69] Dublin, 67–68.
[70] Frederick Green, 1913, quoted in Gunn and Platt, *Voluntary Health Agencies*, 182.
[71] Teller, *Tuberculosis Movement*, 53.
[72] Gunn and Platt, *Voluntary Health Agencies*, vii, 10, 217.
[73] Gunn and Platt, 69, 194–98.
[74] Hiscock, "Opportunities of Voluntary Health Agencies," 55.

federation" would solve the problem.[75] Within cities, Community Chests raised money for multiple charities. By the late 1930s, all but six cities with over 100,000 residents had a Community Chest. By 1961, they raised $478 million a year.[76]

As the Community Chests grew, they sought to include the major disease campaigns, in part because they had unrealistically promised "to stop all other solicitation for health and welfare purposes."[77] Including disease campaigns was also good for fundraising; United Way surveys showed that they would raise more funds if they included health organizations.[78] Yet the most successful health campaigns were uninterested in joining federations.[79] The NTA discouraged local chapters from participating, was unwilling to give up the Christmas Seals drive, and eventually broke with the Community Chests completely.[80] The National Foundation argued that participating in Community Chests would "bury the identity of health agencies and blunt the stimulating impact of individual drives" and "turn all philanthropy into an assembly line project."[81] After finding that participating chapters were raising less money, the ACS pulled out of United Way in 1959.[82]

In the early 1960s, the Rockefeller Foundation funded a study sparked by concern about the "intolerable" conflict between federated and independent fundraising campaigns.[83] In another indication of the dominance of disease campaigns, the report is introduced as a study of "voluntary health and welfare agencies," but it actually focuses primarily on disease organizations.[84] Echoing earlier critics, the report argued that voluntary efforts should be organized more rationally, rather than focusing on a few favored issues.[85] In addition to the familiar concerns that public donations would dry up,

---

[75] Cutlip, Fund Raising, 214.

[76] Blanchard, "Community Chests," 87; Borst, "Community Chests and Councils," 95; Cutlip, Fund Raising, 213.

[77] Cutlip, Fund Raising, 215; see also Thompson, "Community Chests and United Funds," 176.

[78] Ross, Crusade, 204.

[79] Cutlip, Fund Raising, 216.

[80] Cutlip, 217; Shryock, National Tuberculosis Association, 188, 226.

[81] Sills, Volunteers, 55, quoting a Foundation mimeograph.

[82] They relaxed their decision in the late 1970s, again allowing local chapters to cooperate with the United Way. Ross, Crusade, 199, 205.

[83] Hamlin, Voluntary Health and Welfare Agencies, ii.

[84] When the authors list "a sample of national agencies with local chapters and other agencies which solicit contributions on a national or regional basis," a majority (58%) focus on diseases— a supermajority (78%) if we include blindness, deafness, and physical and mental handicaps. Hamlin, 83–87.

[85] Hamlin, 2.

these authors worried that "wasteful competition, if permitted to continue, may well turn the focus of public demand for increased health and welfare services even more toward government."[86] They called for "a new National Commission on Voluntary Health and Welfare Agencies" to evaluate the agencies and promote coordination, to be funded and organized by foundations and endorsed by the US president.[87] To the authors' dismay, the Rockefeller Foundation didn't come through with the money to fund such a commission.[88]

Each of these attempts to rationalize disease campaigns assumed that Americans would be most moved by a single expert-led appeal for public health. The critics imagined that American donors might receive one too many fundraising letters, throw up their hands, and say, "That's it! Nobody gets a penny!" But if they received a letter from the president asking for a donation to an expert-led public health fund, they'd open their wallets. This was a profound misreading of the American public. Donors and volunteers were unexcited by technocratic appeals for public health but willing to give small amounts to fight various diseases. As one health agency official told a researcher, "Whoever heard of anyone dying of United Way? You die of a specific disease."[89] A March of Dimes volunteer reported that when he approached proprietors of "every grocery store, filling station, bank, all the merchants" in his community, "only two people actually said 'No.' . . . This doesn't happen with the Red Cross."[90] Fundraisers also reported that more people were willing to donate to fight polio than to the Community Chest.[91] The reformers assumed that multiple disease campaigns were competing with each other for a fixed pool of health donations. But as an ACS representative pointed out, "almost everyone will give more if he gives four times than if he gives once for four causes."[92] Single-disease campaigns may create windfalls for a few diseases, but in their absence, that pool of money would not flow to other charitable causes.

---

[86] Hamlin, 33.
[87] Hamlin, iii, 35.
[88] Lear, "Business of Giving."
[89] Bakal, *Charity U.S.A.*, 419.
[90] Sills, *Volunteers*, 166.
[91] Sills, 166.
[92] Bakal, *Charity U.S.A.*, 419.

Disease Campaigns and the Federal Government

Just as disease campaigns moved private donors, they inspired policymakers and voters. As the federal government built up its investments in public health and medical research, campaigns against specific diseases attracted the most funds. These disease campaigns conflicted with scientists' preference for basic research and untargeted public health funds.[93] But it was single diseases that aroused the most enthusiasm among policymakers and the public, and they helped build an enormous public health and medical research infrastructure.

Before the turn of the century, there was little government involvement in public health or medical research.[94] As the federal government entered the field of public health in the teens, its programs often favored disease campaigns over broader public health efforts.[95] In the 1910s, the Public Health Service (PHS) received more money for campaigns against pellagra, sexually transmitted infections, and a few other diseases than for all other projects combined.[96] In 1935, the federal government began providing grants to states for public health education, targeted to particular diseases or groups.[97] The Centers for Disease Control and Prevention (CDC)[98] began by fighting malaria and, over the decades, added campaigns against other tropical diseases, then all communicable diseases, and then chronic conditions.[99] When the head of a new CDC division wondered how to set an agenda in 1947, the CDC's main supporter in PHS advised him to "Just stick with diseases. . . . Stay away from milk and food sanitation problems."[100] Not all CDC programs target diseases.[101] Some directors have viewed it as an agency focused on primary prevention efforts, which often cut across disease categories.[102] But over the decades, the CDC's budget and prominence increased through campaigns against polio, flu,

---

[93] Cook-Deegan and McGeary, "Jewel in the Federal Crown?"; Guston, *Between Politics and Science*; Rettig, *Cancer Crusade*; Sampat, "Dismal Science"; Spingarn, *Heartbeat*, 185; Strickland, *Politics, Science, and Dread Disease*.

[94] Fee, "Public Health and the State"; Sealander, "Curing Evils," 235.

[95] Fee, "Public Health and the State," 247.

[96] Harden, *Inventing the NIH*, 54–55.

[97] Fee, "Public Health and the State," 241, 247.

[98] This agency's name changed several times over the years, but it usually retained the acronym "CDC," which I use to refer to it across the decades.

[99] Etheridge, *Sentinel for Health*; Fee, "Public Health and the State," 1, 13, 341.

[100] Mountin 1945, quoted in Etheridge, *Sentinel for Health*, 25.

[101] Etheridge, 224, 228–29, 232, 245, 280–81.

[102] Etheridge, 87, 242.

and emerging infectious diseases; by incorporating PHS divisions fighting venereal diseases and tuberculosis; by launching vaccination campaigns targeting major childhood diseases; and by pushing to eradicate malaria and smallpox.[103]

Federal investments in medical research reflect a related struggle between disease campaigns and basic research. In the 1920s, two senators proposed competing plans for government-sponsored medical research: a cancer campaign or a research institute that "is not limited to any one disease, but takes in all the ills that flesh is heir to." With the founding of the National Institute of Health (NIH) in 1930, the general approach prevailed, but cancer advocates were undaunted.[104] Seven years later, national magazines ran feature stories about cancer, and a public letter-writing campaign urged Congress to act.[105] The ACS joined the chorus, turning to government to supplement fundraising hampered by the Great Depression.[106] A 1937 bill to establish the National Cancer Institute (NCI) was signed by every member of the Senate.[107] Health officials worried about separating out one disease for special attention, but once it became clear that the measure would succeed, they helped draft the bill.[108]

Inspired by the cancer institute, advocates lobbied for institutes for other diseases, often triumphing over the opposition of NIH directors. Putting disease labels on institutes made them more compelling for a public enamored with disease campaigns; since "no one ever died of microbiology," the Microbiology Institute was renamed the National Institute of Allergy and Infectious Diseases in 1955.[109] The institutes developed internal programs that targeted particular diseases.[110] Despite government scientists'

---

[103] Etheridge, 67, 87, 101, 147, 151, 188, 211.

[104] Strickland, *Politics, Science, and Dread Disease*, 9, 28; see also Ginzberg and Dutka, *Financing of Biomedical Research*, 18–19; Harden, *Inventing the NIH*, 129.

[105] Strickland, *Politics, Science, and Dread Disease*, 13.

[106] Casamayou, *Politics of Breast Cancer*, 28–29; Ross, *Crusade*, 29–30; Strickland, *Politics, Science, and Dread Disease*, 14.

[107] Strickland, *Politics, Science, and Dread Disease*, 13.

[108] Strickland, 24–25.

[109] Rettig, *Cancer Crusade*, 12; Strickland, *Politics, Science, and Dread Disease*, 192.

[110] Culliton, "NIH Budget Growth"; Kastor, *National Institutes of Health*, 44, 156; Rettig, *Cancer Crusade*, 23; Strickland, *NIH Grants Programs*, 53, 77, 84, 86; Talley, "Community and Science," 55–58. The NIH's focus on applied research targeting specific diseases was accelerated by the postwar transfer of World War II–related research contracts to the institutes, which increased NIH's budget more than 10-fold and solidified its focus on disease-targeted research. Strickland, *Politics, Science, and Dread Disease*, 27–29, 193.

preference for untargeted basic research, it was becoming accepted that "the main concern [at NIH] should be the conquest of specific diseases."[111]

The conflict between disease categories and untargeted research came to a head in 1970 as advocates and senators called for a "war on cancer."[112] At Mary Lasker's urging, advice columnist Ann Landers supported the campaign, and tens of thousands of letters poured in to policymakers. The 1971 National Cancer Act gave the NCI more money, a presidentially appointed director, and an independent budget submitted directly to the president.[113] This special status for the NCI was "seen by many within NIH and the medical science community as pushing categorization of disease problems to a ludicrous extreme."[114] Yet despite their opposition, "scientists seemingly took the money and ran with their own research agendas."[115] Over the next few years, more disease-focused institutes were added, and an increasing proportion of the budget targeted particular diseases.[116]

Journalists criticized "disease-of-the-month" laws and appropriations, and NIH officials expressed concerns about the "irrational fragmentation" of medical research.[117] And yet, scientists increasingly concluded that "the only really feasible way to get large infusions of new money for research is to tie it to a specific disease."[118] Paul Starr writes that "like the voluntary health organizations, NIH discovered that the way to open wide the public's purse was to call attention to one disease at a time."[119] As with the health charities, disease targeting made it difficult to systematically set priorities, but the increased funding made it worthwhile.

Over time, the federal disease programs became increasingly intertwined with voluntary disease campaigns.[120] While the National Foundation had actively opposed government funding for polio research, calling it

---

[111] Strickland, *Politics, Science, and Dread Disease*, 86; see also Casamayou, *Politics of Breast Cancer*, 35; Cohen, "Conflicting Agendas Shape NIH," 1675; Cook-Deegan and McGeary, "Jewel in the Federal Crown?," 190; Nathan and Schechter, "NIH Support," 2656.

[112] Rettig, *Cancer Crusade*, xv; Spingarn, *Heartbeat*, 40, 183; Strickland, *Politics, Science, and Dread Disease*, 260–67.

[113] Strickland, *NIH Grants Programs*, 78; see also Rettig, *Cancer Crusade*, 279, 291.

[114] Strickland, *NIH Grants Programs*, 79.

[115] Guston, *Between Politics and Science*, 80.

[116] Institute of Medicine, *Scientific Opportunities and Public Needs*, 54.

[117] Culliton, "House Battles," 727; Spingarn, *Heartbeat*, 76.

[118] Suzanne Oparil, quoted in Johnson, *Breast Cancer Research*, 45.

[119] Starr, *Social Transformation of American Medicine*, 343; see also Rettig, *Cancer Crusade*, 11; Sinclair, "Disease Lobbies"; Spingarn, *Heartbeat*, 73; Strickland, *NIH Grants Programs*, 77.

[120] Epstein, "Patient Groups and Health Movements," 506; Fox, "Alzheimer's Disease Movement"; Talley, "Community and Science."

"Communistic" and "un-American,"[121] later disease campaigners increasingly lobbied Congress for medical research funding.[122] Mary Lasker had imagined the cancer fight as a private philanthropic campaign until her husband told her that "the place to get the money is the federal government. . . . There are unlimited funds. I'll show you how to get them."[123] She took his advice to heart, spending years lobbying Congress, making campaign donations, and building relationships with policymakers. Thanks in part to Lasker's efforts, policymakers multiplied the federal cancer research budget 60-fold during the 1940s and 1950s.[124] Following her example, advocates for other diseases lobbied for new institutes and targeted research funding, and in turn, new NIH institutes and funding streams inspired new voluntary associations targeting the disease or diseases.[125] In 1953, Congressman Fogarty asked an institute director whether there was a "coordinating committee" on neurological diseases. The following year, the director reported back that two new organizations now targeted his institute's diseases.[126] Disease crusades helped the federal research budget grow, which in turn inspired more disease campaigns.

Conclusion

The first half of the twentieth century saw the emergence of a vast philanthropic sector and the first major federal investments in public health and medical research. Both were built around fighting dread diseases. The crusaders created a model for disease campaigns: targeting a single disease, framing it as a universal threat, mobilizing millions of volunteers, and calling on all Americans to donate. This organizational repertoire spread across diseases and helped institutionalize mass philanthropy. When we talk about the surge in voluntarism in the middle decades of the twentieth century, [127] we should remember how much of this voluntarism targeted disease campaigns.

---

[121] Oshinsky, *Polio*, 189; see also Etheridge, *Sentinel for Health*, 69.
[122] Cook-Deegan and McGeary, "Jewel in the Federal Crown?," 181.
[123] Mary Lasker, quoted in Ross, *Crusade*, 210.
[124] Carter, *Gentle Legions*, 139; Ross, *Crusade*, 212–14.
[125] Strickland, *Politics, Science, and Dread Disease*, 135.
[126] Strickland, 140.
[127] Hall, "Historical Overview"; Putnam, *Bowling Alone*.

Women typically formed the mass volunteer base for disease campaigns, from the "marching mothers" collecting dimes for polio to the Women's Field Army fighting cancer. The feminine character of mass disease campaigns may have made them easier to dismiss as separate from "real" politics. This impression is likely strengthened by the consensus surrounding disease campaigns; no one could be against curing cancer.

Was this disease fixation specific to the United States? One 1940s-era commentator argued that America's disease campaigns had "no well-developed counterpart" in Europe.[128] Tuberculosis and cancer campaigns did emerge in several Western countries.[129] But they lacked the mass mobilization seen in the United States.[130] According to some scholars, "the politics of funding for health and medical research in the United States is unique in its disease-specific, 'squeaky-wheel-gets-the-grease' character."[131] Lacking universal access to healthcare, Americans may have turned to disease campaigns as an alternative way to fund "health insurance" one disease at a time.

Across the decades, public health experts, journalists, policymakers, and scientists criticized disease crusades' narrow specialization, arguing that they funneled money to only a few favored diseases and distracted government investments from basic research. Again and again, these critics tried to implement plans to spend money more rationally—to make disease charities join forces, and to free the CDC and NIH from categorical funding streams. But while specialized campaigns yield funding distributions that few would consider ideal, it's a mistake to assume that we can choose to distribute that same money more rationally. The campaigns against tuberculosis, polio, cancer, and heart disease did not draw from a pre-existing pool of resources. They created the funding stream with the appeal of their targeted claims.[132]

---

[128] Cavins, *National Health Agencies*, 12.

[129] Cantor, "Introduction"; Cavins, *National Health Agencies*, 84; Gunn and Platt, *Voluntary Health Agencies*, 21; Knopf, *History of the National Tuberculosis Association*, 55; Zunz, *Philanthropy in America*, 47.

[130] Cantor, "Introduction," 10; Davis, *Secret History*, 125–26; Lerner, *Breast Cancer Wars*, 45; Nathanson, *Disease Prevention as Social Change*, 81, 85; Shryock, *National Tuberculosis Association*, 55–57, 308; Tomes, *Gospel of Germs*, 18.

[131] Epstein, *Inclusion*, 333.

[132] This point applies to social movements more generally. While "managerial technocrats" might seek to improve social movements through "rationalization by merger," a large number of specialized organizations may actually mobilize the public more effectively. Zald and McCarthy, "Social Movement Industries," 15.

In addition to their specialization, a key reason for the charitable crusades' success was their universality. As one contemporary observer explained, "no matter how heavy grows the lump in my throat as I sign the check. . . . My gift nourishes science, not handicapped children . . . I have given so as to safeguard and improve human health, including my own."[133] Disease campaigns were special because "[e]very individual is a potential beneficiary of their efforts."[134] The fact that they claimed to benefit everyone may help explain why of all the social problems targeted by Progressive-era reformers, it was disease campaigns that captured the public imagination and dominated modern philanthropy. The other problems were more directly related to poverty, raising thorny questions about redistribution, dependency, and morality. Diseases were conceived of as shared risks in a way poverty never was. Later in the twentieth century, disease campaigns would retain their prominence but with a fundamental difference: the new campaigns would be organized by and for patients and their families. Without universal claims, they would need new ways to mobilize donors and create consensus.

[133] Carter, *Gentle Legions*, 27.
[134] Gunn and Platt, *Voluntary Health Agencies*, 3.

2

Disease Constituencies

The crusades against tuberculosis, polio, cancer, and heart disease had mobilized mass publics around widely shared risks without assuming that volunteers and donors would have any personal connection to the diseases. A new type of disease campaign emerged in the second half of the twentieth century, depicting current patients and their families as constituents.[1] This was a shift from *universalistic* organizing, which claims to benefit everyone, to *constituency-based* organizing, centered around a group of people with shared characteristics and interests.[2] Social scientists have commented on the increasing prominence of patients in disease advocacy[3] and the subsequent proliferation of campaigns against dozens of diseases.[4] But previous studies have been unable to explain when and why disease patients' advocacy took off.[5] This chapter asks how and why patient-focused advocacy emerged, spread, and created a new politics of consensus.

---

[1] Rothman et al., "Health Advocacy Organizations," 603.

[2] I use the phrase "disease constituencies" to refer to constituency-based organizing around disease categories. See Epstein, "Politics of Health Mobilization." I adopt the terms "universalistic" and "constituency-based" from Gamson, *Strategy of Social Protest*, 62; and Clemens, "Organizational Repertoires and Institutional Change," 774. Other social scientists have called the former groups "philanthropic," "public-interest," and "issue-based" and the latter "special-interest" groups. Clemens, 774; Olson, *Logic of Collective Action*, 159–60; Schattschneider, *Semi-Sovereign People*, 22, 26. Confusingly, some scholars call both types "interest groups," while others reserve the term for constituency-based groups. Clemens, *People's Lobby*; Finer, "Anonymous Empire"; Sills, *Volunteers*, 78; Stewart, *British Pressure Groups*; Truman, *Governmental Process*. Meanwhile, some scholars use the term "identity politics" to refer to constituency-based groups when they organize around a common identity. But other researchers have used the phrase to denote advocacy with non-material goals, with various negative connotations. Bernstein, "Identity Politics"; Bernstein, "Analytic Dimensions of Identity."

[3] Arno and Feiden, *Against the Odds*, 243–44; Brown and Zavestoski, "Social Movements in Health," 682; Foreman, "Grassroots Victim Organizations," 34; Kedrowski and Sarow, *Cancer Activism*, 39, 43; Packard et al., *Emerging Illnesses and Society*, 39; Rothman et al., "Health Advocacy Organizations," 603.

[4] Epstein, "Patient Groups and Health Movements," 500; Epstein, "Measuring Success," 260.

[5] Most studies focus on a single disease movement, and many use contemporary data, making it difficult to observe trends in the entire field of disease campaigns. For reviews, see Epstein, "Patient Groups and Health Movements"; Hess et al., "Science, Technology, and Social Movements."

Broad social changes laid the groundwork for patients' activism. As chronic diseases became the biggest killers, patients had more incentive to mobilize. Activism, social movements, interest groups, and the nonprofit sector all expanded dramatically. New patients' groups emerged, many adopting a more contentious approach that challenged medical authority. But these non-universal campaigns faced skepticism from the medical establishment and the government and did not proliferate widely.

In the 1980s, people with AIDS and breast cancer drew on pre-existing identity-based activism to create movements for patients with their diseases. Existing movement communities can incubate new politicized collective identities, connecting people together and providing resources, strategies, and infrastructure that help new movements and organizations get off the ground.[6] But transposing models for organizing from one type of cause (e.g., gender or sexuality) to another (e.g., disease) requires creative work. Without universal beneficiaries, disease constituencies needed to create consensus around a "special interest" and make political demands seem nonthreatening. AIDS activism, especially, started out as a confrontational social movement. But they created a new kind of consensus politics, moving from protests to the AIDS Walk, from Silence=Death pins to red ribbons. Along with breast cancer activists, they created a new model for disease constituencies, combining the reach of a charitable crusade with a focus on promoting patients' interests.

A given type of mobilization often expands quickly once a template becomes institutionalized.[7] People affected by other diseases followed AIDS and breast cancer activists' example, borrowing resources, expertise, and legitimacy from these two enormous movements. Patients and their family members founded thousands of groups targeting hundreds of diseases, launching some of the most powerful citizens' movements of the late twentieth century.

---

[6] Andrews and Biggs, "Dynamics of Protest Diffusion"; Freeman, "Origins of the Women's Liberation Movement"; McAdam, "'Initiator' and 'Spin-off' Movements"; Meyer and Whittier, "Social Movement Spillover"; Minkoff, *Organizing for Equality*; Oliver and Myers, "Coevolution of Social Movements"; Taylor, "Social Movement Continuity"; Walker, "Origins and Maintenance of Interest Groups"; Whittier, "Consequences of Social Movements for Each Other."

[7] Armstrong, *Forging Gay Identities*; Clemens, "Organizational Repertoires and Institutional Change"; Clemens, *People's Lobby*; Clemens and Cook, "Politics and Institutionalism."

1940–1980: Disease Constituencies Face Skepticism

The charitable crusades had targeted infectious diseases and widespread chronic conditions. Since everyone was (or could imagine themselves to be) at risk, tuberculosis, polio, cancer, and heart disease could be framed as universal threats and not as small groups' interests. These conditions lent themselves to charitable crusades but not to patients' activism—it is harder to involve patients in campaigns if they either die or recover quickly, as is the case with many infectious diseases. As the twentieth century progressed, chronic conditions replaced infectious diseases as the leading causes of death.[8] Relatively rare chronic diseases couldn't be framed as widely shared threats, making them poor fits for the charitable crusade model. In contrast, rarer chronic conditions lend themselves to disease constituencies. Patients may be more likely to think of a chronic disease as part of their identity.[9] Since they may live with the disease for a long time, they have more opportunity and incentive to band together to pursue their interests.[10]

The rise of chronic disease intersected with a change in American organizational life: a nationwide upsurge in "small groups" in which people came together to discuss shared interests or problems.[11] Just as disease crusades led the way for modern philanthropy, disease patients' groups were at the forefront of this trend, with many predating the mid-1960s–1980s proliferation of mutual support and self-help groups.[12] The years following World War II saw the formation of associations for patients with several chronic diseases. In 1946, patients and their family members founded the National Multiple Sclerosis Society (NMSS); they gained support from neurologists who were working in "underfunded medical research areas in need of a disease."[13] That same year, parents of children with cerebral palsy found each other through newspaper advertisements and formed what would become United Cerebral Palsy (UCP).[14] In the 1950s, 1960s, and 1970s,

[8] Strauss and Glaser, *Chronic Illness*.

[9] Bury, "Sociology of Chronic Illness"; Charmaz, *Good Days, Bad Days*; Foreman, "Grassroots Victim Organizations"; Kedrowski and Sarow, *Cancer Activism*; Wood, *Patient Power?*

[10] Wood, *Patient Power?*, 44, 46.

[11] Wuthnow, *Sharing the Journey*, 3.

[12] Archibald, *Evolution of Self-Help*, xi, 67; Gussow and Tracy, "Self-Help Clubs," 407; Katz, "Self-Help and Mutual Aid," 131; Katz, *Self-Help in America*, 93, 129; Rabeharisoa, "Experience, Knowledge and Empowerment."

[13] Packard et al., *Emerging Illnesses and Society*, 139; see also Talley, "Community and Science," 43.

[14] Fleischer and Zames, *Disability Rights Movement*, 9.

patients and family members founded organizations to target other chronic conditions.[15]

Mid-century commentators noticed that these new disease associations were different from the charitable crusades: they were "organized in the grief of patients and their families," founded by and for people personally affected by the diseases.[16] A 1970 "guide to volunteer services" listed opportunities for volunteering with the traditional disease crusades—people could handprint cards for the March of Dimes or raise money for the Heart Fund—but then added, "finally, there is a very special kind of volunteer—the afflicted person who has become sufficiently rehabilitated to adjust to his illness or handicap and help others similarly afflicted."[17] The assumption was that volunteers for the former campaigns lacked personal experiences of polio or heart disease and that patient self-help organizations were a different phenomenon. In a telling episode, a Cerebral Palsy Association administrator proposed enlisting philanthropists who were not personally affected by cerebral palsy (CP) in the model of the charitable crusades. The administrator was fired, and as one association member explained, "We can't have this organization taken over by people who don't see CP as we do. *We* are the ones with the CP children."[18] These advocates framed cerebral palsy not as a public health threat affecting everyone equally but as a personal problem affecting them and their families.

To some contemporary observers, patient-centered disease associations seemed nonsensical and likely to be short-lived. In 1958, the president of the American Neurological Association found it absurd to contemplate the emergence of associations targeting every disease:

> Some years ago I was invited to chair a society of amyotrophic lateral sclerosis. Why not one for tuberous sclerosis? And since there is a society for muscular dystrophy, why not another for muscular atrophies, and still

[15] American Diabetes Association, *Journey & and the Dream*, 152; Archibald, *Evolution of Self-Help*, 34; Bell, *DES Daughters*, 122; Cooley's Anemia Foundation, "History"; Crohn's & Colitis Foundation of America, "About"; Katz, "Self-Help and Mutual Aid"; Johnson and Hufbauer, "Sudden Infant Death Syndrome," 65; Kushner, "Construction of Tourette Syndrome," 74; Laffont, "Steady Progress"; Lock, "Biosociality and Susceptibility Genes," 57; Myasthenia Gravis Foundation of America, "About MGFA"; National Kidney Foundation, "History"; National Tay-Sachs and Allied Diseases Association, "Our History"; Parkinson's Disease Foundation, "Parkinson's Disease Foundation 1957–2007"; Tracy and Gussow, "Self-Help Health Groups," 382.

[16] Carter, *Gentle Legions*, 203.

[17] David, *Guide to Volunteer Services*, 37.

[18] Carter, *Gentle Legions*, 208.

others for all the other myopathies and amyotrophies? Not so long ago a society for myasthenia gravis has come into being, for which there is little rhyme and less reason.[19]

This critique of the various neuromuscular disease organizations stems from their specificity: unlike the American Heart Association or the American Cancer Society, they did not gather a group of related diseases into one umbrella organization. Prominent critics predicted that this new organizational form would be short-lived and that associations targeting related diseases would inevitably merge.[20]

If an overly narrow focus threatened the legitimacy of patients' organizations, one possible response would be to affiliate with broader campaigns. Some patients' groups did partner with the major charitable crusades, but their relationships were uneasy. The National Foundation and the American Heart Association began to encourage the formation of patients' support groups,[21] and the American Diabetes Association affiliated with local patient-led associations.[22] The American Cancer Society (ACS) put off calls to incorporate Reach to Recovery, an organization that arranged for breast cancer survivors to visit mastectomy patients, for more than a decade, only coming around when they "realized that cancer self-help programs were growing successfully without them."[23] Worried that Reach to Recovery would "become a crutch," the ACS discouraged the women from staying in touch after the hospital visit.[24] The ACS affiliated with other support groups, including the International Association of Laryngectomees, the Ostomy Rehabilitation Program, I CAN COPE, Candlelighters, and Cansurmount.[25] But in each case, ACS higher-ups felt uneasy about patients organizing among themselves. One ACS official explained that "[w]e don't want colostomates making a social life out of being colostomates . . . we don't want membership drives. We want people leaving us."[26] Local groups

---

[19] Israel S. Wechsler, quoted in Carter, 202.

[20] Carter, 203.

[21] Gussow and Tracy, "Self-Help Clubs," 413; Wuthnow, *Sharing the Journey*, 72.

[22] American Diabetes Association, *Journey & and the Dream.*

[23] Klawiter, *Biopolitics of Breast Cancer*, 118; see also Lerner, *Breast Cancer Wars*, 143–44; Morganstern, "Rehabilitation and Continuing Care," 459.

[24] Kushner, *Breast Cancer*, 211; see also Klawiter, *Biopolitics of Breast Cancer*, 120.

[25] Breslow, *History of Cancer Control*, 834; Klawiter, *Biopolitics of Breast Cancer*, 120; Ross, *Crusade*, 172–76.

[26] Morganstern, "Rehabilitation and Continuing Care," 462; see also Klawiter, *Biopolitics of Breast Cancer*, 120.

bristled when the ACS tried "to control or 'guide' the content of self-help group meetings and newsletters."[27] The bottom-up nature of patients' support groups challenged the disease crusade model.

Like the charitable crusades, some patients' organizations ran mass donation campaigns. The Muscular Dystrophy Association (MDA), which was founded by patients and family members, enlisted the National Association of Letter Carriers and the International Association of Fire Fighters to embark on a door-to-door fundraising campaign and started an annual telethon with celebrities raising money for the disease.[28] Without the presumption of universal beneficiaries, the MDA used demeaning appeals to sympathy to connect to mass publics. The telethon was later criticized for presenting people with disability as objects of pity, rather than advocating for their rights.[29]

While the first disease constituencies tried to partner with or emulate the charitable crusades, social changes in the 1960s and 1970s encouraged patients to mobilize politically and challenge medical authority. This period saw a dramatic increase in Americans' propensity to organize political movements, beginning with the "cycle of protest" of the 1960s and the "advocacy explosion" of the 1970s.[30] These movements inspired others that also focused on rights and identity categories, making claims on the basis of shared interests and using movements to elaborate and valorize new identities.[31] Some of these new movements focused on health issues. The health consumer movement emerged to protect people's rights in healthcare and challenge scientists' decision-making.[32] The women's health movement pushed for women's control over their bodies and their medical care.[33] Other movements promoted occupational and environmental health.[34] These campaigns reflected Americans' increasing willingness to challenge

---

[27] Chesler and Chesney, *Cancer and Self-Help*, 145.

[28] Muscular Dystrophy Association, "MDA—History."

[29] Anspach, "From Stigma to Identity Politics"; Shapiro, *No Pity*.

[30] Minkoff, *Organizing for Equality*, 1; see also Andrews and Edwards, "Advocacy Organizations"; Berry, *Interest Group Society*; Schlozman and Tierney, *Organized Interests and American Democracy*; Walker, "Origins and Maintenance of Interest Groups."

[31] Anspach, "From Stigma to Identity Politics"; Bernstein, "Identity Politics"; Pichardo, "New Social Movements"; Polletta and Jasper, "Collective Identity and Social Movements," 286.

[32] Bastian, "Speaking up for Ourselves," 9; Carpenter, *Reputation and Power*, 337–41; Mintzes and Hodgkin, "Consumer Movement"; Reiser, "Era of the Patient"; Rodwin, "Patient Accountability"; Tomes, "Patients or Health-Care Consumers?"

[33] Morgen, *Into Our Own Hands*; Ruzek, *Women's Health Movement*; Weisman, *Women's Health Care*.

[34] Kedrowski and Sarow, *Cancer Activism*, 39–41.

the authority of physicians and scientists.[35] Despite these challenges to medical authority, Americans continued to report a high level of faith in scientific medicine to heal their problems.[36] This seemingly paradoxical combination of faith in medicine and willingness to challenge expertise created favorable conditions for disease patients' advocacy, inspiring patients to push for changes in medical treatment and research.

This political climate inspired people with mental illness, disabilities, and cancer to form political movements. In the 1970s, former mental patients banded together to challenge psychiatric diagnoses, demand acceptance, and protest involuntary treatment.[37] Disability activists drew on the language of the civil rights movement, rejecting pleas for pity and cures and demanding rights and inclusion.[38] Distrusting a "cancer establishment" that included the ACS, some cancer patients demanded access to Laetrile, an alternative cancer therapy.[39] These movements were more patient-focused than the disease crusades and more political than self-help groups.[40]

As these activist movements joined the early patients' groups, disease constituencies expanded in number and influence. In the 1960s, there were fewer than 10 national voluntary associations that reported having patients or their families as members, and almost no patients or family members testified in congressional appropriations hearings. Their numbers increased moderately in the 1970s, from 11 to 28 national patients' associations and from 3% to 8% of witnesses at Health and Human Services (HHS) appropriations hearings (see Figure 2.1).[41] Commentators began to notice increases in patients' organizations, remarking that "today, almost all

[35] Bell, *DES Daughters*; Carpenter, *Reputation and Power*, 325; Rose, *Politics of Life Itself*, 23; Starr, *Social Transformation of American Medicine*.

[36] Giddens, *Modernity and Self-Identity*, 7; Lupton, *Medicine as Culture*; Pescosolido, "Professional Dominance," 21; Starr, *Social Transformation of American Medicine*, 393; Williams and Calnan, "'Limits' of Medicalization?"

[37] Anspach, "From Stigma to Identity Politics"; Tomes, "The Patient as a Policy Factor," 722–23.

[38] Anspach, "From Stigma to Identity Politics," 766; Shapiro, *No Pity*, 12–24, 112–44. Policymakers also modeled disability legislation after civil rights laws. Skrentny, *Minority Rights Revolution*; Barnartt and Scotch, *Disability Protests*, 20.

[39] Carpenter, *Reputation and Power*, 411–15; Hess, "Antiangiogenesis Research"; Starr, *Social Transformation of American Medicine*, 392.

[40] Anspach, "From Stigma to Identity Politics," 766; Rabeharisoa, "Experience, Knowledge and Empowerment."

[41] This 150% growth in disease patients' associations outpaced the growth of the overall associational sector, which increased by just 50%. See the Appendix for more details on data sources and methods.

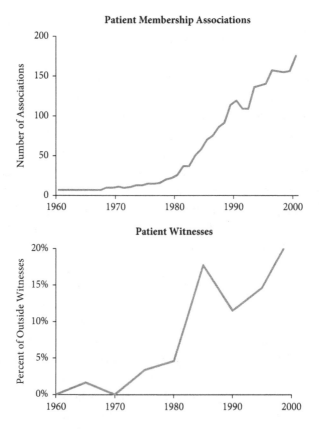

Figure 2.1 The rise of disease constituencies, 1960–2000

Number of national voluntary associations reporting disease patients or families as members; percent of outside witnesses at House appropriations hearings for Health and Human Services, Labor, and Education (pre-1980, Labor, Health, Education, and Welfare) who identified themselves as disease patients or family members.

of the 17 [World Health Organization] disease categories are represented by some form of self-help organization," with the groups "usually run for and by people with a particular health problem."[42]

A few of the new patients' organizations grew large enough to rival the charitable crusades. In 1974, the crusades against tuberculosis, polio,

---

[42] Black, "Self Help Groups and Professionals," 1485; Gussow and Tracy, "Self-Help Clubs," 407.

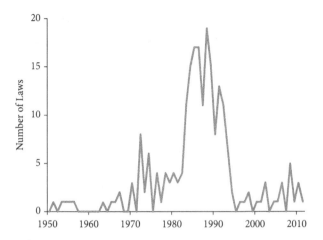

Figure 2.2 Single disease laws, 1950–2011

Number of laws passed by Congress targeting single diseases.

cancer, and heart disease each still raised more money than any other national health agency. But with $20 million raised, the MDA was now the seventh largest (after the National Easter Seal Society for Crippled Children & Adults and the National Association for Retarded Citizens).[43] And the MDA, UCP, the NMSS, and the Arthritis Foundation had joined the list of American charities with the most volunteers, with counts ranging from 450,000 to 1.5 million.[44]

The new patients' associations also had some dramatic policy successes. The NMSS pushed for a research institute for multiple sclerosis, and when the National Institutes of Health (NIH) opposed the idea of a single-disease institute, the advocates successfully campaigned for one targeting neurological diseases.[45] In the 1970s, advocates for patients and their families secured federal earmarks for research on Cooley's anemia, sickle cell disease, sudden infant death syndrome, multiple sclerosis, diabetes, and Huntington's disease, along with federal subsidies for hemophiliacs' medical

---

[43] American Association of Fund-Raising Counsel, "Giving USA," 42.
[44] American Association of Fund-Raising Counsel, 9.
[45] Talley, "Community and Science," 55–57.

supplies and kidney patients' dialysis.[46] Figure 2.2 shows laws targeting single diseases that were passed by Congress over time, with a noticeable bump in the early 1970s.[47] These policy successes yielded criticism of the "Disease of the Month Club," a charge long leveled at the disease crusades revived for the emerging patients' associations.[48]

Legitimizing Disease Constituencies

In the 1980s, two major campaigns accelerated the expansion of patients' activism. To develop a new type of mobilization, group members need a chance to connect with each other.[49] But in the early 1980s, there were few chances for people with the same illness to meet and interact.[50] The gay rights and women's health movements brought together politically active people affected by AIDS and breast cancer. The nesting of one collective identity within another can be a key pathway for the creation of a social movement.[51] The existing gay rights and women's health movements also gave AIDS and breast cancer activists resources, organizational infrastructure, strategies, and a template for identity-based organizing.

Both AIDS and breast cancer activism spun off from the earlier movements, creatively applying interest group politics to disease identities. The new disease campaigns combined the political clout and fundraising prowess of the charitable crusades with constituency-based mobilization. Alongside contentious activism, they forged a new type of consensus politics. Their size and success surpassed any of the existing patients' campaigns, and they sparked an explosive growth of disease patients' activism.

---

[46] Johnson and Hufbauer, "Sudden Infant Death Syndrome," 65; Katz, *Self-Help in America*, 87; Spingarn, *Heartbeat*, 74.

[47] See the Appendix for a detailed description of these data.

[48] Kingdon, *Agendas, Alternatives, and Public Policies*, 52; Spingarn, *Heartbeat*, 76, 88.

[49] Polletta and Jasper, "Collective Identity and Social Movements," 288.

[50] Conrad and Stults, "Internet and the Experience of Illness," 179; Parsons, *Social System*, 321.

[51] Studies of political identity that focus on individuals rather than organizations have difficulty making sense of people's multiple identities. Recognizing that "the same person might seek protection and representation primarily as a Jew, or as a Brooklyn resident, or as a member of a radical socialist party," one study argues that we should ask which identity is "most politically salient." Smith, "Identities, Interests," 304. But these overlaid identities are not just a methodological hurdle to be overcome; intersectionality may actually be a key pathway for the emergence of identity-based movements. Wang, Piazza, and Soule, "Boundary-Spanning in Social Movements," 173; Gamson and Moon, "Sociology of Sexualities," 52.

From Gay Rights to AIDS

Within a decade of the first recognized AIDS cases in the United States, AIDS activists created a powerful model for disease activism that quickly spread to other diseases. The existence of the gay rights movement did not automatically create an AIDS movement: fearing that AIDS would further stigmatize homosexuality, some gay activists distanced themselves from AIDS. However, it was increasingly difficult to maintain this distance as the public at large increasingly defined AIDS as a gay problem and as AIDS stigma threatened to increase anti-gay discrimination.[52] The gay rights movement had a significant organizational infrastructure that could be used for AIDS organizing, including gay organizations that already focused on health or sexually transmitted disease treatment, non-health-related gay organizations that served as incubators for AIDS activism, and alternative media outlets that spread knowledge and rallied support.[53] Eventually, gay activists founded hundreds of organizations to provide services, raise funds for research, develop safe-sex guidelines, and protest delays in drug delivery. The gay rights movement also created a cohort of experienced activists. Their expertise in fighting threats to a group identity translated well into the campaign to reduce the stigma of AIDS, giving AIDS activists a model for identity politics.[54]

The gay rights activists who founded the earliest AIDS organizations did not intend to create a separate social movement.[55] At least initially, the boundaries between gay rights and AIDS activism were blurry. Many early AIDS organizations were explicitly connected to sexuality (e.g., Gay Men's Health Crisis). Even AIDS organizations without explicit gay affiliations often had few non-gay members, and they sometimes organized actions more focused on gay liberation than AIDS.[56] However, as the virus spread

---

[52] Armstrong, *Forging Gay Identities*, 158–60; Epstein, *Impure Science*, 53; Gould, *Moving Politics*, 82–85; Kayal, *Bearing Witness*, 37. The existence of an identity-based social movement does not automatically create a unified response to a disease that disproportionately affects the group. For example, rather than unifying the black community, AIDS created new rifts within it. Cohen, *Boundaries of Blackness*; Kayal, *Bearing Witness*, 65–66; Quimby and Friedman, "Dynamics of Black Mobilization."

[53] ACT UP, "Capsule History"; AIDS Project Los Angeles, "History of APLA"; Armstrong, *Forging Gay Identities*, 161–64; Batza, *Before AIDS*; Cohen, *Boundaries of Blackness*; Epstein, *Impure Science*, 11; Gould, *Moving Politics*, 65.

[54] Armstrong, *Forging Gay Identities*, 162; Epstein, *Impure Science*, 11–12; Gamson, "Silence, Death," 354.

[55] Armstrong, *Forging Gay Identities*, 156.

[56] Gamson, "Silence, Death," 355.

and the people being served were no longer majority gay, many groups redefined themselves as AIDS organizations, rather than gay organizations.[57] The New York ACT UP chapter sent out a standard correction letter whenever newspapers called it a "gay organization." They explicitly defined their constituents across social boundaries, saying that they served everyone from "an entire family with AIDS in Harlem" to "an HIV + gay man in San Francisco."[58] As the field of AIDS organizations became increasingly institutionalized, the number of AIDS organizations without explicit gay affiliations soon dwarfed the number of lesbian/gay AIDS organizations.[59] The gay rights movement had launched the AIDS movement but spun it off into a separate category.[60]

AIDS activists blazed a trail that inspired later disease movements to influence medical research and health policy. They spurred the Food and Drug Administration (FDA) to provide more access to experimental drugs, to approve drugs more quickly, and to change the rules for clinical trials.[61] They also challenged the amount and direction of AIDS research at the NIH.[62] As one NIH director explained, AIDS activists "created a template for all activist groups looking for a cure."[63]

Compared to the charitable crusades, AIDS activism included more contention and protest. ACT UP, especially, emphasized direct action and civil disobedience.[64] And yet other strands of AIDS activism grew to resemble the charitable crusades. In order to provide services to sick and dying people, some AIDS organizations pursued government funding and forged ties to the medical profession, developing organizations that could interface with bureaucracies.[65] The president of Gay Men's Health Crisis explained,

[57] Armstrong, *Forging Gay Identities*, 170–74; Chambré, *Fighting for Our Lives*, 76–77.

[58] Gamson, "Silence, Death," 356–57.

[59] Armstrong, *Forging Gay Identities*, 163; see also Chambré, *Fighting for Our Lives*, 117.

[60] AIDS activists also drew on a variety of other movements, including the peace movement and the women's health movement. Epstein, *Impure Science*, 220; Morgen, *Into Our Own Hands*; Siplon, *AIDS and the Policy Struggle*, 33.

[61] Arno and Feiden, *Against the Odds*; Bix, "Disease Chasing Money and Power"; Carpenter, *Reputation and Power*; Chambré, *Fighting for Our Lives*; Edgar and Rothman, "New Rules for New Drugs"; Epstein, *Impure Science*; Gould, *Moving Politics*; Siplon, *AIDS and the Policy Struggle*.

[62] Arno and Feiden, *Against the Odds*, 232; Epstein, *Impure Science*, 285.

[63] Bernadine Healy, quoted in Gladwell, "Beyond HIV," A29.

[64] Brier, *Infectious Ideas*; Epstein, *Impure Science*; Gould, *Moving Politics*.

[65] Armstrong, *Forging Gay Identities*, 171; Cain, "Community-Based Aids Services"; Chambré, *Fighting for Our Lives*, 25; Epstein, *Impure Science*, 187; Kayal, *Bearing Witness*, 4; Patton, *Inventing AIDS*, 14–20. Formalized social movement organizations tend to receive more funding from foundations and elites. Staggenborg, "Consequences of Professionalization," 597.

"We have created a gay Red Cross. Now we must professionalize it."[66] Some AIDS organizations became larger, more bureaucratic, more focused on courting donors, and less involved in grass-roots activity. Just as the charitable crusades had sought volunteers and donors who were not directly affected by the disease, the AIDS volunteer and donor base expanded far beyond people with AIDS and gay activists.[67] For example, in 1982, women made up only 16% of Gay Men's Health Crisis volunteers, and most donors were gay. By 1990, 33% of volunteers were women, and participation in the United Way and the State Employees Federated Appeal yielded a diverse donor base.[68] As activists decreased the stigma of AIDS in the late 1980s, celebrities could "get publicly involved in AIDS care and fund-raising issues at no reputational risk." AIDS became a "fashionable charity" funded by high-society galas.[69]

To create consensus politics around AIDS, activists needed a symbol that would avoid controversy and allow low-risk participation. Early AIDS activists adopted pink triangles, which had been used by Nazis to identify gay prisoners. This symbol was linked closely to gay activism and was not widely adopted nationwide.[70] At the 1991 Oscars, ACT UP Los Angeles passed out 1,000 Silence=Death pins, but only three celebrities wore them. Searching for a symbol that more people would adopt, activists turned to another type of awareness campaign. According to the director of ACT UP Los Angeles,

The yellow ribbons from the Gulf War were still all around [wrapped around trees]. . . . We noticed that they could mean anything from "I care about young people who have gone overseas" to "I support Bush." We wanted that kind of leeway, too, something that could mean "I hate this Government" or just "I care about people with AIDS."[71]

These multiple possible meanings made ribbons inoffensive, nonthreatening, and easier to wear. When activists distributed single-looped red

---

[66] Paul Popham, 1983, quoted in Chambré, *Fighting for Our Lives*, 25.

[67] From the beginning, it was not exclusively people directly affected who mobilized; for instance, lesbians played an important role in early AIDS activism. Boehmer, *Personal & the Political*, 14; Chambré, *Fighting for Our Lives*, 7.

[68] Chambré, *Fighting for Our Lives*, 64–67.

[69] Kayal, *Bearing Witness*, 60.

[70] McDonnell, Jonason, and Christoffersen, "Seeing Red and Wearing Pink," 6.

[71] Patrick J. O'Connell, quoted in Green, "Year of the Ribbon."

ribbons at the 1991 Tonys and Emmys and the 1992 Grammys, hundreds of celebrities wore them.[72] The non-confrontational symbol allowed crusade-style mass participation (arguably at the cost of diluting the message).

Another consensus-building strategy was the fundraising walk. Activists organized the first American AIDS Walk in Los Angeles in 1984, drawing 4,500 supporters and raising $673,000.[73] Inviting mass participation in fundraising, the AIDS Walk was reminiscent of the Christmas Seals, the March of Dimes, and the ACS's Women's Field Army. Centered on a phys-ical activity, it resembled 1970s fitness fundraisers organized by the March of Dimes, the American Diabetes Association, and the American Heart Association.[74] Compared to a protest, a walk invokes the politics of con-sensus: it need not specify a single set of demands, minimizes disruption, and does not ask participants to risk arrest. AIDS activists had successfully linked patients' activism to the scale and consensus politics of the charitable crusades.

From Women's Health to Breast Cancer

Like the AIDS movement, breast cancer activism drew from a pre-existing identity-based movement but spun off from it. The women's health move-ment laid the groundwork for the breast cancer movement in several ways.[75] First, a key goal of the women's health movement was to educate women about their bodies and encourage them to discuss their health is-sues.[76] The ongoing push for frank discussions of women's health raised the public prominence of breast cancer. In the 1970s and 1980s, feminist writers publicized their experiences with breast cancer, and several influ-ential Republican women followed in their footsteps.[77] These increasingly

---

[72] Green; McDonnell, Jonason, and Christoffersen, "Seeing Red and Wearing Pink," 6.

[73] AIDS Walk Los Angeles, "History." A lower-profile AIDS walkathon had been held in Canada the year before. *Globe and Mail*, "AIDS Walk."

[74] American Diabetes Association, *Journey & and the Dream*, 155; Brenner, "Cast of Thousands"; Hart-Brinson, "Bowling Together."

[75] I focus on the breast cancer movement because of its size and influence over later movements. But breast cancer was not the only health issue targeted by spinoffs from the women's health move-ment. Layne, "Pregnancy and Infant Loss Support"; Taylor, *Rock-a-by Baby*. AIDS activists were also influenced by the women's health movement. Diedrich, *Indirect Action*; Epstein, *Impure Science*, 12.

[76] Epstein, *Inclusion*, 56; Sulik, *Pink Ribbon Blues*, 31; Weisman, *Women's Health Care*.

[77] Anglin, "Working from the Inside Out," 1405; Ferraro, "Anguished Politics of Breast Cancer"; Kedrowski and Sarow, *Cancer Activism*; Kushner, *Breast Cancer*; Lorde, *Cancer Journals*.

open public discussions meant that by the early 1990s, breast cancer organizations received sympathetic media coverage.[78]

Second, the women's health movement created a network of organizations, from health centers to self-help clinics, that incubated the breast cancer movement. These organizations encouraged women to meet and talk about their health concerns, inspiring the growth of breast cancer support groups in the late 1970s and 1980s.[79] Some of these support groups eventually turned to political advocacy.[80]

Third, the women's health movement set precedents for challenging the authority of the medical profession. Some of the movement's key grievances targeted the doctor/patient relationship. Activists claimed that doctors, who were almost all male, treated women with condescension, withheld information from them, and exposed them to risky drugs and devices and unnecessary surgeries.[81] Early breast cancer activism followed in this tradition, pushing for better treatment, more patient-centered decision-making, and less radical surgeries. These efforts contributed to declining rates of radical mastectomies and the passage of breast cancer informed consent laws in 18 states in the 1980s.[82] Later breast cancer advocates also challenged scientists' prerogative to determine the research agenda, arguing that breast cancer and other women's diseases had been systematically underfunded.[83] Breast cancer activist Amy Langer paid homage to earlier movements when she told a reporter, "We grew up in the women's movement and the consumer movement, and to us doctors are not God."[84]

Just as the AIDS movement spun off from the gay rights movement, the breast cancer movement separated from the women's health movement. The first step in the spinoff was narrowing the focus from all women's cancers to breast cancer in particular. In the early 1990s, several feminist activists and

---

[78] Casamayou, *Politics of Breast Cancer*, 60.

[79] Casamayou, 47; Kaufert, "Women, Resistance"; Kedrowski and Sarow, *Cancer Activism*; Sulik, *Pink Ribbon Blues*, 28; Taylor and Van Willigen, "Women's Self-Help"; Weisman, *Women's Health Care*, 76.

[80] Anglin, "Working from the Inside Out," 1406; Kedrowski and Sarow, *Cancer Activism*, 24; Moffett, "Moving Beyond the Ribbon," 289.

[81] Weisman, *Women's Health Care*.

[82] Anglin, "Working from the Inside Out," 1405; Casamayou, *Politics of Breast Cancer*, 50–52; Kedrowski and Sarow, *Cancer Activism*, 23; Leopold, *Darker Ribbon*; Lerner, *Breast Cancer Wars*. These efforts marked a break with mainstream cancer advocacy; the American Cancer Society opposed breast cancer informed consent laws in the 1980s. Klawiter, *Biopolitics of Breast Cancer*, 109; Montini, "Resist and Redirect."

[83] Casamayou, *Politics of Breast Cancer*, 137–40; Weisman, *Women's Health Care*, 79.

[84] Quoted in Belkin, "Charity Begins at . . ."

organizations had turned their attention to all types of cancer, founding advocacy organizations and publishing a series of "feminist cancer anthologies." Of the seven organizations that founded the National Breast Cancer Coalition (NBCC), four were feminist organizations focused on all women's cancers.[85] But these broader organizations sometimes came into conflict with leaders who sought to clarify the NBCC's focus on breast cancer.[86]

In addition to drawing on the women's health movement, breast cancer advocacy was influenced by AIDS activism. According to Fran Visco, the NBCC "was formed to offer breast cancer what AIDS activists had offered AIDS,"[87] and the director of the National Alliance of Breast Cancer Organizations learned from AIDS activists that "if you want your disease to be dealt with, you go and you talk about it and you market it and you visit and you stomp and you write letters and you do it."[88] Another advocate recalled that "the AIDS activists were our model. . . . They showed that if the populace became very concerned, then politicians would respond."[89] Like AIDS activists, breast cancer campaigners developed scientific expertise and gained representation on panels distributing federal research funds.[90]

Just as some threads of AIDS activism came to resemble the charitable crusades, mainstream breast cancer advocacy moved toward consensus politics and mass participation. The largest breast cancer charity, the Susan G. Komen Foundation, distanced itself from lesbians and feminists, embraced traditional femininity, and rejected the women's health movement's critiques of medical authority.[91] As a nonthreatening women's issue, breast cancer faced a favorable political climate in the early 1990s. After the Clarence Thomas/Anita Hill controversy, one senator noted that "a lot of male colleagues don't want to be on the wrong side of any women's issue."[92] However, many women's issues were politically risky, tied up with

---

[85] Klawiter, *Biopolitics of Breast Cancer*, 282.

[86] For instance, when NBCC president Fran Visco proposed a bylaw specifying how many board members must represent national and breast cancer–specific organizations, a representative of the Women's Community Cancer Project was left with the impression that "Fran wants us off the board." Women's Community Cancer Project Archives, "Report from Jean Powers."

[87] Kedrowski and Sarow, *Cancer Activism*, 26; see also Kaufert, "Women, Resistance," 298.

[88] Amy Langer, quoted in Belkin, "Charity Begins at . . ."; see also Casamayou, *Politics of Breast Cancer*, 78; Ferraro, "Anguished Politics of Breast Cancer"; Klawiter, *Biopolitics of Breast Cancer*, 285.

[89] Francine Kritchek, quoted in Ferraro, "Anguished Politics of Breast Cancer"; see also Epstein, "Politics of Health Mobilization," 250.

[90] Dresser, *When Science Offers Salvation*, 25–26.

[91] Brinker, *Winning the Race*; Klawiter, *Biopolitics of Breast Cancer*, 139, 144.

[92] Tom Harkin, quoted in Casamayou, *Politics of Breast Cancer*, 141; see also Bix, "Disease Chasing Money and Power," 11–12; Weisman, *Women's Health Care*, 78.

the politics of abortion or feminism. Supporting breast cancer funding was a politically attractive option for members of Congress seeking to demonstrate sympathy for women's issues while avoiding controversy.[93] Advocates knew this and strategized accordingly; one NBCC board member noted that breast cancer research funding was "a chance for the Republicans to make some points with women. It is not an abortion issue."[94] Breast cancer's unique combination of links to and distance from women's identity politics fostered consensus and expanded advocates' political influence.

Mainstream breast cancer advocacy's strategies for fundraising and mass participation grew to resemble the charitable crusades.[95] The Komen Foundation's "grassroots network of committed volunteers—the Komen Foundation Affiliate Network" recalls the mid-century marching mothers and Women's Field Army.[96] In a campaign reminiscent of the Tuberculosis Association's Christmas Seals, advocates convinced the federal government to issue postage stamps with a price markup that funded federal breast cancer research.[97] Breast cancer activists, led by Komen Foundation founder Nancy Brinker, sought out corporate sponsors for their events and pioneered the use of "cause marketing," in which companies donate some of their proceeds to a particular charity. Breast cancer organizations were among the first to adopt this strategy, and they have attracted more cause-marketing dollars than any other cause.[98] Corporations were initially wary; when Brinker asked bra manufacturers to promote mammograms in 1982, they refused, saying it would be "negative marketing."[99] But nowadays, breast cancer organizations don't have to go hunting for sponsors; corporations seek out breast cancer organizations to work with.[100] The corporate popularity of the breast cancer cause indicates the successful creation of consensus since corporations tend to seek out "safe" issues.[101] Like the Christmas Seals and the March of Dimes, cause-marketing campaigns

---

[93] Gross, "Turning Disease into Political Cause"; Kedrowski and Sarow, *Cancer Activism*, 145. Breast cancer lay at the intersection of several policy arenas, and in each one, it was arguably the least controversial option. It was a women's issue but not identifiably "feminist"; it was a "safe" disease to support, unlike AIDS; and it was a health issue that would not attract organized opposition, unlike healthcare reform. Casamayou, *Politics of Breast Cancer*; Stabiner, *To Dance with the Devil*, 470.

[94] Kay Dickersin Papers, "Board of Directors Meeting."

[95] Leopold, *Darker Ribbon*, 271.

[96] Brinker, *Winning the Race*, 79.

[97] King, *Pink Ribbons, Inc.*, 61–70.

[98] Brinker, *Winning the Race*, 76; Strach, *Hiding Politics in Plain Sight*, 3, 13.

[99] Brinker, *Winning the Race*, 76.

[100] Strach, *Hiding Politics in Plain Sight*, 38.

[101] Lofland, *Polite Protesters*, 69.

involve millions of Americans making tiny donations to a disease campaign. But unlike the earlier campaigns, the contemporary version funnels more money to corporations than causes.[102]

Breast cancer advocates also adopted ribbon symbols and fitness fundraisers that allowed unconfrontational mass participation. Around the same time AIDS activists designed the red ribbon symbol,[103] breast cancer advocates began producing pink ribbons. Evelyn Lauder, founder of the Breast Cancer Research Foundation, recalls that another advocate "had the idea to take the loop pin, from AIDS, and to make it pink. I said, 'We could give away these pink ribbons at all the Estee Lauder counters all over the country.'"[104] They also began using fitness fundraising around the same time that AIDS activists did. The Susan G. Komen Foundation's first Race for the Cure was held in Dallas in 1983; the trademarked races now occur annually in 136 locations and draw 1.5 million participants.[105] The ribbons and races allow mass participation and provide a non-contentious way to signal commitment to the cause.

As they developed a consensus politics of breast cancer, advocates further increased the political legitimacy of disease constituencies. In the early years of the movement, grass-roots breast cancer advocates struggled to get meetings with congressional staffers. From 1990 to 1992, they launched letter-writing campaigns and brought busloads of advocates to Washington, where they faced initially cool reactions from members of Congress and from President Bush, who vetoed a breast cancer funding increase in 1991.[106] When the movement secured funding increases for breast cancer research in 1992, it was criticized for promoting "junk science."[107] But a decade later, members of Congress were "anxious to meet with them personally and . . . to attend NBCC events,"[108] and the media published glowing descriptions of breast cancer advocacy.[109]

---

[102] Rothman et al., "Health Advocacy Organizations," 603; Strach, *Hiding Politics in Plain Sight*, 31.

[103] The Komen Foundation states that it gave out pink ribbons to participants in the Race for the Cure in 1990, suggesting that it may have adopted the symbol before AIDS advocates. Sulik, *Pink Ribbon Blues*, 47. These ribbons do not seem to have used a single-loop design. McDonnell, Jonason, and Christoffersen, "Seeing Red and Wearing Pink," 7. Others state that the pink ribbons first appeared at Komen's Race for the Cure in 1991. King, *Pink Ribbons, Inc.*, xxiv; Ley, *From Pink to Green*, 118; Strach, *Hiding Politics in Plain Sight*, 148.

[104] Quoted in Belkin, "Charity Begins at . . ." Others attribute the pink ribbon to Charlotte Haley or to the Susan G. Komen Foundation. Kedrowski and Sarow, *Cancer Activism*, 59; McCormick, *No Family History*, 44–45.

[105] Strach, *Hiding Politics in Plain Sight*, 145–48; Sulik, *Pink Ribbon Blues*, 50.

[106] Casamayou, *Politics of Breast Cancer*, 122–27, 151.

[107] Anglin, "Working from the Inside Out," 1410.

[108] Kedrowski and Sarow, *Cancer Activism*, 145.

[109] Sulik, *Pink Ribbon Blues*.

AIDS and breast cancer activists had drawn on pre-existing identity-based movements to crystallize a new model for disease advocacy. This creative work was facilitated by the fact that pre-existing movements around gender and sexuality brought together activists affected by the diseases. The new model for disease constituencies was more patient-focused than the charitable crusades but also adopted crusade-style symbols and strategies that cultivated consensus and encouraged mass participation.

A Ribbon for Every Disease

Disease constituencies expanded rapidly in the 1980s. This timing belies descriptions of patients' activism as a response to the emergence of the Internet or the expansion of genetic diagnosis.[110] In the 1980s, there were no mass browsers and search engines, few Americans had Internet access, and few patients met each other online.[111] The expansion of disease patients' activism in the 1980s predates the genomic revolution, meaning that we cannot attribute it to new techniques for diagnosing genetic risks.[112] The Internet, genetic diagnoses, and risk monitoring have created new disease constituencies and accelerated the expansion of patients' activism; but they cannot explain its beginnings. To truly understand why disease constituencies expanded, we need to look to spillovers across movements. The AIDS and breast cancer movements had done significant cultural work in developing a model for disease constituency politics—a new organizational repertoire.[113] It was quicker and easier for other diseases to follow in their

---

[110] Epstein, "Patient Groups and Health Movements," 514–15.

[111] Conrad and Stults, "Internet and the Experience of Illness," 180–82.

[112] Rabinow, "Artificiality and Enlightenment," 244. Other scholars of "biosociality" have expanded beyond genetic risks to study how a broader set of changes in medicine and science—an increased focus on monitoring and reducing risks, on improving (not just healing) bodies, and on molecular science—encourage the formation of new identities and collectivities. Clarke et al., "Biomedicalization"; Klawiter, *Biopolitics of Breast Cancer*, 27; Rose, *Politics of Life Itself*. These scholars recognize that disease advocacy did not appear out of nowhere in the 1990s, and yet many implicitly argue that genetic diagnosis and risk monitoring are responsible for the rise of disease advocacy. Gibbon and Novas, "Biosocialities," 2; Rabinow, "Concept Work," 188; Rose, *Politics of Life Itself*, 134; Wood, *Patient Power?*, 37.

[113] Clemens, *People's Lobby*; Clemens, "Organizational Repertoires and Institutional Change"; McAdam, "'Initiator' and 'Spin-off' Movements"; Meyer and Whittier, "Social Movement Spillover"; Minkoff, *Organizing for Equality*; Taylor, "Social Movement Continuity"; Tilly, "Contentious Repertoires."

footsteps, demonstrating the relative ease with which an existing model can be adapted to similar categories.[114]

Some disease advocates were inspired by ACT UP's contentious politics.[115] Muscular dystrophy activists staged theatrical protests.[116] One group of breast cancer activists borrowed ACT UP's strategy of tying up phone lines with a barrage of calls and collaborated with AIDS activists to blockade a drug company's headquarters.[117] But other disease advocates drew distinctions between their own more "respectable" advocacy and the AIDS movement.[118] Large, mainstream breast cancer organizations benefited from presenting themselves as a less controversial alternative to AIDS activism.[119] Similarly, while some chronic fatigue syndrome advocates adopted contentious tactics, the Chronic Fatigue and Immune Deficiency Syndrome Association sought "mainstream respectability" and avoided "sit-ins or noisy street protests."[120]

The symbols and strategies that spread fastest were those associated with a politics of consensus. Campaigns for various diseases adopted breast cancer advocates' use of cause marketing and corporate sponsorship.[121] Once AIDS and breast cancer activists publicized single-looped ribbons and walks, advocates for other diseases could adopt a ribbon or schedule a walk and feel confident that their actions would be intelligible, even without a major promotional campaign. Now, hundreds of diseases have ribbon symbols.[122] Fitness fundraisers also diffused widely and remained tightly linked to diseases. In 2012, a website attempting to compile an exhaustive list of charitable walks listed events in 46 categories, 38 of which were diseases.[123] The wide reach of ribbons and walks indicates their social safety; these are symbols corporations feel comfortable printing on

---

[114] Haveman, Rao, and Paruchuri, "Winds of Change"; Skrentny, *Minority Rights Revolution*; Strang and Meyer, "Institutional Conditions for Diffusion."

[115] Epstein, "Politics of Health Mobilization," 250.

[116] Epstein, *Impure Science*, 348.

[117] Anglin, "Working from the Inside Out."

[118] Epstein, "Politics of Health Mobilization," 250. Their success is reminiscent of the way moderate civil organizations benefited from the existence of the movement's "radical flank," attracting more funding because they were viewed as a less threatening alternative. Haines, "Black Radicalization."

[119] King, *Pink Ribbons, Inc.*, 109.

[120] Barrett, "Illness Movements," 160; Foreman, "Grassroots Victim Organizations," 42–43.

[121] Strach, *Hiding Politics in Plain Sight*, 13. Of 381 cause marketing campaigns identified by Strach, more than one in five targeted diseases, and an additional one in six targeted other health issues.

[122] craftsnscraps.com, "Awareness Ribbon Colors."

[123] Charity Walks Blog, "Charity Walk Events."

their products and fundraisers people feel free to ask their colleagues and neighbors to contribute to.

Previous movements' successes open doors for new movements, creating political opportunities and legitimacy.[124] New disease organizations often explicitly drew parallels to AIDS or breast cancer. For instance, an early prostate cancer group called "US TOO!" derived its name from the breast cancer organization "Y-ME," and advocates formed the National Prostate Cancer Coalition based on the National Breast Cancer Coalition.[125] Chronic fatigue syndrome activists called their disease "AIDS junior" and "non-HIV positive AIDS" and pushed to add "immune dysfunction" to the name to invoke "an association with AIDS."[126] Advocates cited AIDS and breast cancer as precedents when they pushed for research funding and access to FDA and NIH meetings.[127] They used systems the FDA had developed under pressure from AIDS activists to gain access to experimental drugs and followed ACT UP's example to challenge drug pricing.[128] Once breast cancer activists convinced Congress to earmark Department of Defense (DOD) funds for breast cancer research, advocates for other diseases successfully pushed for DOD funds for their diseases.[129]

Reading disease advocates' congressional testimony across the years reveals the increasing legitimacy of patients' perspectives. In the 1960s and 1970s, most congressional witnesses who spoke about diseases were doctors, scientists, or leading philanthropists.[130] They argued for their diseases with universal claims, as when a tuberculosis campaigner argued that failing to control the disease could be "dangerous to the community."[131] Powerful members of Congress occasionally sought out patients as "window dressing" to justify funding increases for diseases they considered important, but disease associations almost never brought patients to testify

[124] McAdam, "'Initiator' and 'Spin-off' Movements"; Minkoff, "Sequencing of Social Movements"; Skrentny, "Policy-Elite Perceptions"; Tarrow, *Power in Movement*.

[125] Kedrowski and Sarow, *Cancer Activism*, 32.

[126] Barrett, "Illness Movements," 160–61.

[127] Dresser, "Public Advocacy"; Johnson, *Disease Funding and NIH Priority Setting*; Saguy and Riley, "Weighing Both Sides," 909.

[128] Arno and Feiden, *Against the Odds*, 239, 244; Dresser, *When Science Offers Salvation*, 49.

[129] Kedrowski and Sarow, *Cancer Activism*, 160; Stabiner, *To Dance with the Devil*, 472–73; see Chapter 5 in the present volume.

[130] Many of these professionals were "managed" by Lasker and other disease crusaders. Strickland, *Politics, Science, and Dread Disease*, 151.

[131] US House of Representatives, "Appropriations for 1970, Part 7," 1399.

before Congress.[132] In an exception that proves the rule, Mike Gorman incorporated personal experiences into his 1959 testimony for the National Committee Against Mental Illness. After completing his official testimony about federal funding for mental health, he announced that he would also like to discuss federal efforts to fight cancer, which had recently killed his wife. He insisted that despite his personal experience with cancer, he was not allowing his testimony to be polluted by private concerns, saying, "I do not mean to invoke any personal emotion" and "I don't point this out for a personal reason."[133] These disavowals of personal motivations signal that the experiences of patients and families were not yet thought of as legitimate bases for congressional testimony.

By the mid-1980s, personal motivations were no longer something to apologize for—they now seemed *more* important than professional expertise. In 1986, a doctor told Congress, "I might tell you I am the President of the Cystic Fibrosis Foundation, but more importantly, the father of a child with the disease."[134] Instead of making universal claims, advocates described themselves as representing disease constituencies, as when two psoriasis patients and advocates declared that "we are here on behalf of all psoriatics" and asked Congress to "make a difference in the lives of those of us afflicted with psoriasis."[135] By the end of the 1980s, patients and their family members made up one-fifth of the witnesses at the HHS appropriations hearings (see Figure 2.1).[136] This is an extraordinarily high proportion, given that these hearings cover all of health and human services, labor, and education. The prominent place of patients in congressional hearings and their unapologetic claims on behalf of affected subpopulations demonstrate the new political legitimacy of disease constituencies.

As disease constituencies became increasingly legitimate, patients' organizations proliferated. In the 1980s, the number of disease patients' associations tripled, far outpacing the overall 25% growth of the associational sector (see Figure 2.1). By 2000, there were 175 national disease patients' associations. Congress passed dozens of laws targeting single diseases (see

---

[132] Kingdon, *Agendas, Alternatives, and Public Policies*, 36; Strickland, *Politics, Science, and Dread Disease*, 139–41.

[133] US House of Representatives, "Appropriations for 1960," 263–64.

[134] US House of Representatives, "Appropriations for 1987, Part 9," 220.

[135] US House of Representatives, 435–36.

[136] Figure 2.1 shows associations in the *Encyclopedia* that specified having patients and/or families as members and congressional witnesses who identified themselves as patients and/or family members of patients. See the Appendix for a fuller discussion of data sources and methods.

Figure 2.2). By 2003, there were over 1,000 single disease nonprofits, and their share of the health nonprofit field doubled to 15%.[137]

Conclusion

At the close of the twentieth century, campaigns against single diseases remained at the center of American public life. As they had for decades, millions of Americans contributed money and time to fight diseases. But in a departure from the earlier charitable crusades, many of the new disease advocates were patients and families coming together to promote their interests. The late twentieth-century prominence of disease patients' advocacy reflects the continued power of disease campaigns to capture the public imagination, wedded to the rise of social movements and identity politics.

The shift from universalistic to constituency-based organizing was made possible by major social changes. Chronic diseases replaced infectious ones as the biggest killers, and declining deference to physicians and scientists combined with increasing faith in medicine and science, creating incentives to mobilize around diseases. Meanwhile, the overall growth of social movements and interest groups encouraged political activism. These changes set the stage for disease patients' advocacy and inspired various health movements. But since they happened over decades, they cannot explain why patients' advocacy increased so rapidly in the 1980s and 1990s. This pattern only makes sense once we supplement these long-term social changes with an understanding of spillovers between movements and the diffusion of organizational forms. These complex interactions between movements mean that we should not expect a deterministic relationship between structural conditions and political mobilization.[138] Instead, movements build on each other in ways that are serendipitous and path-dependent.

The charitable crusades had created consensus by imagining everyone as a potential beneficiary. Rarer chronic diseases needed another route to inspire mass participation and avoid being derided as "special interests."

[137] See Appendix for detailed discussions of the data, including which nonprofits are included in the counts.
[138] Walder, "Political Sociology and Social Movements."

They pursued consensus through strategic selection of symbols and the creation of mass participation events with open-ended meanings that allowed for apolitical participation. The success of the AIDS and breast cancer campaigns, and the subsequent disease campaigns that adopted their model, proves that patient-focused campaigns can still evoke mass appeal. But this option is not equally available to all diseases. The next chapter explores inequalities across diseases, demonstrating that various types of stigma inhibit organizing.

3

Deserving Patients

Since the start of the twentieth century, single-disease campaigns have funneled more attention and resources to some diseases than others. But there have been changes over time in the types of diseases that are favored. In the early twentieth century, the charitable crusades targeted major infectious and chronic diseases, arguing that everyone was at risk. In the late twentieth century, patients and family members formed disease constituencies, mobilizing around their shared interests. But not all patients are equally willing or able to mobilize, and not all patients are viewed as equally deserving of help. By presenting patients (and not the general public) as the campaigns' beneficiaries, constituency-based activism tends to disadvantage stigmatized diseases in favor of those that create valorized identities.

Analyzing data on 92 diseases in the late twentieth and early twenty-first centuries, this chapter reveals the powerful role of stigma in determining which diseases get the most attention and which are neglected.[1] This analysis overcomes two methodological problems that have made it difficult to test theories about why some problems attract more attention and advocacy than others. Many studies of advocacy organizations look at a single issue, making it difficult to determine what features of issues help them attract attention.[2] Comparing dozens of diseases allows for statistical tests of the relationship between mobilization and other variables. Meanwhile, studies of mobilization often sample on the dependent variable, only studying issues targeted by active movements.[3] By sampling diseases instead of movements,

---

[1] These 92 diseases are the conditions for which I have data on both disease burden and level of advocacy. See the Appendix for a fuller description of the data and methods.

[2] Baumgartner and Leech, *Basic Interests*; Giugni, "How Social Movements Matter," xxiv; Heaney and Rojas, "Hybrid Activism," 1053; Larson and Soule, "Sector-Level Dynamics," 293; McAdam and Scott, "Organizations and Movements," 9; Minkoff, *Organizing for Equality*, 5. In recent years, increasing numbers of scholars have studied multiple problems, but the literature is still overly focused on case studies. Bearman and Everett, "Structure of Social Protest"; Clemens, *People's Lobby*; Gamson, *Strategy of Social Protest*; Hojnacki et al., "Studying Organizational Advocacy," 390; Larson and Soule, "Sector-Level Dynamics"; Soule and King, "Competition and Resource Partitioning."

[3] Burstein, "Interest Organizations," 54; Leech, "Lobbying and Influence," 540; Olzak, "Analysis of Events," 121; for notable exceptions, see Biggs and Andrews, "Protest Campaigns and Movement Success"; Gamson, *Strategy of Social Protest*; King, Bentele, and Soule, "Protest and Policymaking."

I include diseases targeted by little or no advocacy, permitting stronger conclusions about the determinants of mobilization. These methodological choices help me test two main predictions about which problems will attract the most attention.

Prior to the "interpretive turn" in social movement scholarship, much mainstream research assumed that political and economic structures matter more than culture for explaining mobilization.[4] Relatedly, "objectivist" approaches to social problems focus on their real-world severity.[5] These theories suggest that severe problems, problems that affect socially advantaged groups, and problems that attract sponsorship and funding will be targeted by the most advocacy. But in the case of disease campaigns, there is surprisingly little relationship between the amount of death and disability inflicted by a disease and the amount of advocacy it attracts. There is no systematic relationship between the amount of mobilization and patients' race and gender, key axes of inequality that affect people's motivation and opportunities to organize. Corporate funding is also only weakly related to the amount of advocacy.

In contrast, more recent social movement theorists turn to cultural and subjective factors—identities, meanings, emotions—to explain mobilization.[6] And "constructionist" approaches to social problems focus on how culture and ideas shape which issues come to be *perceived* as serious problems.[7] The patterning of disease campaigns lends support to these theories. The amount of advocacy targeting a disease is best explained by various types of stigma. When diagnoses are met with exclusion, negative stereotypes, discrimination, and loss of status,[8] people may keep them private, hampering mobilization. Diseases marked by the stigma of contagion, preventability, or mental illness see much less advocacy. Meanwhile, patients who do mobilize around these conditions face further barriers in arguing that their condition is important and their patients are deserving. The claims advocates can make and how those

[4] Armstrong and Bernstein, "Culture, Power, and Institutions," 75; Minkoff, *Organizing for Equality*, 23; Walder, "Political Sociology and Social Movements," 394.

[5] Best, *Threatened Children*, 10.

[6] Armstrong and Bernstein, "Culture, Power, and Institutions"; Benford and Snow, "Framing Processes and Social Movements"; Goodwin and Jasper, *Rethinking Social Movements*; Klandermans, "Social Construction of Protest"; Polletta and Jasper, "Collective Identity and Social Movements."

[7] Best, *Threatened Children*; Rochefort and Cobb, "Agenda Access"; Spector and Kitsuse, *Constructing Social Problems*.

[8] Pescosolido and Martin, "Stigma Complex," 91.

claims will be received depend on culture, stigma, and constituents' perceived deservingness.[9]

Many movements do target stigmatized identities, and extreme levels of stigma can provide a powerful impetus to mobilize. Fighting back against deadly stigma, AIDS activists formed arguably the most influential disease constituency. But less extreme stigma tends to dissuade potential participants. Since constituency-based activism depends on public affiliation with a movement, the shift from charitable crusades to disease constituencies disadvantaged stigmatized diseases.

Objective Conditions: Severity, Demographics, and Corporate Funding

Social scientists sometimes assume that bigger problems motivate bigger social movements and more interest group activity.[10] And yet others argue that grievances don't matter much to explain mobilization: almost any problem meets the minimum threshold needed to inspire advocacy, grievances can be manufactured, and public responses rarely seem proportionate to severity.[11] This debate has remained unsettled because researchers struggle to quantify which issues affect more people.[12] How would you determine, for example, whether more people are affected by housing insecurity or by racial discrimination in the labor market and which experience is more severe? Because they can be compared by deaths and disability-adjusted life years (DALYs), diseases offer a good opportunity to see whether more serious problems inspire more advocacy.

These measures of disease severity are imperfect. Mortality statistics can be biased by conventions about which causes of death are primary and by over- or underreporting of particular causes.[13] They ignore the disability

[9] Best, *Threatened Children*, 17, 176–77; McCammon et al., "Movement Framing."

[10] Baumgartner and Leech, "Interest Niches and Policy Bandwagons"; Brown et al., "Embodied Health Movements," 74; Eckstein, *Pressure Group Politics*, 158; Gurr, *Why Men Rebel*; Smelser, *Theory of Collective Behavior*; Turner and Killian, *Collective Behavior*.

[11] Armstrong, *Conceiving Risk, Bearing Responsibility*, 3; Funkhouser, "Issues of the Sixties"; Gusfield, *Culture of Public Problems*; Jones and Baumgartner, *Politics of Attention*; Kingdon, *Agendas, Alternatives, and Public Policies*; McCarthy and Zald, "Resource Mobilization and Social Movements."

[12] Halpin, "Explaining Policy Bandwagons," 216.

[13] Anderson, "Coding and Classifying Causes of Death"; Modelmog, Rahlenbeck, and Trichopoulos, "Accuracy of Death Certificates"; Lloyd-Jones et al., "Accuracy of Death Certificates," 1024; Timmermans, *Postmortem*.

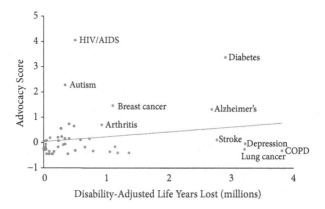

Figure 3.1 Weak relationship between advocacy and disease burden

The *y*-axis shows the advocacy score, an index of standardized measures of lobbying expenditures, organizations, and congressional testimony. The *x*-axis shows the number of disability-adjusted life years lost to a disease each year, in millions. Both variables are means for 2005–2015. COPD, chronic obstructive pulmonary disease.

and hardship inflicted by non-fatal diseases, and they weight timely and premature deaths equally. DALYs include consideration of disability and age, but their calculation rests on subjective decisions about how to weigh the costs of dying at different ages and how to weigh the severity of various disabilities.[14] The next chapter discusses the difficulty in choosing a single metric to rank diseases. Despite these drawbacks, deaths and DALYs capture a lot of information about the burden of disease. We might expect major differences in mobilization between diseases that kill dozens of people and those that kill tens of thousands.

Diseases that kill and disable more people tend to have slightly more advocacy, but the differences are surprisingly small.[15] In Figure 3.1, the *x*-axis shows the number of DALYs lost to a disease each year. The *y*-axis shows the advocacy score, which takes into account the number of associations, nonprofits, lobbying expenditures, and congressional witnesses.[16] Figure 3.1

[14] Ashmore, Mulkay, and Pinch, *Health and Efficiency*, 89–105; Callahan, *What Price Better Health?*, 71–73; Daniels, "Four Unsolved Rationing Problems"; Gold, Stevenson, and Fryback, "HALYS and QALYS and DALYS"; Morrow and Bryant, "Measuring and Valuing Human Life."

[15] See the Appendix for details on data.

[16] The advocacy index is the mean of standardized measures of organizations, lobbying, and congressional witnesses for the years 2005–2015; see the Appendix for details. For example, the score of 4

also shows a regression line to summarize the linear relationship between DALYs and advocacy. The regression line is not very steep, indicating that diseases that inflict more disability do not tend to be targeted by dramatically more advocacy. The relationship between mortality and advocacy is similarly small and not statistically significant (see Appendix, Table A.3 and Figure A.1). In this case, at least, attention to a problem (a particular disease) is not strongly related to the scope of the problem (mortality or DALYs).

If not deaths and disability, what *does* explain why some diseases attract more attention than others? The characteristics of affected groups may shape how much mobilization develops. Some research suggests that traditionally excluded groups are more likely to mobilize for change.[17] Other studies suggest that socially advantaged people mobilize more since they have more resources, influence, and access to decision-makers.[18] But in most cases, it's difficult to systematically compare problems based on the demographics of the affected populations. Diseases again provide a good opportunity for theory-testing because there are concrete data on the race and gender of the people they kill.

In the case of disease advocacy, Phil Brown and colleagues argue that diseases that affect more minorities and women might see more mobilization since these patients are "most likely to view their illness in terms of previous injustices," but they also might be "least likely to have access to the resources necessary to transform their politicized collective illness identity into an efficacious social movement."[19] Overall, there is little systematic relationship between patients' race and gender and the amount of advocacy targeting a disease. Regression analyses show small and non-significant relationships between black- and female-dominated diseases and the level of advocacy (see Table A.3).[20] Patients' race and gender likely shape the *type*

for HIV/AIDS indicates that on average this disease was four standard deviations above the mean for each advocacy variable.

[17] Berry, *New Liberalism*; Lofland, *Social Movement Organizations*; Loomis and Cigler, "Interest Group Politics"; McAdam, *Political Process*; Piven, *Challenging Authority*; Radcliff and Saiz, "Labor Organization and Public Policy."

[18] Edwards and McCarthy, "Resources and Social Movement Mobilization"; Hacker and Pierson, "Winner-Take-All Politics"; Schattschneider, *Semi-Sovereign People*; Schlozman et al., "Inequalities of Political Voice"; Verba, Schlozman, and Brady, *Voice and Equality*.

[19] Brown et al., "Embodied Health Movements," 74.

[20] The Appendix includes details about the race and gender analyses, including alternate ways of coding these variables.

of advocacy that develops and how policymakers and the public react to disease campaigns, but they do not determine the *amount* of advocacy.[21]

One reason for the weak relationship between patients' race and the amount of advocacy is that compared to other collectivities people might form (e.g., professions, neighborhood residents, victims of police violence) diseases are less segregated by racial lines. Racial minorities face an increased risk of most diseases, and these disparities are more dramatic for some conditions than others. And yet for almost all diseases, risks cross social boundaries. When societies distribute resources by disease category, race doesn't become the main axis of inequality the way it does for problems that affect more racially homogeneous groups.

Another concrete determinant of advocacy is the ability to attract resources.[22] For disease advocacy, one major source of resources is the corporate sector. While pharmaceutical companies were generally suspicious of 1960s and 1970s patient advocacy organizations,[23] they now fund many or most disease organizations.[24] Disease campaigns have also increasingly sought out other corporate sponsors.[25] I found a positive but small and non-significant relationship between corporate funding and the amount of advocacy targeting a disease.[26] And even a strong relationship would not prove that the corporate sector determines the amount and direction of disease advocacy. While corporate money can encourage the formation of organizations and give them more money to spend on lobbying, funding also tends to flow to established organizations.

Severity, demographics, and corporate funding don't tell us much about why some diseases attract more attention than others. What can explain the remaining variation across diseases? Why do diseases rise above or fall below the regression line in Figure 3.1? Figure 3.2 focuses on the diseases with the largest gaps between their actual advocacy and what we'd expect

---

[21] Mortality and patients' demographics go further in explaining media coverage of diseases. Armstrong, Carpenter, and Hojnacki, "Whose Deaths Matter?"

[22] Jenkins, "Resource Mobilization Theory"; McCarthy and Zald, "Resource Mobilization and Social Movements."

[23] Batt, "A Community Fractured"; Henderson, "Drug Firms' Funding of Advocates"; Lofgren, "Pharmaceuticals and the Consumer Movement," 231–32.

[24] Baggott, Allsop, and Jones, *Speaking for Patients and Carers*; Hemminki, Toiviainen, and Vuorenkoski, "Patient Organisations and the Drug Industry"; Hughes and Minchin, "Drug Giants"; O'Donovan, "Corporate Colonization of Health Activism?"

[25] Strach, *Hiding Politics in Plain Sight*, 13.

[26] An important limitation of these analyses is that my data only include grants that corporations choose to disclose.

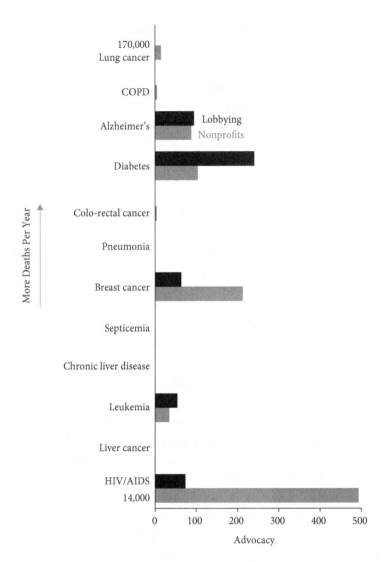

Figure 3.2 Mismatches between mortality and advocacy

The diseases listed have the largest residuals when using mortality to predict advocacy (see Appendix). From top to bottom, diseases are ordered from most to fewest deaths (*y*-axis is not to scale). "Lobbying" is tens of thousands of 2013 dollars. "Nonprofits" is the number of nonprofits targeting the disease with budgets of at least $25,000 in 2013 dollars. All variables are means for 2005–2015. COPD, chronic obstructive pulmonary disease.

based on how many people they kill. Diseases are ordered by mortality, with the biggest killers at the top of the graph. The black and gray bars show the average lobbying expenditures and number of nonprofits targeting each disease. Why is there so little advocacy for lung cancer, chronic obstructive pulmonary disease, and colorectal cancer and so much for Alzheimer's and diabetes? Across all diseases, are there general patterns that can explain why some diseases have more advocacy than others?

The Power of Stigma: Neglecting Preventable, Infectious, and Mental Illnesses

To truly understand the patterns in mobilization, we need to consider the features of diseases that make people more or less likely to publicly identify themselves as patients. When conditions are stigmatized—devalued, discrediting, or shameful[27]—patients are less likely to mobilize, and if they do, they face limitations in the claims they can effectively make. Preventable diseases, infectious diseases, and mental illnesses all tend to have less advocacy than other conditions (see Figure 3.3). Holding mortality, demographics, and corporate funding constant, these differences are all statistically significant (see Table A.3).[28]

On average, more preventable diseases have substantially less advocacy (see Figure 3.3).[29] Looking at the diseases with the biggest advocacy deficits (see Figure 3.2) suggests that some types of preventability matter more than others. Skin cancer doesn't make the list of undermobilized diseases, even though many cases can be prevented by limiting sun exposure. Instead, most of the highly preventable diseases with the biggest advocacy deficits can be caused by smoking or drinking. Some of these diseases are targeted by broader campaigns (e.g., organizations fighting all lung diseases, liver diseases, or all cancers). And they are also targeted by public campaigns and policies to discourage smoking and drinking. But given their burden

[27] Pescosolido and Martin, "Stigma Complex," 92.

[28] The regression models (shown in detail in Table A.3—see Appendix) control for mortality instead of DALYs since mortality data are available for more diseases. The results are similar when I control for DALYs instead.

[29] I use preventability scores from Phelan et al., "'Fundamental Causes.'" The scores range from 1 (least preventable) to 5 (most preventable), and I classify diseases with scores of 4.5 or 5 as highly preventable.

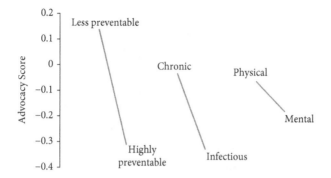

Figure 3.3 Less advocacy for preventable, infectious, and mental illnesses

Mean advocacy scores for diseases in each category, 1986–2015, excluding AIDS and breast cancer. Advocacy score is an index of standardized measures of lobbying expenditures, organizations, and congressional testimony. Scores do not average to zero because AIDS and breast cancer are excluded. Differences are statistically significant in multivariate models (see Appendix, Table A.3).

of deaths and DALYs lost, they have surprisingly small single-disease campaigns. Lung cancer—the biggest killer in my study[30]—kills 170,000 Americans per year.[31] It's targeted by a few organizations[32]—by 2010, three organizations in the *Encyclopedia* and 16 nonprofits—but they reported only $5,000 per year in lobbying. Chronic obstructive pulmonary disease (COPD), which kills 140,000 Americans a year and is responsible for more DALYs lost than any other disease, has even less advocacy—never more than one association in the *Encyclopedia* or seven nonprofits and no reported lobbying expenditures. Compare that to Alzheimer's and diabetes. Each kills about 80,000 Americans per year and each has about 100 nonprofits and $1–$2 million in annual lobbying expenditures.[33] Like lung cancer and COPD, chronic liver disease and liver cancer are each targeted by one or two nonprofits and no lobbying. Meanwhile, leukemia kills a comparable number of Americans but averages 35 nonprofits and half a million dollars of lobbying per year (see Figure 3.2).

---

[30] These analyses exclude heart disease, which can be thought of as a collection of multiple different diseases.

[31] Mortality figures in this section are means for 2005 through 2015.

[32] See the Appendix for a detailed discussion of how associations and nonprofits were identified.

[33] While a recent *New York Times* headline called Alzheimer's disease a "neglected epidemic," it is in fact another of the most highly mobilized diseases. Bellafante, "Alzheimer's."

If disease advocacy is primarily targeted toward solving mysteries and discovering cures, it may make sense to focus on diseases we don't know how to prevent. But ignoring preventable diseases is troubling for two reasons. First, much disease advocacy focuses on raising awareness, which improves health outcomes most if individual actions can prevent the disease. Second, compared to other conditions, preventable diseases disproportionately affect the poor, who have fewer resources to respond to them.[34] These factors suggest that the neglect of preventable diseases is not simply a rational allocation of scarce resources.

With the notable exception of HIV/AIDS, infectious diseases also tend to have much less advocacy than chronic conditions (see Figure 3.3).[35] This may be due in part to the fact that most infectious diseases have an acute course—people have the disease for a relatively short amount of time and then either recover or die. Compared to chronic conditions, these illness experiences are less likely to become part of people's identities,[36] a crucial step in building a social movement.[37] For example, pneumonia kills 10,000 more Americans per year than breast cancer but is targeted by no large nonprofits, associations, or lobbying expenditures. Septicemia, another big killer,[38] has a handful of nonprofits and no lobbying. In contrast, breast cancer, responsible for a comparable number of deaths, is targeted by over 200 nonprofits and $650,000 in lobbying (see Figure 3.2).

Mental illnesses are also targeted by less advocacy than physical illnesses (see Figure 3.3).[39] Depression ranks second in DALYs lost, behind only COPD. There are a few depression associations and about a dozen nonprofits, reporting lobbying expenditures of around $50,000 per year—some advocacy but not in proportion to the burden of disease.

---

[34] Phelan et al., "'Fundamental Causes.'"

[35] Besides HIV/AIDS, the only infectious disease that received more advocacy than expected (based on mortality) is leprosy. It kills only a few people per year in the United States but is targeted by advocacy organizations with Christian missions and an international focus.

[36] Bury, "Sociology of Chronic Illness"; Foreman, "Grassroots Victim Organizations"; Kedrowski and Sarow, *Cancer Activism*; Wood, *Patient Power?*

[37] Brown et al., "Embodied Health Movements"; Polletta and Jasper, "Collective Identity and Social Movements"; Taylor and Whittier, "Collective Identity in Social Movement Communities."

[38] Septicemia's ranking in Figure 3.2 reflects an average of 41,000 deaths per year, as reported by the CDC. As for all diseases, these numbers can be disputed. The American Sepsis Alliance reports that sepsis kills over 250,000 Americans per year. One complication is that some deaths may be classified based on the initial infection (e.g., pneumonia) and others by the eventual widespread infection.

[39] The regression models control for mortality, which is not a good measure of the burden of mental illnesses. But models controlling for DALYs show a similar significant negative coefficient for mental illnesses.

Schizophrenia also ranks high in DALYs lost but has only a handful of nonprofits and no reported lobbying expenditures. Like diseases with behavioral causes, mental illnesses are often stigmatized,[40] which may make patients reluctant to mobilize or donors reluctant to support them. However, the relatively small campaigns for specific mental illnesses do not include organizations targeting mental illness in general. We should not conclude that mental illnesses are entirely neglected—just that they have not developed large single-disease campaigns.

Looking at these determinants of advocacy, a broader pattern emerges, suggesting that various forms of stigma inhibit the formation of disease constituencies.[41] Infectious diseases, preventable conditions, and mental illnesses are often stigmatized: their patients tend to face exclusion, negative stereotypes, discrimination, and/or loss of status.[42] People with infectious diseases may be viewed as tainted or dangerous and face a stigma of contagion.[43] People with preventable conditions may be blamed for their illness and judged for moral failings.[44] These two forms of stigma overlap for infections acquired through sex and/or drug use. People with mental illnesses, too, are often viewed as different or threatening, even when not believed to be responsible for their conditions.[45]

People faced with any kind of stigma may adopt a strategy of "passing," keeping their status as secret as they can to avoid the negative consequences of stigma.[46] "Closeted" patients will find it difficult to make political claims on the basis of a disease category.[47] As one bioethicist explained, "urinary incontinence is a big problem, but you don't see anybody lobbying for

---

[40] Pescosolido and Martin, "Stigma Complex."

[41] There are no systematic data on the level of stigma targeting large numbers of diseases. And any effort to collect such data would be hampered by the fact that different scholars focus on different aspects of stigma. Most studies measure one aspect of stigma for one condition; a few compare three or four diseases. Pescosolido and Martin.

[42] Pescosolido and Martin, 91.

[43] Davis, *Passage Through Crisis.*

[44] Lebel and Devins, "Stigma in Cancer Patients"; Leichter, "'Evil Habits' and 'Personal Choices'"; Rush, "Affective Reactions"; Weiner, Perry, and Magnusson, "Reactions to Stigmas."

[45] Pescosolido et al., "'A Disease Like Any Other'?"; Pescosolido and Martin, "Stigma Complex"; Phelan, "Geneticization of Deviant Behavior."

[46] Goffman, *Stigma*, 41–104.

[47] Beard, "Advocating Voice"; Carpenter, "Is Health Politics Different?," 290; Kedrowski and Sarow, *Cancer Activism*; Siplon, *AIDS and the Policy Struggle.* "Closeted" patients could participate more easily in charitable crusades, with their participation framed as philanthropic, as in Franklin D. Roosevelt's polio philanthropy. Patients with stigmatized diseases can avoid the risk of disclosure when they form online communities. Conrad and Stults, "Internet and the Experience of Illness," 183; Dumit, "Illnesses You Have to Fight to Get," 588. Internet-based activism may decrease some of the disparities in mobilization between stigmatized and non-stigmatized diseases.

more funds for that" because it's "embarrassing."[48] Social movements need to overcome the "collective action problem": they must motivate people to participate even though any benefits ultimately secured will be shared with non-participants.[49] For non-stigmatized diseases, the benefits of publicly adopting a valorized identity (e.g., "breast cancer survivor") may help overcome collective action problems. For stigmatized diseases, the reverse is true: in addition to the regular costs of investing time and resources in the movement, participants face the cost of having to "come out." What may be a rational individual-level decision to minimize the consequences of stigma by staying "closeted" can have problematic consequences on the collective level, if no movement emerges to challenge the stigma.

The mobilization deficit for stigmatized diseases may be even more severe than it appears. People may avoid seeking treatment for stigmatized conditions, leading to lower rates of diagnosis. When diagnosed with stigmatized conditions, patients may hesitate to mention them in surveys. In response to families' concerns, physicians may substitute less stigmatized causes on death certificates.[50] Therefore, mortality and DALY statistics likely underestimate the death and disability caused by stigmatized diseases, and the disparities between health burden and advocacy may be even larger than they appear.

Paradoxically, while stigma often discourages activism, it can also inspire powerful campaigns. In the 1950s and 1960s, sociologists assumed that social movement participants were trying to ameliorate a "spoiled identity."[51] Some more recent scholars still describe movements, especially identity politics, as a response to stigmatization.[52] To predict whether stigma will encourage or discourage activism, we need to consider the amount of stigma and the severity of its consequences. Powerful movements emerged around disabilities and mental illnesses, two cases in which stigma helped justify imposing major limitations in people's lives, up to and including forced institutionalization.[53] Arguably the most influential contemporary

---

[48] Arthur Caplan, quoted in Havemann, "Crusading for Cash," 5.

[49] Olson, *Logic of Collective Action*.

[50] Lenfant, Friedman, and Thom, "Fifty Years of Death Certificates," 1066. This pattern may not be widespread; for example, social desirability has less influence on medical examiners' determinations of suicide than the examiners' professional motivations. Timmermans, "Suicide Determination."

[51] Gamson, "Social Psychology of Collective Action," 56.

[52] Bernstein, "Identity Politics," 52; Britt and Heise, "From Shame to Pride"; Piore, *Beyond Individualism*.

[53] Anspach, "From Stigma to Identity Politics"; Rabeharisoa, "Experience, Knowledge and Empowerment."

disease campaign targets AIDS, which first affected gay men and intravenous drug users. The stigma these groups faced limited the initial government response to AIDS, and people infected and at risk faced death while
the government stood by. Stigma also created the real possibility of repres-
sive state action: proposals to identify and even tattoo HIV carriers aroused
little moral outcry outside gay circles. The Supreme Court upheld a law
criminalizing gay sex. The resulting crisis forced action. As sociologist and
early Gay Men's Health Crisis volunteer Philip Kayal explained, "because
PWAs [people with AIDS] were being left to die unfed and uncared for, the
community had to respond and create a specific, often militant, gay/AIDS
agenda. . . . The alternative was abandonment and collective death." This
extreme stigma that threatened life and liberty inspired some of the most
influential activism of the late twentieth century.[54]

While the stigma more commonly attached to preventable, infectious, and
mental illnesses also has important consequences for people's lives,[55] it is on
an entirely different scale than the deadly contempt faced by people with
AIDS in the 1980s or the forcibly institutionalized mentally ill in the 1960s.
While those stigma-fueled emergencies propelled action, stigma impedes
activism in the case of diseases like hepatitis and lung cancer. Without the
extreme neglect, life-or-death urgency, and threat of repression, the negative
consequences of publicly claiming an illness identity hold people back.[56]

As the previous chapter showed, the AIDS movement helped inspire the
current wave of disease constituencies. This pattern suggests an ironic relationship between AIDS activism and attention to stigmatized diseases.
AIDS activists fought valiantly against the stigma of HIV infection.[57] But
for the wave of disease constituencies they inspired, stigma was a hurdle
to clear, and the later campaigns focused disproportionately on non-
stigmatized conditions.[58] Ironically, these movements inspired by AIDS

[54] Arno and Feiden, *Against the Odds*; Chambré, *Fighting for Our Lives*, 119; Epstein, *Impure Science*; Kayal, *Bearing Witness*, 5, 9, 35, 43, 48, 63, 88; Brier, *Infectious Ideas*, 36; Gould, *Moving Politics*, 121–23.

[55] Pescosolido and Martin, "Stigma Complex."

[56] In fact, this process may have temporarily slowed AIDS organizing in the early days of the epidemic, when some gay activists tried to distance their cause from AIDS to avoid further stigmatizing homosexuality. Armstrong, *Forging Gay Identities*, 158–60; Epstein, *Impure Science*, 11, 53; Gould, *Moving Politics*, 82–85; Kayal, *Bearing Witness*, 37.

[57] Donovan, *Taking Aim*; Epstein, *Impure Science*.

[58] In a more general statement of this phenomenon, Clemens argues that disadvantaged groups sometimes fare well in politics by innovating new organizational forms. But there's nothing to prevent those forms from being subsequently adopted by advantaged groups. Clemens, *People's Lobby*.

advocacy may actually have expanded the influence of disease stigma on health policy.[59]

Stigma and the Claims Disease Advocates Make

When advocates do mobilize around stigmatized conditions, stigma constrains their claims for sympathy and resources. Because they were imagined to benefit everyone, the charitable crusades didn't need to justify the worthiness of tuberculosis, polio, cancer, or heart disease patients. In contrast, since policies and laws tend to disadvantage, punish, or impose restrictions on stigmatized groups and/or distribute benefits to positively constructed groups,[60] disease constituencies face pressures to present their patients as deserving. Their claims are constrained by widely shared assumptions that some patients deserve less help than others.[61] Advocates for non-stigmatized diseases have more options available to convince people that their diseases should receive attention and resources. These dynamics play out as disease advocates speak to Congress.[62] Fewer witnesses testify about preventable, infectious, and mental illnesses. But even when advocates for stigmatized diseases do testify, their claims are constrained.

Advocates can make claims on the basis of values and emotions and/ or on the basis of rationality and data.[63] Witnesses for non-stigmatized diseases often do the former, taking their patients' perceived deservingness for granted and focusing their testimony on their suffering and its effects on their families. For example, one mother spoke about her 13-year-old

---

[59] Best, "Disease Politics and Medical Research Funding."

[60] Best, *Threatened Children*; Gilens, *Why Americans Hate Welfare*; Lieberman, *Boundaries of Contagion*; Schneider and Ingram, "Social Construction of Target Populations"; Skrentny, "Policy-Elite Perceptions"; Steensland, "Moral Classification and Social Policy."

[61] When activists engage in strategic framing, the "discursive opportunity structure" constrains their choices by determining which claims seem "sensible," "realistic," and "legitimate." Claims are more likely to be successful when they align with dominant ways of thinking. Benford and Snow, "Framing Processes and Social Movements"; Best, *Threatened Children*, 17, 176–77; Brown, "Anti-Immigration Mobilization"; Ferree, "Resonance and Radicalism"; Koopmans and Statham, "Conceptions of Nationhood"; McCammon et al., "Movement Framing"; Paschel, "Right to Difference"; Skrentny, "Policy-Elite Perceptions."

[62] I examine disease advocates' testimony before the House Appropriations Subcommittee for Labor, Health and Human Services, and Education. See Appendix for a description of this data source.

[63] Best, *Threatened Children*, 43–44.

son, saying that "Michael is not comfortable as he sits here strapped to his wheelchair. If you look into his beautiful brown eyes, he has no vision. . . . It is horrible what Batten's disease does to a normal healthy child."[64] These witnesses also made claims on scientific and economic grounds, but their most common strategy was to evoke sympathy.

In contrast, witnesses with stigmatized diseases seem less confident that their stories will evoke sympathy. Instead, they often reach for universal beneficiaries by using economic arguments to justify funding increases.[65] For example, a former drug user emphasized that research and treatment allowed her to go from "tax burden to tax payer," and an American Lung Association official noted that "lung diseases cost the U.S. economy an estimated $84.4 billion annually."[66] This rhetorical strategy has a long history. For example, in 1960, a representative of the American Social Health Association testified that "It costs $12 million a year to maintain the syphilitic blind, and $46 million a year for hospitalization of syphilitic psychotics. That is tax money."[67]

In addition to their constrained use of emotional claims for sympathy, advocates for stigmatized diseases must fight back attacks on their deservingness. Sometimes advocates for non-stigmatized diseases explicitly argue that as innocent victims they deserve more support.[68] A pancreatic cancer advocate told Congress, "This is a disease you cannot protect yourself against. . . . It just comes like a thunderbolt out of the blue." He then asked that the government "help protect us from the things that we cannot protect ourselves from."[69] In a letter to Representative Porter, a muscular dystrophy advocate attacked funding for research on drug abuse and alcoholism, saying that "it is shocking that over $754 million is devoted to address the health problems of people whose irresponsible behavior causes those problems, while less than 1 percent of that sum helps children dying of Duchenne muscular dystrophy."[70]

In response, advocates for stigmatized diseases often focus on deserving subgroups, implying that while some patients may be blameworthy,

[64] US House of Representatives, "Appropriations for 1991, Part 8a," 701.
[65] Advocates for non-stigmatized diseases also use economic arguments and other quantitative ways to rank diseases, but they do so less frequently than advocates for stigmatized diseases. Too few witnesses testified about stigmatized diseases to test the statistical significance of this difference.
[66] US House of Representatives, "Appropriations for 1998, Part 7a," 318, 143.
[67] US House of Representatives, "Appropriations for 1961," 168.
[68] As Best notes, "blameless victims offer rhetorical advantages to claims-makers" since they elicit the most sympathy. Best, *Threatened Children*, 34.
[69] US House of Representatives, "Appropriations for 2009, Part 7," 155–56.
[70] Havemann, "Crusading for Cash," 4.

others are not. Juvenile diabetes advocates emphasize the differences between their disease and type 2 diabetes, which has more behavioral risk factors.[71] Lung cancer advocates focus public awareness campaigns on types of lung cancer not caused by smoking, emphasizing cancers with genetic links that affect "younger, nonsmoking women" and protesting government awareness campaigns that overemphasize "the role of tobacco in promoting lung cancer."[72] A sexually transmitted disease advocate testified that "thousands of babies will be born with these diseases and some will die."[73] A congressional witness with liver disease emphasized that he did not drink or smoke, "never experimented with drugs," and "had one sexual partner and continue to have one sexual partner in my whole life, my wife."[74] A witness with hepatitis C, which can be transmitted between intravenous drug users, emphasized non-stigmatizing modes of infection, claiming the disease can be transmitted by "sharing a toothpaste tube." He went on to say, "My mother was a teacher, my sister that died was a teacher. We did not lead lives that, you know, we do not drink or smoke and things like that."[75]

Focusing on the patients who are perceived to be the most deserving can lead to policies that only benefit favored subgroups. For instance, juvenile diabetes advocates pushed for the Special Diabetes Program, a major earmark for research focusing on type 1 diabetes (and not type 2).[76] Congress focused on children with AIDS in order to pass the Ryan White Act.[77] The law imposed some burdens on the most stigmatized subgroups and emphasized benefits for the most sympathetic populations. But all AIDS patients received benefits that might not have been politically feasible without the focus on a child with hemophilia, indicating that benefits achieved from a focus on "deserving" subgroups can sometimes spill over to other patients.[78]

---

[71] Type 2 diabetes affects 20 times as many people as type 1, but they tend to be older, poorer, less white, and more overweight. Perez-Pena, "Beyond 'I'm a Diabetic.'" Type 1 advocates worry that their children will face a spillover stigma and work to remind policymakers and the public of the differences between the two conditions. This pattern suggests that if the data on advocacy and burden were split between the two types, type 1 diabetes would be even more of an outlier.

[72] Griffith, "Lung Cancer Patients Fight Societal Neglect."

[73] US House of Representatives, "Appropriations for 1990, Part 8," 1442.

[74] US House of Representatives, "Appropriations for 1998, Part 7a," 132.

[75] US House of Representatives, "Appropriations for 2000, Part 7a," 1188, 1196.

[76] Juvenile Diabetes Research Foundation, "JDRF Advocacy"; National Institute of Diabetes and Digestive and Kidney Diseases, "Special Diabetes Program"; Perez-Pena, "Beyond 'I'm a Diabetic.'"

[77] Donovan, Taking Aim, 54–55, 60–65, 90.

[78] Donovan, 54–55, 60–68, 90; see also Oliver, "Politics of Public Health Policy," 202.

Conclusion

The move from charitable crusades to disease constituencies created a double disadvantage for stigmatized diseases. Since the stigma of contagion, preventability, or mental illness makes it unappealing or risky to publicly claim an illness identity, these conditions are targeted by fewer advocacy organizations, meaning that stigmatized patients have less access to supportive communities and valorized identities. When advocates do mobilize against stigmatized diseases, they face limitations in the claims they can effectively make for sympathy and resources. These inequalities in mobilization and claims-making may put stigmatized diseases at a disadvantage in the competition for government resources, creating inequalities in service provision, access to care, and the discovery of cures.[79] This is particularly problematic because disease stigma tends to line up with other social inequalities. Since the rich have more resources to use to protect themselves, preventable diseases disproportionately affect the poor.[80] Patients suffering from diseases that afflict richer, whiter patients are likelier to be classified as "deserving."

This chapter showed that, on average, stigmatized diseases have smaller campaigns than non-stigmatized diseases, especially in the context of constituency-based claims. This does *not* imply that if there were no disease constituencies, we would see more public attention to stigmatized diseases. The reverse is true: the handful of organizations targeting stigmatized diseases would probably not exist in the absence of a broader field of disease campaigns. When noting imbalances between the advocacy targeting stigmatized and non-stigmatized diseases, we should not falsely assume that one detracts from the other. Chapter 5 addresses this question directly, asking whether disease campaigns compete with one another for federal research funding.

This chapter also showed that two commonly used metrics of severity—mortality and DALYs—tell us little about how much advocacy a disease will receive. While metrics don't shape mobilization, the next chapter shows that the reverse is true: mobilization helps determine which metrics of severity shape medical research policy. Advocacy helps determine which metrics matter in political debates and how they affect the distribution of resources.

---

[79] Best, "Disease Politics and Medical Research Funding."
[80] Link and Phelan, "Social Conditions"; Phelan et al., "'Fundamental Causes.'"

4

Ranking Diseases

We see medical research differently through the lens of disease campaigns. Disease campaigns shaped the terms of the debate over medical research funding, changing how policymakers think about whether funds are being distributed fairly.[1] Deborah Stone argues that "every policy issue involves the distribution of something." When judging these distributions, we ask "who are the recipients," "what is being distributed," and "what are the social processes by which distribution is determined?"[2] Disease campaigns encourage policymakers to think of medical research funding as a benefit distributed to patients, judge the distribution of funding across disease categories, and search for ways to objectively rank the severity of various diseases. These ways of conceptualizing medical research funding and judging the fairness of the funding distribution have concrete effects on where the money goes.

When they lobbied for more funding for particular conditions, disease advocates asserted that diseases are the relevant categories across which to judge the National Institutes of Health (NIH) funding distribution. That is, they depicted medical research as a benefit distributed to the patients and potential patients of various diseases—not to universities in different states or to scientists at different stages of their careers. Advocates then ranked diseases by health burden and economic effects, choosing the metrics most favorable to their own condition.

In response, policymakers searched for formal tools to rank and prioritize diseases that would provide a seemingly rational and objective way to weigh competing claims from advocates for various diseases. Over the years, Congress pressured NIH officials to justify their priority-setting and advocates critiqued them for "underfunding" high-mortality diseases. NIH officials worried that a focus on health burden might distract from other important metrics for comparing diseases, including scientific opportunity

---

[1] Some of the findings in this chapter were previously discussed in Best, "Disease Politics and Medical Research Funding."

[2] Stone, *Policy Paradox*, 53.

and market failure. They also warned that being held accountable for funding to particular diseases might siphon funds from untargeted research and basic biomedical research that cuts across disease categories. As the NIH budget grew, there were slight declines over time in the percent of the budget devoted to basic and untargeted research. But the *total* funding for basic and untargeted research increased dramatically. Disease campaigns expanded funding for applied and targeted research but not at the expense of basic and untargeted research. When specialized campaigns allocate resources to narrow priorities, these gains need not come at the expense of broader goals.

Disease campaigns do seem to have redistributed funds across disease categories. While Congress never required the NIH to standardize funding by disease severity, the ongoing pressure changed where the money went. Over the years, the distribution of funds at the NIH began to match up better and better with mortality. By shaping the categories across which the funding distribution was judged and inspiring a search for metrics to compare diseases, disease campaigns changed the terms of the debate over medical research funding, affecting how political decisions are made and which outcomes are favored. These results demonstrate that advocacy's political effects go beyond securing benefits for constituents: advocates can also change the rules of the game.

Non-Disease Categories

To understand how a disease focus changes medical research politics, it's important to consider the alternatives. Diseases are not the only lens through which to view the NIH budget. While the institutes' overarching goal has always been to improve the nation's health, debates about the NIH have often framed scientists and universities as the beneficiaries of medical research funding. Testifying before Congress in 1963, NIH Director Shannon defended the large research budget by arguing that the scientists and universities that received the money deserved it: "the national figures are very large. . . . But when you go from a national picture to a State . . . and begin to recognize institutions and scientists, you begin to understand the role they play in the community life."[3] In mid-century debates about the

---

[3] US House of Representatives, "Appropriations for 1964, Part 3," 30.

effectiveness of NIH research, some members of Congress felt that "whether or not disease was in fact being conquered, medical schools were being financially helped."[4] Officials in other government agencies have sometimes accused the NIH of being "more concerned about the budgetary headaches of scientists than the health needs of the public."[5]

When we conceptualize medical research funding as a benefit given out to scientists, it makes sense to ask what kinds of scientists are receiving grants. In the mid-twentieth-century, congressional critiques asked whether unqualified researchers were being funded.[6] The NIH director emphasized the importance of "picking the right man to do the right research" to defend against claims that the funding distribution was elitist and geographically unbalanced.[7] More recent discussions have centered on the correct balance of funding to intramural and extramural researchers and to scientists at different stages of their careers. These debates have sometimes led to policy changes, including giving early-career scientists a leg up in the competition for grants.[8] Other critics focus on grants' success rates, with metrics including pay lines.[9] At congressional hearings over the years, NIH officials and members of Congress have suggested various targets for the percent of grants funded (e.g., 45%–50% or 35%–40%).[10] When the NIH budget stabilized or declined after rapid growth (see Chapter 5), researchers raised concerns about declining success rates. Other researchers focus on the number of grants or trainees the NIH will fund.[11] These measures are important for individual scientists, determining how many grants they will need to write and how predictable their funding streams will be.

A related perspective sees scientific funding as an economic benefit to be distributed to regions, states, and educational institutions. In 1967, a congressional committee criticized the NIH for "concentrating grants in a small group of institutions and by doing so widening the gap in the biosciences between 'rich' and 'poor' schools."[12] President Johnson favored broadening

---

[4] Strickland, *Politics, Science, and Dread Disease*, 190.

[5] Palca, "Emphasizing the Health in NIH," 23.

[6] Guston, *Between Politics and Science*, 74; Strickland, *Politics, Science, and Dread Disease*, 220.

[7] Strickland, *Politics, Science, and Dread Disease*, 220.

[8] Zerhouni, "NIH in the Post-Doubling Era," 1089.

[9] Zerhouni.

[10] US House of Representatives, "Appropriations for 1985, Part 4a," 9199; US House of Representatives, "Appropriations for 1995, Part 4," 24.

[11] Insel, Volkow, and Li, "Research Funding," 2043; US House of Representatives, "Appropriations for 1985, Part 4a," 60–63, 115–46, 182; Zerhouni, "NIH in the Post-Doubling Era."

[12] Strickland, *Politics, Science, and Dread Disease*, 219; see also Guston, *Between Politics and Science*, 74.

the funding geographically and spreading it to a wider range of universities.[13] More recently, an NIH advisor complained that policymakers were "even questioning the sanctity of peer review since it includes no provision for distributing funds on a geographical basis, obviously important for their constituencies."[14] In 1993, the NIH responded to these concerns by establishing the Institutional Development Award program, which seeks to spread NIH funding more evenly around the country.[15]

Unsurprisingly, the advocates pushing these metrics tend to be scientists and representatives of research institutions. Their voices used to be more prominent in NIH policymaking. In the 1960s and 1970s, more than 15% of the witnesses testifying at the House Labor, Health, Education, and Welfare appropriations hearings represented health institutions like medical schools, research institutes, and hospitals (see Figure 4.1). As the groups most likely to receive money directly from the NIH, they were a natural constituency for NIH policy. During those decades, fewer witnesses represented disease organizations and/or were disease patients.

Beginning in the 1980s, the proportion of witnesses representing health institutions dropped by more than half. They were replaced by disease organizations and patients,[16] who made up about one-third of the witnesses by the 1990s (see Figure 4.1).[17] This percentage is astonishingly high, given that the denominator includes witnesses testifying about the appropriations for all of Health and Human Services (HHS), Labor, and Education, from labor unions to librarians. In their testimony, disease advocates portrayed patients as the beneficiaries of research funding. For instance, in 1992, one

[13] Strickland, *Politics, Science, and Dread Disease*, 219.

[14] Edward Benz, chair of the Advisory Board for Clinical Research, Clinical Center, quoted in Kastor, *National Institutes of Health*, 39–40.

[15] EPSCoR/IDeA Foundation, "National Institutes of Health." Congress also sometimes addresses these critiques by earmarking funds for research at particular universities. De Figueiredo and Silverman, "How Does the Government (Want to) Fund Science?," 37; Payne, "Earmarks and EPSCoR."

[16] Figure 4.1 differs from Figure 2.1. Since Chapter 2 focused on the rise of patients as constituents of disease advocacy, Figure 2.1 included only patients who were witnesses, excluding representatives of disease organizations who did not identify as patients or family members. Since this chapter focuses on disease categories in general, not patient constituencies in particular, Figure 4.1 includes all disease witnesses, regardless of whether they have a personal connection to the disease. In a previously published version of Figure 4.1, I only included witnesses with organizational affiliations; see Best, "Disease Politics and Medical Research Funding," 791. Here, I combine them with witnesses identified only as disease patients and apply a lowess smoother.

[17] A similar change occurred at the Food and Drug Administration (FDA). In the 1960s, the FDA's main external critics were scientists, industry, medical professionals, and Congress; this changed in the 1970s and 1980s as cancer and AIDS patients began to challenge the FDA's practices. Carpenter, *Reputation and Power*, 322, 395.

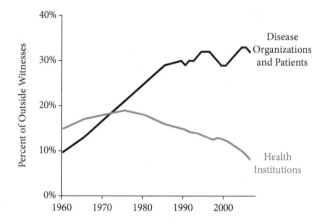

Figure 4.1 Disease witnesses replace health institutions, 1960–2006

Percent of outside witnesses at House appropriations hearings for Health and Human Services, Labor, and Education (pre-1980, Labor, Health, Education, and Welfare) representing disease organizations and/or patients and health institutions (e.g., hospitals, medical schools). Lowess smoother applied.

breast cancer advocate argued that "my daughter Jody, the women in this room, and women everywhere deserve no less" than increased funding for breast cancer research. Another asked, "Is this too much to ask for your wife, your sister, your mother?"[18] These advocates depict breast cancer patients and potential patients, not scientists, as the beneficiaries of breast cancer research funding.

People organized around disease categories don't care as much about early-career or late-career scientists (except to the extent that it will affect the quality of the research produced). When discussing the distribution of research funds, their primary concern is which *diseases* receive more research funding. Over the decades, they have promoted various criteria for weighing one disease against another. These political debates encouraged policymakers to judge the NIH funding distribution across disease categories and search for ways to rank diseases. While the NIH resisted the push to use metrics to rank diseases, these debates encouraged them to match funding more closely to mortality.

[18] US House of Representatives, "Rising Influence of Breast Cancer," 31, 59.

Advocates Rank Diseases

Diseases can be ranked according to health burden, economic effects, the extent to which each is the target of private sector research, and the level of scientific opportunity in research on the disease. Different criteria put different diseases on top, and advocates tend to select the metrics that are most advantageous for their diseases.

Health Effects

The most common way to rank diseases is by quantifying their health effects. As early as 1944, Mary Lasker and colleagues criticized the emerging federal research bureaucracy, arguing that "the bulk of [Public Health Service] research funds were going to health problems, such as rickets, other than those causing the highest percentage of deaths and greatest physical and financial disablement."[19] That same year, a congressional witness argued that federal research funds "should be distributed equitably . . . according to the number of yearly deaths in the United States from these diseases."[20] The trouble was that no one really knew how many people most diseases killed or sickened.[21] And so the Lasker Foundation funded a committee to track the medical and economic costs of various diseases.[22] Over time, advocates became more and more likely to use mortality and prevalence to justify a disease's importance. In the 1960s and 1970s, about 60% of disease advocates testifying before Congress mentioned health burden; by the early 2000s, over 80% did so (see Figure 4.2).

Advocates tend to choose the measure of health burden that makes their disease look the most serious. One common tactic is to compare research dollars per death. For example, in 1995, a representative of the American Heart Association noted that "in fiscal year 1993, HHS spent 36 times more on research funding per death of an AIDS victim than was spent per death of a heart disease victim."[23] While most focus on US mortality and prevalence statistics, advocates for diseases more common abroad sometimes

---

[19] Strickland, *Politics, Science, and Dread Disease*, 34.
[20] Dr. Henry S. Sims, 1944, quoted in Strickland, 39.
[21] Strickland, 102.
[22] Strickland, 137.
[23] US House of Representatives, "Appropriations for 1995, Part 7," 129.

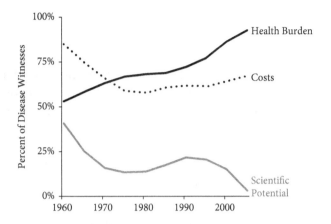

Figure 4.2 How advocates promoted their diseases, 1960–2005

Percent of disease advocates testifying at House appropriations hearings for
Health and Human Services, Labor, and Education (pre-1980, Labor, Health,
Education, and Welfare) who justified the importance of their diseases by
referring to health burden (e.g., mortality or prevalence), economic costs, and
potential for scientific discoveries. Lowess smoother applied.

use international statistics, as when one advocate reported that "Hepatitis
B kills more people worldwide in one day than AIDS does in one year."[24]
While most use raw mortality rates, others emphasize years of life lost,
which prioritizes diseases that kill the young—for example, "when compared to cancer or heart disease, AIDS receives the lowest amount of federal funds per years of potential life lost."[25] In turn, advocates for non-fatal
diseases base their claims on prevalence rather than mortality, comparing
dollars per patient. For instance, the American Brittle Bone Society testified in 1979 that "the National Institute of Health spends about 85 cents per
person on these diseases, whereas you very well know, about 10 times that
much or more is spent on equally substantial diseases."[26]

These competing measures of health burden reflect a fundamental
truth: there is no single metric that can capture everything about the
burden of disease. Death can be measured less subjectively than other

[24] US House of Representatives, "Appropriations for 1993, Part 8a," 148.
[25] US House of Representatives, "Appropriations for 1995, Part 7," 608.
[26] US House of Representatives, "Appropriations for 1980, Part 8," 724.

health outcomes (though the classification of deaths still depends on diagnostic practices and coding rules),[27] but mortality statistics ignore disability and age at death. Researchers have developed additional measures to attempt to capture these other aspects of disease severity. For instance, disability-adjusted life years (DALYs) account for disability and weigh deaths occurring at younger ages more heavily.[28] But DALYs and related measures also rely on contestable choices about how to rank the severity of various types of disability and how to weigh the impact of deaths at various ages.[29] There is no perfect measure; each reflects some aspects of disease burden and obscures others.[30]

Policymakers and advocates (like all humans) tend to pay more attention to some metrics than others, often "locking onto" a particular indicator.[31] Despite the development of other measures of disease burden, mortality remained the most visible metric for ranking diseases. Counts of the number of deaths are compiled by federal agencies, giving them an aura of official respectability. They are also non-technical and easy to understand. Perhaps for this reason, advocates almost never discuss DALYs; instead, they tend to use personal stories to describe the disability and hardship their diseases inflict. Some policymakers adopt mortality metrics to advocate for a favored disease and/or attack AIDS spending. In the House, Representatives Istook (R-OK) and Nethercutt (R-WA) echoed advocates' claims that some diseases were being underfunded compared to AIDS.[32] Representative Bonilla (R-TX) also picked up the dollars-per-death frame

---

[27] For example, compared to autopsies and expert reviews, death certificates attribute many more deaths to heart disease, suggesting that "physicians may use coronary heart disease as a 'default' cause" of death. Lloyd-Jones et al., "Accuracy of Death Certificates," 1024; see also Modelmog, Rahlenbeck, and Trichopoulos, "Accuracy of Death Certificates"; Timmermans, *Postmortem*. Consequently, mortality statistics that rely on death certificates will tend to overestimate the number of deaths due to heart disease. Classification rules also matter; revisions to the *International Classification of Diseases* changed how many deaths were attributed to particular causes. Anderson, "Coding and Classifying Causes of Death," 477–78. A majority of deaths have more than one cause listed; historically specific coding rules govern the choice of a single underlying cause. Anderson, 474.

[28] Murray and Acharya, "Understanding DALYs."

[29] Ashmore, Mulkay, and Pinch, *Health and Efficiency*, 89–105; Callahan, *What Price Better Health?*, 71–73; Daniels, "Four Unsolved Rationing Problems"; Gold, Stevenson, and Fryback, "HALYS and QALYS and DALYS"; Morrow and Bryant, "Measuring and Valuing Human Life."

[30] Even though I recognize the incompleteness of any one metric, I also rely on these data to perform my analyses—asking, for instance, how closely NIH funding aligns with mortality and DALYs.

[31] Jones and Baumgartner, *Politics of Attention*, 57, 128.

[32] Dresser, "Public Advocacy"; Istook, "Research Funding on Major Diseases"; Marshall, "Lobbyists."

to push for more money for diabetes research.[33] As early as the 1970s, "match[ing] funds to total deaths" was referred to as "Congress's rule."[34]

Economic Costs

A majority of disease advocates also discuss diseases' economic costs in their congressional testimony (see Figure 4.2). They sometimes refer to the costs of medical care, as when the National Psoriasis Foundation told Congress that "the cost of this skin disease in care and treatment has been estimated to be $1 billion annually."[35] They also discuss non-healthcare spending, as when the American Rheumatism Association reported that "in 1973, social security disability payments to arthritics were running at an annual rate of $660,000,000. Fifteen-percent of all disability payments go to arthritis victims."[36] Sometimes advocates discuss lost economic productivity, as when the AIDS Action Council pointed out that "people with AIDS died at a young age, cutting off many years of productive life, of work, of paying taxes, of contributing to society."[37] Often they discuss all costs together, as when a mental health advocate stated that mental illnesses cost "over $1 billion for direct care" and "$2 billion . . . from loss of work and so forth."[38] Sometimes advocates imply that diseases should receive research funding in proportion to their economic costs, as when a representative of the National Foundation for Ileitis and Colitis testified that "more dollars are spent for medical purposes by individuals afflicted with digestive disease than any other class of disease . . . despite the enormity of the problem, only one-tenth of 1 percent of Federal funds for research on disease—1/1000—is spent for digestive disease research."[39]

Rather than comparing diseases to each other, other advocates compare research funding to the money lost to the disease. In 1974, the Arthritis Foundation reported that "the economic cost of [rheumatic] diseases is calculated at $9–$10 billion annually. Yet this year . . . [the NIH] is spending

---

[33] Marshall, "Lobbyists."

[34] Mushkin, *Biomedical Research*, 364.

[35] US House of Representatives, "Appropriations for 1975, Part 7," 75.

[36] US House of Representatives, 97.

[37] US House of Representatives, "Appropriations for 1995, Part 7," 608.

[38] US House of Representatives, "Appropriations for 1960," 256.

[39] US House of Representatives, "Appropriations for 1975, Part 7," 465.

only $14 million on its arthritis program."[40] Twenty years later, the Juvenile Diabetes Foundation International noted that "diabetes is estimated to cost this country nearly $92 billion in 1994, yet we spend less than $30 million in diabetes research."[41] These comparisons implicitly assume that research expenditures could bring costs down. An Alzheimer's Association witness explained that "if we were able to delay the disease for only five years, we would . . . cut the Nation's health and long-term care costs by as much as $60 billion in a year."[42] This calculation assumes that whatever preventive intervention researchers discovered would be cost-free.[43] But more plausibly, we might replace spending on current treatments with spending for a newly discovered drug. And since there is no definitive way to tell who is about to develop Alzheimer's, scores of people who might never have developed the disease would also be prescribed the new drug. Delaying the onset of Alzheimer's for five years would have tremendous non-economic benefits for patients and their families. But it might just as easily increase healthcare spending as decrease it.

The claim that medical research will bring down healthcare costs is heavily promoted by both the NIH and the pharmaceutical industry.[44] It may have been true for an earlier generation of research on infectious diseases that new discoveries could prevent. But now, most research targets chronic conditions, most advances ameliorate symptoms with long-term treatments rather than producing cures, and medical research is more likely to increase costs than decrease them.[45] And so claims that we should prioritize diseases based on healthcare spending make little sense unless we respond with the types of research with the potential to contain healthcare costs instead of increasing them—research on prevention, social determinants of health, and health service delivery.[46]

[40] US House of Representatives, 91.
[41] US House of Representatives, "Appropriations for 1995, Part 7," 173.
[42] US House of Representatives, 118.
[43] Academic studies sometimes make the same problematic assumption; see Brookmeyer, Gray, and Kawas, "Projections of Alzheimer's Disease."
[44] Callahan, *What Price Better Health?*, 223–25.
[45] Callahan, 224; Mushkin, *Biomedical Research*, 315–17; Okunade and Murthy, "Technology"; Orzag, "Growth in Health Care Costs"; Smith, Newhouse, and Freeland, "Income, Insurance, and Technology." Claims based on diseases' "indirect" costs—lost wages, etc.—are similarly problematic. These calculations often include lost future earnings, falsely assuming, for example, that everyone who survives a heart attack will return to the workforce and none will remain disabled. They also exclude the costs of the other diseases people will eventually get if they survive. Callahan, *What Price Better Health?*, 230.
[46] Callahan, *What Price Better Health?*, 223–33; Martin, "Research in Biomedicine"; Mushkin, *Biomedical Research*, 315–16, 365; Sampat, "Mission-Oriented Biomedical Research," 1739.

Congress Pushes for Data

As advocates made competing claims about diseases' health and economic burdens, commentators noted that "the public is increasingly confronted with 'duelling' statistics—which disease is worse, has higher mortality and is harder to treat."[47] A Congressional Research Service report lamented the "vast and sometimes confusing array of charts and tables comparing disease-specific research funding with statistics on morbidity, mortality, and health care costs."[48] The confusion stemmed from two sources: advocates selected both the *metrics* and the *data sources* that were most favorable to their diseases. In response, members of Congress repeatedly sought more authoritative and systematic data on various measures of disease severity.[49] They were searching for an official way to "commensurate" diseases—a way to adjudicate between different disease advocates' competing claims by ranking all diseases on some common metric.[50] Turning to the numbers was appealing because it gave the appearance of impartiality.[51]

Some policymakers turned to commensuration as a way to respond to single-disease advocacy without inserting earmarks in the NIH budget. After World War II, many federal policymakers concluded that scientists should be given more autonomy than other recipients of government funding. In the following decades, influential members of Congress worked to avoid earmarks and preserve NIH control over research funding decisions.[52] Faced with competing claims from disease advocates but seeking to avoid earmarks, policymakers embraced metrics as a reasonable way to prioritize diseases. Turning to the numbers also promised to achieve the decades-old goal of rationalizing the distribution of attention to

[47] Brower, "Squeaky Wheel," 1014.

[48] Johnson, *Disease Funding and NIH Priority Setting*.

[49] In an earlier article, I argued that disease advocates introduced metrics for commensuration which were adopted by policymakers. Best, "Disease Politics and Medical Research Funding." This chapter looks across a longer time period and shows that while disease advocates introduced metrics to support their claims rhetorically, they were not the main proponents of formally commensurating diseases. More often, it was policymakers who, in response to advocacy, searched for a single, standard metric.

[50] Espeland and Stevens, "Commensuration as a Social Process"; Lamont, "Valuation and Evaluation"; Timmermans and Epstein, "A World of Standards."

[51] Porter, *Trust in Numbers*, 8; Starr, "Sociology of Official Statistics," 56.

[52] Dresser, "Public Advocacy"; Epstein, *Inclusion*; Frickel and Moore, "Prospects and Challenges"; Guston, *Between Politics and Science*; Hess, "Antiangiogenesis Research"; Spingarn, *Heartbeat*; Strickland, *Politics, Science, and Dread Disease*.

diseases, correcting the unbalanced funding distributions that result from disease campaigns.

In the early 1970s, Representative Tim Lee Carter (R-KY) introduced legislation that would require that appropriations requests prioritize diseases based on mortality, morbidity, and economic effects.[53] Other members of Congress simply pushed the NIH to provide more systematic data. In 1979, Representative Obey (D-WI) told the NIH director, "We have every group in the world coming in here with a disease which they think is more important to attack than any other disease in the world. They have a whole list of diseases which they think are short-changed in terms of research." Looking for a way to adjudicate these claims, he asked for data across diseases on NIH funding, deaths per year, the number of people suffering from the disease, new cases per year, and hospital days per year.[54]

But the NIH couldn't say precisely how much research funding each disease was receiving since some grants address multiple diseases and others focus on basic research that might or might not have implications for a particular disease. In 1974, the NIH commissioned a study "to determine the feasibility of developing a methodology by which funds for national health research could be classified by disease problem."[55] The researchers were able to classify 82% of extramural grants,[56] and the NIH gave Congress information on funding to broad categories including digestive diseases and neurological disorders.[57] In the mid-1970s, the NIH funded several studies of the costs attributable to various diseases and published a report comparing grant funding to various measures of mortality, morbidity, and economic costs.[58] The efforts to track funding by disease categories continued over the years. In the early 1990s, the NIH's chief financial officer told a journalist that the agency might "calculate each year the amount of money being spent on each disease, and publish these numbers in the agency's annual budget request" in order to "tell advocacy groups what NIH is already doing."[59]

In 1994, Congress sought further data on NIH funding. The Congressional Research Service produced a report of NIH funding and

[53] Mushkin, *Biomedical Research*, 15.
[54] US House of Representatives, "Appropriations for 1980, Part 4," 131, 95.
[55] Mushkin, *Biomedical Research*, 197.
[56] Mushkin, 199.
[57] US House of Representatives, "Appropriations for 1975, Part 4," 6.
[58] Mushkin, *Biomedical Research*, 14–15, 191, 363.
[59] Anderson, "Opponents of Earmarks," 4.

mortality rates for the leading causes of death.[60] The same year, the Senate appropriations committee ordered the NIH to submit a report of funding by death rates, medical spending, and indirect economic costs of diseases.[61] The NIH responded in 1995 with data on 66 diseases and conditions.[62] By the late 1990s, the NIH was collecting funding data on about 250 programs (many of which were specific diseases) and publicly providing data on about 50.[63]

Next, Congress asked the Institute of Medicine (IOM) to issue recommendations on how to improve priority setting at the NIH. The study was motivated in part by the desire to avoid earmarks, proposed "in re-sponse" to "the offering of amendments to fund specific disease research."[64] Published in 1998, the IOM report was largely deferential to the NIH, [65] but it did suggest that the NIH develop better mechanisms for responding to public health needs. The authors noted that the NIH was collecting "data on disease burden and costs . . . rather informally," with different institutes using "different databases and methodologies."[66] They called for the NIH to develop "metrics for spending according to disease burden (e.g., inci-dence, mortality, disability, and cost) . . . because not doing so leads some to conclude, incorrectly I believe, that NIH cares more about curiosity than cure."[67] This phrasing assumes that the NIH is already adequately targeting funding to disease burden and suggests that data would be most useful for increasing public support.

In the late 1990s and early 2000s, the data struggles briefly calmed down. The NIH director reassured Congress that the NIH was looking into the IOM report and working on a response; members of Congress acknowl-edged the NIH's efforts.[68] This period coincided with the doubling of the NIH budget (see Chapter 5). This rapid funding growth lowered the stakes for between-disease struggles.[69]

---

[60] Johnson, AIDS and Other Diseases.

[61] Agnew, "Body-Count Budgeting."

[62] Institute of Medicine, Scientific Opportunities and Public Needs, 31.

[63] Institute of Medicine, 21.

[64] Frist, "Setting Biomedical Research Priorities"; see also Institute of Medicine, Scientific Opportunities and Public Needs, 26, 71.

[65] Callahan, What Price Better Health?, 249.

[66] Institute of Medicine, Scientific Opportunities and Public Needs, 5, 22.

[67] Institute of Medicine, viii.

[68] US House of Representatives, "Appropriations for 2000, Part 4a," 74, 86.

[69] Growing budgets reduce the demand for "reallocative financing." Steuerle, "Financing the American State," 415.

In the following decade, Congress continued to push the NIH to provide more data. The NIH Reform Act of 2006 required the NIH to report funding by disease to Congress every other year.[70] The act also required that the NIH formalize its coding system. In response, the NIH developed the Research, Condition, and Disease Classification (RCDC) system, which uses computerized text mining to classify grants. Before RCDC, different institutes coded grants differently—for instance, if a grant dealt with more than one disease, some institutes would prorate it, assigning some of the funds to one disease and some to another, and some would double-count it. RCDC does the latter—for instance, if a grant targets diabetes and hypertension, 100% of the funding is counted for diabetes and 100% for hypertension.[71] Double-counting is more politically advantageous for the NIH since it maximizes each disease's funding tally.[72]

NIH Pushes Back

NIH officials and scientists worried that these calls to align funding with various measures of the burden of disease would compromise their autonomy and force them to neglect important scientific goals. Social scientists sometimes assume that standardization and expert authority increase together.[73] But, in fact, quantification and standardization tend to challenge the autonomy of experts, forcing them to justify their decisions on the basis of objective standards instead of expert judgment.[74] Rejecting advocates' and policymakers' focus on health burden and economic effects, NIH officials suggested alternate criteria for prioritizing diseases, often focusing on scientific opportunity and market failure. They also questioned the feasibility of prioritizing diseases and planning science.

[70] Gillum et al., "NIH Disease Funding," 1.

[71] National Institutes of Health, "August Crosswalk"; Studwell, "NIH Launches New System."

[72] I interviewed one NIH staffer who raised concerns about this change, noting that, for instance, the computerized system does not distinguish "non-lymphoma" from "lymphoma." She preferred her institute's previous system, which used human coders and prorated grants, but noted that the new system seemed popular with smaller institutes that lacked staff to do the coding.

[73] Weber, *General Economic History*, 200.

[74] Espeland and Stevens, "Commensuration as a Social Process," 328–31; Guston, *Between Politics and Science*; Porter, *Trust in Numbers*, 8, 89–90; Timmermans and Epstein, "A World of Standards," 71.

Scientific Opportunity

Arguing against an exclusive focus on the health and economic burdens imposed by diseases, NIH officials often highlight the importance of investing in areas with high potential for important discoveries.[75] In 1974, NIH director Robert Stone argued that one reason that "constituencies and pressure groups and concerned individuals who back the disease-of-the-month approach" should not have undue influence over priority setting was that "perceptions of nonscientists about where the money can best be spent are often emotional or ill-informed, and they don't represent, in many ways, the scientist's most objective view of where it is possible to make research findings."[76] Similarly, in 1997, NIH director Harold Varmus argued that "not all problems are equally approachable, regardless of their importance for the public health."[77] Representative John Porter (R-IL) agreed, saying "I think scientific opportunity, as judged by scientists, not politicians, should be the guiding principle in NIH resource allocation decisions."[78] This criterion was less popular with advocates; fewer than one in five disease witnesses discussed scientific potential, and the percentage has decreased over time (see Figure 4.2).

Although they emphasize the importance of scientific opportunity, NIH researchers certainly do not want to quantify it. Rather, they view scientific opportunity as best left up to expert judgment and as a reason for rejecting standardized priority setting. Occasionally, policymakers and academics attempt to quantify scientific opportunity. For instance, in 1979, Representative Obey (D-WI) asked the NIH director whether "the number and quality of grant applications that come to NIH is a good indicator of what research opportunities there are in a particular disease."[79] He also asked whether equalizing paylines (the peer review scores above which grant applications were funded) across institutes could help assure that funds "would go where the best science would indicate they ought to go."[80] Academic researchers have also quantified scientific opportunities by

---

[75] Lichtenberg, "Allocation of Biomedical Research"; Sampat, "Mission-Oriented Biomedical Research," 1730.

[76] US House of Representatives, "Appropriations for 1975, Part 4," 52.

[77] US Senate, "Biomedical Research Priorities," 8.

[78] US House of Representatives, "Appropriations for 1998, Part 4b," 2431.

[79] US House of Representatives, "Appropriations for 1980, Part 4," 133.

[80] US House of Representatives, 139.

counting numbers of disease-specific patents or articles published in high-impact journals.[81]

But scientific opportunity cannot be thought of as truly independent of NIH funding. As Representative Porter put it in an appropriations hearing, scientific opportunity and research dollars create a "chicken-and-egg situation" since research funding attracts students and researchers to specialize in fields, develop expertise, begin projects, and make discoveries.[82] If "scientific potential" reflects previous years' NIH funding, then using potential to set priorities would widen the gaps between well-funded and neglected diseases. Instead, some scholars have argued that in addition to funding the areas that currently seem to have the most potential, the NIH should "do more to create scientific opportunity in the most burdensome disease areas by channeling funds to those areas."[83]

Market Failure

NIH officials, scientists, and academics also occasionally suggest another criterion for priority setting: the degree to which a disease is neglected by private industry. Private companies tend to underinvest in drugs for rare diseases, prevention, and health education.[84] Companies also tend to focus on applied research, viewing the payoffs of basic research as too uncertain.[85] Varmus noted that "[s]uch considerations may, for example, favor the expenditure of NIH dollars on relatively rare diseases . . . for which there is little incentive for research and development in the private sector."[86] Ideally, a market failure approach would minimize the extent to which NIH research subsidizes the pharmaceutical industry by paying for studies it would otherwise have funded.[87]

---

[81] Gillum et al., "NIH Disease Funding."

[82] US House of Representatives, "Appropriations for 1998, Part 4b," 2471; see also Brooks, "Problem of Research Priorities," 179–80; Moses et al., "Financial Anatomy of Biomedical Research," 1338.

[83] Dresser, *When Science Offers Salvation*, 80.

[84] Mukherjee, *Emperor of All Maladies*, 418, 436; Resnik, "Setting Biomedical Research Priorities," 184. Market failure justifications have been most explicit in arguments about public funding for "orphan diseases." In policy debates, an "orphan drug" was initially defined as an unprofitable one but eventually came to be understood as the related (but not identical) category of a drug to treat a rare disease. Huyard, "Uncommon Disorders," 466.

[85] Institute of Medicine, *Scientific Opportunities and Public Needs*, 16; Kastor, *National Institutes of Health*, 32–34; Resnik, "Setting Biomedical Research Priorities," 185.

[86] Varmus, "Evaluating the Burden of Disease," 1914.

[87] Gerth and Stolberg, "Drug Firms."

One barrier to using market failure considerations to set research priorities is that the market responds to government actions. Pharmaceutical companies' conception of what research is profitable and/or necessary for them to do depends on what the NIH is funding. For instance, after the passage of laws designed to promote licensing of federally funded discoveries, pharma companies started spending less of their budgets on preclinical stages of research.[88]

For this metric as well, NIH officials and scientists were not actually interested in formally ranking diseases. The 1998 IOM report suggested that the NIH collect data on private research spending.[89] So far, the NIH has not collected systematic data on private companies' research spending by disease, market failure is rarely used as a metric to judge the funding distribution, and there is no evidence that the NIH systematically considers it in setting priorities.[90]

Rejecting Rankings

In addition to providing alternative metrics, the NIH pushed back against the very idea of ranking diseases. One strategy was to discourage policymakers and the public from taking the numbers too seriously. At a 1997 Senate hearing on NIH priority setting, NIH director Harold Varmus rejected diseases as the appropriate categories for judging the funding distribution and opposed formal commensuration as a priority-setting tool. He argued that "numbers are suspect" and "assessing or designing a research portfolio from numbers alone is a very tricky, indeed a hazardous enterprise."[91] In a 1997 report, the NIH argued that priority setting by the numbers would be foolhardy because there are too many different ways to measure health needs, including mortality, prevalence, years of life lost, amount of disability caused, economic and social costs, and potential for rapid spread.[92]

---

[88] Angell, *Truth About the Drug Companies*; Gerth and Stolberg, "Drug Firms"; Moses et al., "Financial Anatomy of Biomedical Research," 1336.

[89] Institute of Medicine, *Scientific Opportunities and Public Needs*, 5, 33; see also Kastor, *National Institutes of Health*, 32–39; Marks, "Rescuing the NIH."

[90] Sampat, "Dismal Science," 157.

[91] US Senate, "Biomedical Research Priorities," 9, 8.

[92] National Institutes of Health, *Setting Research Priorities*, 8.

In addition to questioning the numbers, NIH officials repeatedly emphasized the unpredictability of science.[93] In 1967, NIH director Shannon argued that targeting medical research would be foolhardy since medical advances are

> dependent upon empirical approaches, serendipity, and the brilliance of too few gifted individuals. Therefore, the hope of major advances lies in sustaining broad and free-ranging inquiry into all aspects of the phenomena of life, limited only by the criteria of excellence, the scientific importance, and the seriousness and competence of the investigator.[94]

Thirty years later, Director Varmus told the Senate that "important discoveries often come from totally unexpected directions."[95] An NIH report similarly noted that "[t]here are limits to planning science" since "it is impossible to know with certainty which area will produce the next important discovery."[96] If science is unpredictable, they argued, it would be foolhardy to target research funding to particular disease categories.

Critics call this "the myth of unfettered research" or "the serendipity hypothesis": the argument "that any line of basic research is as likely to lead to societal benefit as any other" and that serendipitous results cannot come from targeted or applied research.[97] There is surprisingly little evidence to support these claims, beyond examples of major innovations that resulted from basic research.[98]

NIH officials and scientists also emphasized the importance of basic research into biological processes, in addition to applied and clinical research into treatments for particular diseases. An NIH report argued that "basic research projects may appear initially to be unrelated to any specific disease, but might prove to be a critical turning point in a long chain of discoveries

---

[93] One exception to this rule was Bernadine Healy, who served as NIH director from 1991 to 1993. During her brief tenure, she began work on a strategic plan to set broad goals for the NIH and allocate funding targets to them. The plan angered biomedical researchers. Cohen, "Conflicting Agendas Shape NIH," 1679; Fallows, "Political Scientist," 69; Marshall and Rubinstein, "Under the Microscope," 788; Palca, "Emphasizing the Health in NIH," 23.

[94] Shannon, "Advancement of Medical Research," 104–5.

[95] US Senate, "Biomedical Research Priorities," 9.

[96] National Institutes of Health, *Setting Research Priorities*, 3, 5.

[97] Greenberg, *Science, Money, and Politics*, 10; Sampat, "Mission-Oriented Biomedical Research," 1730; Sarewitz, *Frontiers of Illusion*, 34, 38.

[98] Mukherjee, "Fighting Chance"; Sampat, "Mission-Oriented Biomedical Research," 1739; Sarewitz, *Frontiers of Illusion*, 34.

leading to improved health."[99] Harold Varmus and Marc Kirschner made a similar case in the *New York Times* in 1992, arguing that

> the most effective long-term approach to improving health lies in fostering the research that increases understanding of genes and tissues. Basic biomedical science cannot promise specific cures in a defined time, but a general understanding of cells will lead to cures for many diseases. . . . What works best is a system in which the choice of research projects is not imposed by Congress and is free of specified methods, materials and goals.[100]

These arguments about the importance of serendipity and basic research propose that as much of the NIH budget as possible should be untargeted (with scientists following their instincts and curiosity) and basic (as opposed to clinical or translational).

Historically, the NIH has argued for a focus on basic research by drawing on a "linear model" of science and technology development, in which basic research comes first, followed by technology. This model, popularized by Vannevar Bush in his influential report *Science: The Endless Frontier*, was designed to secure for scientists "the holy grail of money without interference."[101] In fact, the relationship between basic science and applied development is more complicated and can run in the other direction; sometimes applied problems move basic science forward.[102]

Powerful lawmakers echoed NIH officials' arguments, opposing attempts to formalize priority setting. Representative Obey told NIH officials that Congress should "increase your ability to withstand political pressure, rather than decrease it," and Senator Kennedy argued that "the final judgment on the direction of biomedical research must be left largely to NIH."[103] Respecting scientific expertise meant avoiding strict metrics. Representative Obey noted that "we ought to be very careful before we take the simple-minded approach of looking at only one index by which to measure what we

---

[99] National Institutes of Health, *Setting Research Priorities*, 9.

[100] Varmus and Kirschner, "Don't Undermine Basic Research," A23.

[101] Greenberg, *Science, Money, and Politics*, 44–45.

[102] Brooks, "Problem of Research Priorities," 182; Greenberg, *Science, Money, and Politics*, 45; National Academy of Sciences, *Allocating Federal Funds for Science and Technology*, 5; Sarewitz, *Frontiers of Illusion*, 37; Stephan and Ehrenberg, "Introduction," 4–6.

[103] US House of Representatives, "Appropriations for 1998, Part 4b," 2432; US Senate, "Biomedical Research Priorities," 6.

are spending," and Senator Frist argued against "setting research priorities in such a prescriptive manner."[104] These powerful defenders have made the NIH more successful than other federal agencies at maintaining autonomy over its funding decisions.[105] Throughout decades of discussions of how to rank diseases, the NIH never formalized its priority-setting procedures, continuing to rely on a list of unranked criteria—a process so vague that it is "really not quite a priority setting procedure at all."[106]

Effects on the Funding Distribution

NIH officials and their congressional defenders worried that pressure to fund particular diseases would crowd out basic research (since it often doesn't target a particular disease) and untargeted research project grants (as opposed to targeted research, in which institutes allocate money to a particular research topic before grant applications come in).[107] Figure 4.3 shows that basic and untargeted research did decline slightly in proportional terms.[108] From 1984 to 2015, the percent of the NIH budget devoted to basic research dropped from 62% to 52%. From 1997 to 2017, the percent of new research project grant (RPG) funding that was untargeted declined from 88% to 74% (see Figure 4.3, top panel). But since these proportional declines occurred as the budget was growing dramatically, the actual amount of money devoted to basic research and the amount of new RPG funding that was untargeted both more than doubled, even when adjusted for inflation (see Figure 4.3, bottom panel). Basic and untargeted research did not increase quite as fast as applied and targeted research, but they were not being crowded out, either.

Yet despite the NIH's success in avoiding mandates to "commensurate" diseases and increasing funds for basic and untargeted research, the decades

---

[104] US House of Representatives, "Appropriations for 1998, Part 4b," 2474; US Senate, "Biomedical Research Priorities," 2.

[105] While some members of Congress have pushed the NIH to fund more targeted and applied research, others have long emphasized basic research. Strickland, *Politics, Science, and Dread Disease*, 119, 179, 189–90, 202–3.

[106] Callahan, "Shaping Biomedical Research Priorities," 121.

[107] National Institutes of Health, "NIH Data Book."

[108] Data for Figure 4.3 come from Lauer, "NIH's Commitment to Basic Science"; National Institutes of Health, "REPORT"; Zerhouni, "NIH in the Post-Doubling Era."

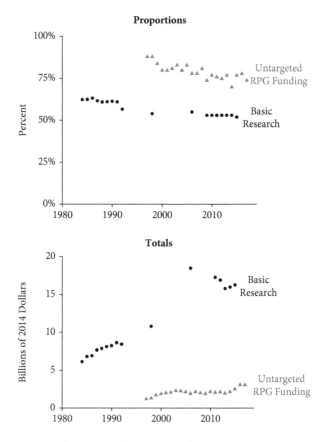

Figure 4.3 Basic and untargeted research at the NIH, 1984–2017: Percentages decline but amounts increase

Top panel: Basic research as a percent of the NIH budget and untargeted funds as a percent of new research project grant (RPG) funds. Bottom panel: Total basic research funding and total new untargeted RPG funds.

of critiques had concrete effects on NIH funding distribution. Although Congress never required that the NIH use any particular metric to set priorities, as the NIH was increasingly critiqued on the basis of dollars per death, mortality gradually became a better predictor of NIH funding. In the late 1980s, there was only a weak relationship between dollars and deaths. Mortality explained less than one-tenth of the variation in funding,[109] and

---

[109] The gray line in Figure 4.4 shows the R^2 values from regressions of NIH funding to diseases on mortality in the previous year. See Appendix for details.

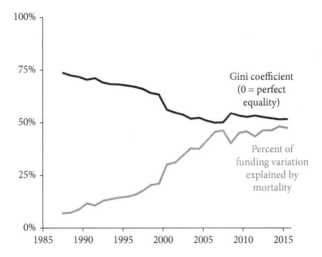

Figure 4.4 Equalizing dollars per death, 1987–2015

Gray line shows R^2 statistics from regressions of NIH funding to diseases on mortality (lagged by one year). Black line shows the Gini coefficient, a measure of inequality in dollars per death. If NIH funding were distributed solely on the basis of mortality, the Gini coefficient would equal zero. Both calculations are based on the same 29 diseases in each year.

the Gini coefficient[110] indicated substantial inequality in dollars per death (see Figure 4.4). But during the 1990s, as the NIH faced increasing criticism over unequal dollars per death, the funding distribution began to line up more closely with this standard. Twenty years later, mortality explained almost half the variation in research funding, and the Gini coefficient had declined substantially (see Figure 4.4). The increasing influence of mortality was particularly dramatic in the late 1990s and early 2000s (after the debates about NIH priority setting and during the doubling of the NIH budget, discussed in the next chapter). NIH funding also moved closer to equalizing dollars per DALY, but the changes were less dramatic because DALYs were already a reasonably good predictor of NIH funding (see Appendix, Figure A.2).

---

[110] The Gini coefficient is traditionally used to measure income inequality between individuals. For this analysis, I assigned each person who died from a particular disease an equal share of that disease's research funding and measured inequality in research funding across the people who died from these 29 diseases. If each disease received exactly the same number of dollars per death, the Gini coefficient would equal zero.

Academic researchers have examined the question of how well NIH funding lines up with disease burden, generally finding strong relationships between the NIH funding distribution and various measures of the burden of disease.[111] My results suggest that this relationship is historically specific, a result of decades of struggles over disease priority setting. Even though NIH officials vigorously resisted efforts to standardize the funding distribution by deaths or disability, they faced increasing pressure to correct presumed funding imbalances based on these measures. Disease comparisons and the political prominence of health burden metrics created powerful incentives for the NIH to align deaths and dollars.[112]

Conclusion

Over the years, advocates, policymakers, and researchers approached metrics in distinct ways. Disease campaigners encouraged policymakers to think of the NIH budget as divided up among diseases and strategically used numbers and statistics to highlight the severity of their problems.[113] Policymakers sought more systematic ways to determine which diseases deserved the most funding, pressing for data and encouraging the NIH to formalize its priority setting. NIH officials pushed back against attempts to quantify the severity of various diseases and use these metrics to determine funding. But despite this resistance, NIH funding to diseases increasingly lined up with measures of the burden of disease.

In seeking trustworthy data on the burden of disease, policymakers were trying to ensure that the funding distribution would be based on principled arguments, rather than interest group power. They turned to statistics to avoid being unduly swayed by lobbying. But ironically, in their attempt to rise above lobbying, policymakers accepted the advocates' definition of the problem, focusing on the funding distribution *across diseases*. This is not the

---

[111] Gillum et al., "NIH Disease Funding"; Gross, Anderson, and Powe, "Funding and the Burden of Disease"; Sampat, Buterbaugh, and Perl, "New Evidence."

[112] Daniel Carpenter describes a similar case of a metric for evaluation changing the actions of a federal agency. In the 1970s, academics and advocates criticized the FDA for being too slow to approve new drugs. They evaluated the FDA based on the number of new chemical entities approved per year and the average lag between drug approvals in Europe and the United States. After facing public criticism on the basis of these metrics, the FDA began keeping data on them, discussing them in reports, and considering them when making decisions. Carpenter, *Reputation and Power*, 377–78.

[113] Benford and Snow, "Framing Processes and Social Movements," 615; Best, *Threatened Children*, 29; Rochefort and Cobb, "Emerging Perspective," 17–21.

only way to judge the NIH funding distribution. The choice to focus on disease categories was itself an effect of disease advocacy—one that had concrete effects on the funding distribution, favoring high-mortality diseases.

When researchers study the political outcomes of advocacy, they tend to focus on the extent to which movements secure benefits for their constituents.[114] This chapter reveals that advocacy can also change the structures, systems, or schemas of political decision-making, including the relevant categories for comparison and the dominant metrics for commensuration.[115] Since these changes affect all participants in political fields, outlast the advocates who introduced them, and contribute to institutional change, they may be the most sweeping and durable effects of advocacy. These findings suggest a more subtle role for social movement framing, which researchers often describe primarily as an instrumental way for individual social movement organizations to achieve their goals.[116] The subtle push to "rationalize" the NIH funding distribution in a way that favored high-mortality diseases wasn't necessarily what the advocates wanted—as the previous chapter showed, the biggest killers don't tend to have the most advocacy. When disease advocates used various metrics to push for more funding for their diseases, the pressure to formalize NIH priority setting and the increasing influence of mortality were field-defining side effects. Advocacy's effects on policymaking may be unintended and cultural, as well as consciously sought and concrete.

This chapter asked a somewhat unusual question about how advocacy affects policy, focusing on the categories and metrics used to judge funding distributions. But we shouldn't lose sight of the more traditional question of whether advocacy organizations secure gains for their constituents.[117] Disease advocates changed the terms of the debate. But did they also get what they wanted? Did lobbying pay off? The next chapter explores these

[114] Burstein, Einwohner, and Hollander, "Success of Political Movements"; Gamson, *Strategy of Social Protest*; Amenta and Young, "Making an Impact"; Andrews and Edwards, "Advocacy Organizations"; Amenta et al., "Political Consequences of Social Movements," 201; Baumgartner and Leech, *Basic Interests.*

[115] Best, "Disease Politics and Medical Research Funding."

[116] Amenta et al., "Political Consequences of Social Movements"; Benford and Snow, "Framing Processes and Social Movements"; Burstein and Hirsh, "Interest Organizations"; Cress and Snow, "Outcomes of Homeless Mobilization."

[117] Amenta et al., "Political Consequences of Social Movements"; Andrews and Edwards, "Advocacy Organizations"; Baumgartner et al., *Lobbying and Policy Change*; Baumgartner and Leech, *Basic Interests*; Burstein, "Social Movements and Public Policy"; Giugni, "How Social Movements Matter"; Smith, "Interest Group Influence."

questions by asking whether highly mobilized diseases received bigger funding increases.

This chapter and the next also address related questions about whether specialized claims hamper the achievement of broad goals. NIH officials worried that targeting funds to particular diseases would disadvantage basic and untargeted research. These concerns were overblown: applied and targeted research expanded faster, but the basic and untargeted research budgets also grew dramatically. Specialized claims and broad goals do not compete in a zero-sum game. The next chapter addresses a related concern: that specialized claims for particular diseases would slow the growth of the NIH budget.

5

Budget Battles

Critics have often worried that disease campaigns skew the health budget and misallocate money. At mid-century, experts hoped that the money donated to fight polio or tuberculosis could be bundled into a public health budget and distributed more rationally. They falsely assumed that there was a set amount of money that people were ready to donate to improve health— that if the money wasn't going to fight polio, it would have been donated for another health cause. Later in the twentieth century, policymakers searched for systematic ways to rank the importance of diseases and set medical research priorities. They "rationalized" the research budget somewhat but could not overcome the drive for scientific autonomy and the power of single-disease campaigns. As the field of disease advocacy expanded in the 1990s, these criticisms heated up. Policymakers, government officials, and critics described a crisis in science policy. A rabid pack of disease advocates were fighting a zero-sum game, aggressively stealing resources from one another.

Congressional aides and National Institutes of Health (NIH) staffers complained that while biomedical research advocates used to "close ranks behind a common goal: to increase the overall pot of money for biomedical research," disease lobbies had begun "making aggressive public appeals for a larger slice of NIH's pie for their own areas."[1] A journalist argued that new disease advocates, targeting "dozens of ailments, from Lyme's disease to leukodystrophy," were "bypassing the public and heading straight to Congress. This strategy pits one disease group—and its associated researchers—against another in a lobbying war for research funds."[2] The Institute of Medicine agreed that in the past, disease advocates had "avoided open competition with each other" and instead "worked together to seek increased overall funding for NIH, the proverbial 'rising tide that lifts all the boats.'" But the success of AIDS and breast cancer advocates had "put pressure on all groups

---

[1] Marshall, "Lobbyists," 344; see also Heinz et al., *Hollow Core*, 50.
[2] Anderson, "Opponents of Earmarks," 4.

to make more specific demands and to compete openly with other groups for more resources."[3] The head of the Parkinson's Action Network claimed that her organization had recently decided to stop being "self-sacrificing." Similarly, a representative of the Juvenile Diabetes Foundation claimed that "there was a time when we were very good citizens and really went up to the Hill with one message—overall [funding] for NIH. But it becomes hard as you see other disease areas advance far beyond where we are."[4]

Observers worried that the advocates would compete in a zero-sum game, with gains for any one disease invariably coming at the expense of other diseases. The Institute of Medicine reported that "specific advocacy efforts can succeed in gaining large increases in funding for certain diseases (e.g., AIDS and breast cancer) at the expense of funding for others."[5] They argued that slower NIH budget growth in the early 1980s and 1990s, combined with rising numbers of earmarks, meant that the NIH was forced to take money from some diseases to give to others.

Others warned that specialized disease advocacy would prevent overall increases in the NIH budget. National Institute of Allergy and Infectious Diseases director Anthony Fauci argued that "jockeying for more money by constituencies of a certain disease . . . doesn't help" achieve funding increases.[6] And Representative John Porter, chair of the House appropriations subcommittee with jurisdiction over the NIH, worried that "the fighting between diseases, this 'siblicide,' . . . could provoke ugly battles that result in NIH funding being cut overall."[7] "[C]ompetition between disease interest groups has always diluted the research community's ability to 'move the needle' when it comes to funding," according to a public relations firm promoting research funding increases.[8] "It'll be a disaster if the research communities start attacking each other to get more of the money for themselves," said a representative of the American Society of Clinical Oncology.[9]

These critics assumed that competitive disease advocacy was something new. There certainly were a lot more disease advocates in the 1990s than

[3] Institute of Medicine, *Scientific Opportunities and Public Needs*, 24, 56.
[4] Marshall, "Lobbyists."
[5] Institute of Medicine, *Scientific Opportunities and Public Needs*, 54; see also Wachter, "AIDS, Activism," 132.
[6] Quoted in Cohen, "AIDS," 345.
[7] US House of Representatives, "Appropriations for 1998, Part 4b," 2432.
[8] Stapleton, "Lobby for Labs."
[9] Anderson, "Opponents of Earmarks," 4.

there had been twenty years earlier, and they had become more likely to focus on patients as constituents than to make universal claims to benefit everyone. But fears about single-disease campaigns stretch back to the beginning of the twentieth century. There was nothing new about advocates promoting one disease over another and critics worrying that this competition would misallocate funds.

The critics also assumed that 1) disease advocates were successfully attracting government money; 2) this money was invariably taken from one disease to fund another; and 3) without a unified science lobby, the NIH budget would stagnate. But nobody examined the data to see if advocacy really was paying off, if money was really moving from one disease to another, and if disease advocacy was stunting the growth of the NIH budget. This chapter looks at the numbers and finds that disease advocacy was successful but only when the NIH budget was growing. Rather than being taken from other diseases, these research funding increases competed with other priorities, like expanding social spending or reducing federal deficits. And rather than stalling the growth of the NIH budget, disease advocacy seems to have accelerated it.

These findings address three major questions for social scientists. First, social scientists often ask whether advocacy affects policy. But instead of asking *whether* advocacy pays off, we should ask *when* and *why* it does.[10] Since beneficiaries invariably protest budget cuts, it's difficult to set priorities by moving money around. It's much easier to give new money to something you favor, meaning that advocacy is most influential when budgets are increasing.[11] The largest gains for the NIH came during a federal budget surplus, and within the NIH budget, disease lobbying paid off most when the NIH budget was increasing—when there was new money to move around.

Second, some social scientists reflexively assume that similar priorities are more likely to compete with each other—that is, that political gains for one issue come at the expense of related issues. Others emphasize the

[10] Baumgartner and Leech, *Basic Interests*, 134.

[11] Because interest groups "can be counted on to come to the defense of a threatened program, they reduce the flexibility of budget decision makers, who find it difficult to cut programs with strong interest-group backing." Rubin, *Politics of Public Budgeting*, 14. When cuts are too politically difficult, policymakers can set priorities by dividing up budget increases, "budgeting by addition rather than subtraction." Wildavsky, *New Politics of the Budgetary Process*, 159; see also Jones and Baumgartner, *Politics of Attention*, 97; Kamlet and Mowery, "Budgetary Base"; Padgett, "Bounded Rationality in Budgetary Research"; Rubin, "Demise of Incrementalism"; Smith and McGeary, "Don't Look Back."

opposite pattern: political attention to one issue attracts attention to similar issues.[12] Instead of asking whether policy outcomes are zero-sum, we should ask *when* and *why* particular priorities compete. Which trade-offs are made depends on budgetary strategies and political institutions. In this case, a series of budgeting rules tried to make the NIH compete with all other domestic spending priorities. Other policymakers maneuvered around these rules, drawing NIH funding increases from the Department of Defense, the federal budget surplus, and economic stimulus funds.

Third, scholars debate whether smaller, specialized, or identity-based movements are less likely than large, general movements to achieve broad goals. Some worry that specialized groups may fail to pursue larger agendas.[13] Others suggest that the proliferation of specialized advocacy organizations may lead to better political outcomes.[14] In this case, while critics worried that specialized disease advocacy would stunt the growth of the NIH budget, it actually coincided with major increases. These findings show that diversity, specialization, and identity politics do not necessarily undermine broad goals.

NIH in the 1980s: Overruling Reagan, Fighting AIDS, and Increasing the Deficit

Biomedical research advocates worried that the NIH budget would stagnate as the Reagan administration sought to shrink the federal government. But the AIDS crisis and the NIH's bipartisan popularity in Congress overpowered Reagan's efforts to limit research spending. The NIH budget grew, with much of the new money earmarked for AIDS. The funding for AIDS rarely came from other diseases, and the funding for the NIH rarely

---

[12] Hilgartner and Bosk, "Rise and Fall of Social Problems," 68; Kingdon, *Agendas, Alternatives, and Public Policies*, 201–2; McCombs, *Setting the Agenda*; Skrentny, "Policy-Elite Perceptions"; Skrentny, *Minority Rights Revolution*; Zhu, "Issue Competition."

[13] Collins, *Black Feminist Thought*; Gamson, "Hiroshima"; Gitlin, "From Universality to Difference"; Gitlin, *Twilight of Common Dreams*; Hobsbawm, "Identity Politics and the Left"; hooks, *Talking Back*; McAdam, *Political Process*; Mushaben, "Struggle Within"; Piore, *Beyond Individualism*; Putnam, *Bowling Alone*; Rorty, *Achieving Our Country*; Skocpol, *Diminished Democracy*; Turner, "Intersex Identities."

[14] Armstrong, *Forging Gay Identities*; Bernstein, "Celebration and Suppression"; Bernstein, "Identity Politics"; Berry, *New Liberalism*; Bickford, "Anti-Anti-Identity Politics"; Ghaziani and Baldassarri, "Cultural Anchors"; Haines, "Black Radicalization"; Levitsky, "Niche Activism"; Minkoff, *Organizing for Equality*; Minkoff, "Sequencing of Social Movements"; Minkoff, Aisenbrey, and Agnone, "Organizational Diversity"; Polletta, "Strategy and Identity."

came from other federal programs. Instead, the federal deficit grew to record levels.

As policymakers gradually recognized the political and moral necessity of using federal funds to fight AIDS, they explicitly argued over where the money would come from. Focused on reducing the federal deficit, the Reagan administration sought to fund AIDS programs by transferring money from other domestic spending. In the early 1980s, NIH officials avoided directly asking the Reagan administration for additional money to fight AIDS, concerned that they would be told to take it from elsewhere in their budget. But since Congress generally preferred to add new funds, the AIDS crisis actually "opened up a substantial source of new funds for biomedical research."[15] This new money often took the form of supplemental appropriations to the NIH, ranging from $500,000 to $10 million dollars from FY 1982 to 1984.[16] An amendment to the FY 1985 Health and Human Services appropriations bill added almost $15 million specifically to fight AIDS; the FY 1986 appropriations added $70 million in AIDS funding through the NIH director's office.[17] Rather than transferring money from existing NIH priorities, Congress tended to pair AIDS earmarks with increases in the NIH budget. From 1982 onward, Congress approved annual budget increases for the NIH, usually appropriating more money than Reagan had requested.[18]

The Reagan administration responded with budgetary strategies to halt the "burgeoning growth of biomedical research," but Congress was usually able to continue to grow the NIH budget.[19] After Congress approved a 14% increase for FY 1985, Reagan's Office of Management and Budget (OMB) tried to require the NIH to fund all three years of some new grants from the 1985 budget. After the US comptroller general ruled the OMB directive illegal, the NIH was able to initiate more grants, creating pressure to maintain the new high funding levels over the next two years.[20] Next, the Gramm-Rudman-Hollings Balanced Budget and Emergency Deficit Control Act

[15] Kolata, "Congress, NIH," 436; see also Stoto et al., "Federal Funding for AIDS Research," 409–10; Culliton, "AIDS Amendment"; Norman, "AIDS Funding Transfusion"; Norman, "More of the Same," 1987; Panem, "AIDS"; White, "Budgeting and Health Policymaking," 65.

[16] Stoto et al., "Federal Funding for AIDS Research," 409.

[17] Culliton, "AIDS Amendment," 1056; Stoto et al., "Federal Funding for AIDS Research," 413.

[18] Culliton, "Congress Passes Generous NIH Budget"; Marshall, "'Burgeoning Growth of Biomedicine.'"

[19] Marshall, "'Burgeoning Growth of Biomedicine,'" 847.

[20] Culliton, "Who Runs NIH?"; Culliton, "NIH to Award 2200 New Grants"; Culliton, "OMB Raid"; Norman, "Congress Votes."

of 1985 (GRH) laid out a plan to eliminate the deficit over eight years and threatened sequestration—automatic cuts to discretionary spending—if the deficit missed its annual targets. These cuts were triggered in FY 1986, and the NIH budget was cut by over $200 million that year. The cuts made NIH's victory over OMB the year before a mixed blessing: still responsible for all the grants initiated in 1985, the NIH had to cut other programs.[21] For FY 1987, Congress approved another enormous budget increase for the NIH, but the OMB proposed that the NIH wait until 1988 to spend about one-third of the increase. After being threatened with another lawsuit, the OMB backed down and the full increase stood.[22] The large funding increase in 1987 created another boom/bust cycle, with low success rates for grants in FY 1989 and 1990.[23]

These political machinations ensured that AIDS funding increases did not come at other diseases' expense.[24] If AIDS had never existed, the NIH budget would likely have continued its earlier trajectory of slower growth (see Figure 5.1) or, given the budget-cutting proclivities of the Reagan administration, stagnated entirely. As a Centers for Disease Control and Prevention (CDC) official remarked, "AIDS has been one of the only things that Congress has been willing to bust the budget on."[25]

In fact, AIDS funding may have spilled over into other diseases' budgets.[26] Some commentators have suggested that NIH officials used creative accounting to count some research projects as AIDS-related. One analysis found that 15% of the grants covered by an AIDS earmark did not refer to the disease in their titles or abstracts.[27] In the long run, AIDS funding may

[21] Culliton, "NIH Faces Budget Cut," 444; Dodge, "Doomed to Repeat," 841; Franklin, *Making Ends Meet*, 34–35; Marshall, "Research and the 'Flexible Freeze,'" 1368; Norman, "NIH Gets a Friendly Hearing," 1364.

[22] Culliton, "Congress Boosts NIH Budget"; Culliton, "Battle over NIH Funds," 1129; Norman, "More of the Same," 1987, 151.

[23] Crawford, "Science and Congress," 404; Palca, "Hard Times at NIH," 988.

[24] There were occasionally trade-offs between funding for AIDS and for other diseases, but these were exceptions rather than the rule. For instance, in 1984, Congress instructed the NCI to increase its AIDS spending by $7.9 million, of which only $2 million was added during appropriations; some scientists protested that AIDS research was coming at the expense of cancer research. Culliton, "AIDS Amendment," 1056. Despite scattered exceptions, AIDS funding rarely increased more than the overall NIH budget.

[25] James Bloom, assistant director for AIDS activities at the CDC, quoted in Booth, "No Longer Ignored," 858.

[26] Similarly, when looking at international health spending, researchers have found that AIDS may have encouraged funding increases for other infectious diseases. Shiffman, Berlan, and Hafner, "Aid for AIDS."

[27] Kaiser, "What Does a Disease Deserve?," 902.

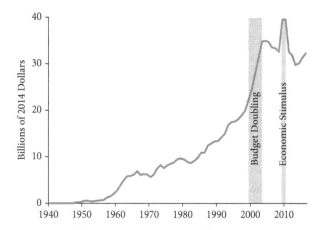

Figure 5.1 NIH budget, 1940–2016

Adjusted for inflation; includes funding from the American Recovery and Reinvestment Act of 2009.

provide an even bigger boost to research on other conditions. By the early 1990s, AIDS research made up about 10% of the NIH budget. Lawmakers informally agreed to keep it at that level and began including language to that effect in the reports accompanying NIH appropriations bills. At a 2015 hearing, NIH director Francis Collins suggested that AIDS funding would no longer necessarily grow "in lock-step" with the rest of the NIH budget, and the appropriations bill report dropped the language instructing NIH to spend 10% of its budget on AIDS.[28] The AIDS crisis had shifted billions of dollars into the NIH budget, some of which might now flow to other research programs.

1990–1997: Funding Breast Cancer and Struggling with Budget Rules

Budget politics remained central in the 1990s, creating further battles about where disease funding would come from. Like Reagan, President George H. W. Bush adopted legislative strategies to limit government spending. The

[28] Kaiser.

Budget Enforcement Act of 1990 (BEA) introduced caps on discretionary spending, with firewalls between defense spending, domestic spending, and foreign aid. This meant that, for instance, defense spending cuts could not be transferred to the domestic budget—within each category, programs would compete in a zero-sum game.[29] Several Bush administration budgets suggested modest increases for the NIH budget, matched by cuts to popular domestic programs. Facing these trade-offs, Congress tended to approve smaller increases than Bush had proposed.[30] Budgetary maneuvers to meet the BEA caps further limited NIH spending. In FY 1992, the Bush administration ordered the NIH to wait until the last day of the fiscal year to approve almost $400 million in grants (6% of the year's budget) so that they would count in FY 1993. The following year, the administration proposed holding back over $600 million. After being approved by Congress, the FY 1993 budget was cut by 0.8% to meet the BEA's spending limits.[31]

A decade earlier, Congress had found new money for AIDS. Now, it did the same for breast cancer. Senator Tom Harkin (D-IA) proposed taking $200 million from the Department of Defense (DOD) and using it to fund breast cancer research at the NIH, which would have breached the BEA's firewall between defense and domestic spending. Unable to transfer money *out* of the DOD to pay for breast cancer research, Harkin introduced an amendment to the 1993 defense appropriations bill earmarking $210 million for breast cancer research *within* the DOD.[32] Despite protests from the OMB director and the *New York Times*, which called it "an openly cynical maneuver," the amendment passed the Senate and the House and created the Department of Defense Congressionally Directed Medical Research Program (DOD-CDMRP).[33] For FY 1994, President Clinton proposed transferring the DOD breast cancer program to the NIH, which would have avoided the need for a parallel system to review grants. But instead of moving the program, Congress essentially duplicated it, adopting Clinton's proposal to increase breast cancer research at the National Cancer Institute

[29] Dodge, "Doomed to Repeat"; Penner and Steuerle, "Budget Rules"; Poterba, "Federal Budget Policy"; Thurber, "Congressional Budget Reform."
[30] Cowen, "Federal R&D Budget"; Cowen and Raloff, "Bush's '93 Budget"; Marshall and Hamilton, "R&D Budget"; Norman, "Growth Amid Red Ink," 1991, 616.
[31] Cowen, "Federal R&D Budget"; Marshall and Hamilton, "R&D Budget"; Norman, "Selective Growth," 1992; Palca, "NIH Grants."
[32] Casamayou, *Politics of Breast Cancer*, 148; Johnson, *Breast Cancer Research*.
[33] Casamayou, *Politics of Breast Cancer; New York Times*, "Medical Madness."

(NCI) by over $200 million, without eliminating the defense program.[34] Harkin's strategy had prevented breast cancer from competing with other domestic priorities by broadening the boundaries of the funding competition to include the defense budget.

In fact, rather than siphoning funds from other diseases, breast cancer's bounty spilled over to other diseases. For FY 1996, breast cancer research received $75 million through the DOD-CDMRP, and prostate cancer received $5 million. Prostate cancer activists pushed to equalize funding. Some breast cancer advocates worried that the competition would spell the end of the DOD-CDMRP; Fran Visco, head of the National Breast Cancer Coalition, argued that "If we pit one against the other then we're all going to lose."[35] They needn't have worried: the prostate cancer advocates secured a $45 million prostate cancer program, and breast cancer funding also increased, topping $100 million. This process continued over the years; the DOD-CDMRP now earmarks $400–$500 million to 25 research areas, including 15 diseases.[36]

As the NIH increased its spending on breast cancer, critics worried that this money was coming from other diseases. In 1993, Congress directed the NCI to increase its spending on breast cancer by $60 million but only increased the institute's budget by $40 million. Journalists suggested that breast cancer funding would logically need to be taken from other priorities. On the other hand, since the NCI's own budget had requested an $80 million increase for breast cancer, there's no indication that the earmark caused it to redirect money it had planned to spend on another cancer.[37] At other times, breast cancer advocacy benefited the NCI overall. In the early 1990s, breast cancer advocates and Congress negotiated directly with the NCI, which agreed to target more funds for breast cancer research in exchange for an increase in its budget.[38]

Budget fights continued after Republicans took over Congress, promising to cut taxes, reduce spending, and balance the budget within seven years.[39]

---

[34] Anderson, "NSF Wins, NIH Loses," 25; Mervis, Anderson, and Marshall, "Better for Science," 837. Congress appropriated a smaller amount to the DOD for breast cancer research for fiscal years 1994 and 1996, but in all other years, the appropriation remained above $100 million.

[35] Fran Visco, quoted in Weiss, "War Between Sexes."

[36] Department of Defense, "Funding History."

[37] Burd, "Scientists Worry," A23.

[38] Kaufert, "Women, Resistance," 301.

[39] Pierson, "Deficit and Domestic Reform"; Rosenbaum, "It's the Economy Again"; Thurber, "Republican Roles."

As a step toward this goal, the House and the Senate approved budget resolutions outlining FY 1996 spending cuts. For the NIH, the House proposed a 5% cut followed by a spending freeze. A vaguer Senate proposal required either a 10% or 20% cut.[40] Ultimately, the NIH's bipartisan popularity and supporters on the appropriations committees saved it from these cuts, but the reprieve came at the expense of other domestic discretionary spending. The NIH's 5.7% increase for FY 1996 was paid for with cuts to other health, education, and jobs programs.[41] In the next two years, the NIH received similar funding increases matched by cuts to other domestic programs.[42] Thus, despite the deficit hawks, the NIH usually beat inflation through budget maneuvers and bipartisan agreement. But these weren't boom times, and the NIH's budget increases didn't match the 10%–15% annual increases of previous decades (see Figure 5.1).

During these budget struggles, and in this time of slow increases for the NIH, was disease lobbying effective? Figure 5.2 shows the estimated effects of lobbying in each year, beginning with FY 1991.[43] Positive numbers indicate years when diseases that lobbied more tended to receive bigger funding increases. The lobbying coefficient is statistically significant in years when the confidence intervals, indicated by vertical lines, do not cross zero.

From 1991 through 1997, there was little relationship between lobbying expenditures by a disease's advocates and funding increases for that disease (see Figure 5.2). The lobbying coefficients were statistically significant in 1991 and 1994, but these results are entirely attributable to AIDS and breast cancer (see Appendix, Figure A.3).[44] When we look beyond these two diseases, advocacy was not paying off in terms of funding increases for particular diseases during this time of relatively slow budget growth.

This was the time period when the journalists, policymakers, and academics quoted at the beginning of this chapter were arguing that

[40] Lawler, "GOP Plans"; Lawler and Mervis, "House Panel."

[41] Lawler, "Research Knows No Season"; Marshall, "Senate Restores NIH Funding Cut," 1271; Marshall and Lawler, "R&D Budget Takes Shape," 471; Mervis and Marshall, "When Federal Science Stopped."

[42] Lawler, "Congress Targets Fusion," 303; Marshall, "Last-Minute Deal Gives NIH 7.1% Raise"; Marshall and Lawler, "Biomedical Research Wins Big."

[43] These analyses begin when the quantitative data become available in 1991. For each year, I ran a regression predicting changes in NIH and DOD funding for a disease. The key independent variable is the previous year's lobbying index. The models control for changes in mortality. Results are similar when controlling for DALYs instead of mortality and when excluding AIDS and breast cancer. See details in Appendix.

[44] These years were also linked to budget increases—the NIH budget increased 9.6% in 1991, and 1994 saw a major increase for the breast cancer program at the DOD.

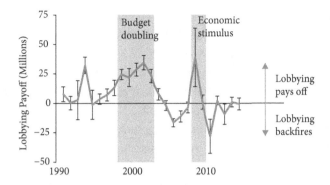

Figure 5.2 Lobbying only sometimes pays: Predicted funding increase per standard deviation increase in lobbying, 1991–2015

Lobbying coefficients and 95% confidence intervals from regressions of NIH and DOD funding changes in millions on lobbying and mortality changes. Lobbying variable is standardized. Both independent variables are lagged by one year.

cutthroat and effective disease lobbyists were stealing money from one another. But there is no evidence that such trade-offs were occurring. AIDS and breast cancer funding had increased dramatically, but these increases were almost always "new" money, not pulled from other diseases. Congress funded AIDS research first by increasing deficits and second by cutting other domestic spending; breast cancer research competed with domestic discretionary spending and, through the DOD-CDMRP gambit, with defense spending. For other diseases, there was little payoff to lobbying.

1998–2015: Big Leaps and Hard Landings

In addition to worrying about a zero-sum competition between diseases, critics warned that disease activism would stunt the growth of the NIH budget. In fact, the opposite occurred: disease advocates joined a powerful coalition that doubled the NIH budget.[45] Concerned that Republicans were getting all the credit for prioritizing medical research, Clinton started

---

[45] Greenberg, *Science, Money, and Politics*, 443–48; Kastor, *National Institutes of Health*, 143.

requesting bigger budget increases for the NIH.[46] The chairs of both the House and Senate appropriations subcommittees responsible for the NIH, John Porter (R-IL) and Arlen Specter (R-PA), were strong NIH supporters. In 1997, the Senate unanimously adopted a resolution to double the NIH budget over 5 years.[47] Research!America, a coalition of universities, researchers' professional associations, pharmaceutical and healthcare companies, and disease advocates, announced that its primary goal was to double the NIH budget.[48] A complementary campaign, called NIH2, campaigned for NIH budget increases.[49] So did the Ad Hoc Group for Medical Research Funding, a lobbying association of medical schools, scientific societies, universities, and other research advocates with links to the NIH bureaucracy.[50]

With this powerful constellation of allies, it would be naive to attribute the push to double the NIH's budget solely to disease advocacy. But the proliferating disease campaigns helped make the case. A representative of Research!America framed its effort as an attempt to "deal with the infighting and competition among diseases by making enough money available so that research on all could grow."[51] A congressional staffer reported that Congress decided to double the NIH budget based "on the hope that this policy would eliminate some of the intense competition for funds among advocates for particular diseases."[52] In support of the budget doubling, Senator Ted Kennedy (D-MA) argued that "we cannot afford to pit the suffering of one group of patients or the interests of one branch of science against those of another."[53] Rather than constraining NIH funding, disease advocates' claims provided an extra incentive for budget increases.

By 1998, the president and Congress agreed on the goal of doubling the NIH budget, but they disagreed on where the money should come from. Still constrained by the BEA, the Senate Budget Committee favored funding the NIH increases out of the existing domestic discretionary budget.[54]

---

[46] Lawler, "Science Catches Clinton's Eye"; Teitelbaum, *Falling Behind?*, 61.

[47] Greenberg, *Science, Money, and Politics*, 438; Mervis, "Senate Bills Back Huge Increases," 608; Teitelbaum, *Falling Behind?*, 61.

[48] Stapleton, "Lobby for Labs"; Teitelbaum, *Falling Behind?*, 60.

[49] Stapleton, "Lobby for Labs."

[50] Greenberg, *Science, Money, and Politics*, 197–98.

[51] Havemann, "Crusading for Cash."

[52] Kedrowski and Sarow, *Cancer Activism*, 208.

[53] US Senate, "Biomedical Research Priorities," 6.

[54] Lawler, "Senate Panel," 2035.

House Republicans also proposed paying for NIH increases through cuts to domestic programs, including jobs programs and energy subsidies, a trade-off that one congressional staffer summarized as "science versus poor people."[55] Representative Nancy Pelosi (D-CA) hoped "that any increase in the NIH would not come at the expense of other lambs in our lamb-eat-lamb allocation," such as job training and Head Start.[56] Clinton proposed another way around the trade-offs required by the BEA: his budget specified that the increases for the NIH would be funded by a settlement with the tobacco industry.[57]

Meanwhile, there was a budget surplus—the first in decades.[58] What would the government do with the money? Some policymakers proposed tax cuts; others wanted to spend it on federal discretionary programs; Clinton wanted to "save Social Security."[59] In the end, the surplus provided another way around the BEA. The BEA had been designed to reduce the deficit; now there was none, but spending caps were still in place. Making use of a loophole, Congress declared an "emergency" that let them use the surpluses to fund additional discretionary spending.[60] The surplus meant that NIH funding could increase without any visible cuts to other programs. There were still trade-offs, of course, since the stimulus money could have been spent elsewhere. But the surplus made those trade-offs less visible and painful. The NIH budget increased by 15% for FY 1999, the first step in the five-year doubling plan. As the surplus continued, Congress officially raised the BEA spending limits, and the NIH received a 14.7% increase for FY 2000 and a 14% increase for FY 2001.[61] As FY 2002 approached, the federal budget's four-year streak of surpluses came to an end. But the NIH doubling was underway; stopping it would seem like a cut. With the support of newly elected President George W. Bush, the NIH completed the five-year budget doubling with a 15% increase for FY 2002 and a 16% increase for FY 2003 (see Figure 5.1).[62]

[55] Marshall and Lawler, "Political Football."
[56] US House of Representatives, "Appropriations for 1998, Part 4b," 2498.
[57] Marshall, "Science Funding," 974; Smith, "Washington Watch," 79.
[58] Congressional Budget Office, "Historical Budget Data."
[59] Marshall, "Science Funding," 974; Stevenson, "Surplus Dreams."
[60] Malakoff and Marshall, "NIH Wins Big," 598; Weiner, "Congress Chafing at Spending Caps."
[61] Malakoff, "Another Record Year"; Malakoff, "NIH Gets $2.5 Billion More"; Marshall, "Plan to Reduce"; Weiner, "Senate Approves Budget Package."
[62] Malakoff, "Science Lobbyists," 1882; Malakoff, "Biomedicine," 24.

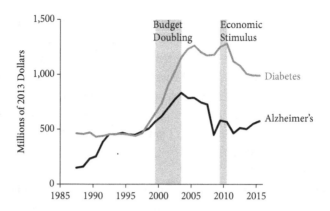

Figure 5.3 Funding for mobilized diseases rises and then declines

NIH funding for diabetes and Alzheimer's disease, adjusted for inflation, 1987–2015

Journalists suspected that advocacy was particularly influential as the NIH budget ballooned. *Science* reported that "virtually every NIH interest group has shared in the doubling bonanza—from patient groups advocating more research on 'their' disease to scientists urging greater spending on the agency's intramural program."[63] Quantitative data confirm that lobbying paid off during these flush years. During the FY 1999–2003 budget doubling, disease lobbying was rewarded with larger funding increases (see Figure 5.2). During the budget doubling, a one standard deviation increase in lobbying (equal to about $200,000) was associated with a $20–$35 million[64] increase in NIH funding—a hundredfold payoff.[65] Figure 5.3 shows the funding trajectories for diabetes and Alzheimer's disease, which were second only to HIV/AIDS in their lobbying expenditures. Each shows

---

[63] Malakoff, "NIH Prays for a Soft Landing," 1992.

[64] The estimates vary from year to year and depending on whether I control for mortality or DALYs. In all models, though, the estimated payoffs to lobbying during the doubling are large and statistically significant. Excluding AIDS and breast cancer, the predicted increases would be between $10 and $25 million (see Figure A.3).

[65] In an earlier article about the effects of disease advocacy, I looked at a shorter time period (1989–2007). I found that diseases tended to secure funding increases the year after lobbying by their advocates. But I noted that these "funding increases occurred in the context of an expanding NIH budget," and I suggested that "advocacy's effects might be smaller during times of austerity." Best, "Disease Politics and Medical Research Funding," 794. In this chapter, I look at a longer time period and confirm that advocacy was primarily effective during the doubling of the NIH budget from 1999 to 2003 (and then again during the economic stimulus of 2009–2010).

a dramatic bump for fiscal years 1999–2003, the era of budget doubling. Disease advocacy hadn't been particularly effective in the earlier part of the 1990s. But just as it was easier for Congress to funnel money to the NIH when it wouldn't have to be visibly taken away from another priority, it was easier for the NIH to funnel money to diseases with mobilized patients when there was new money to go around.

Darker times were coming; 2003 was the end of an era for the NIH. With the exception of briefly flat budgets in the late 1960s and early 1980s, funding had grown for half a century, culminating with the budget doubling (see Figure 5.1). But the federal government was no longer flush with surplus money; an economic slump, tax cuts, and war had produced record deficits. The Bush administration pushed to limit domestic discretionary budget increases to 1% in FY 2005. In FY 2006, Congress approved a 1% across-the-board cut in all discretionary spending. In FY 2007, Bush continued to push for flat budgets, prioritizing war spending and further tax cuts. And in FY 2008, Bush set a cap on domestic spending and threatened to veto any bills that exceeded it, leading to repeated cuts in the appropriations committees.[66]

In this climate of austerity, and after the massive ramp-up in the NIH budget, policymakers viewed biomedical researchers' requests for funding increases skeptically.[67] Some congressional allies continued to push for large increases in the NIH budget. But with renewed fiscal constraints and so soon after the budget doubling, they could not achieve the supermajorities needed to get around budget rules.[68] From 2004 to 2008, the NIH budget failed to keep up with inflation. In 2006, it was even cut slightly for the first time since 1970.[69]

The end of this remarkable period of growth was greeted with alarm by scientists and science advocates. Journalists reported that a "chilling" and "paralyzing" funding climate left a "dark shadow" hanging over scientists, with researchers feeling "under assault" and young scientists at risk of being forced out of the field.[70] We should take scientists' claims of a funding crisis

[66] Kaiser, "NIH Set for Tiny Spending Hike"; Kaiser et al., "2005 Budget"; Kintisch and Mervis, "Big Winners and Losers," 762; Lawler et al., "Science Agencies"; Mervis, "Promising Year"; Mervis et al., "NIH Shrinks," 28.

[67] Bishop and Varmus, "Editorial"; Kastor, National Institutes of Health, 157; Teitelbaum, Falling Behind?, 67.

[68] Kaiser, "Bid to Boost NIH Budget."

[69] Mervis et al., "NIH Shrinks."

[70] Couzin and Miller, "Boom and Bust," 357, 359; Kaiser, "Bumpy Landing for Cancer Research," 936.

with a grain of salt. During the half-century of increasing budgets, and even during the flush years of the 1990s, science lobbyists had repeatedly announced funding crises, seeking a return to an imagined "golden age."[71] And while the NIH budget had stopped growing in 2003, this stasis was at an extraordinarily high level: over $30 billion (in today's dollars), more than any other country in the world spent on biomedical research, five times as much as the entire European Union.[72]

One reason for the angst was structural. When budgets increase, scientists take on more graduate students and postdoctoral researchers; a few years later, they apply for grants of their own. Meanwhile, universities and medical schools expand their facilities and encourage faculty to rely more heavily on grants to fund their salaries. And so bountiful budget increases lead to perceived funding shortages a few years later.[73] The insatiable scientific enterprise demands constant growth; an appropriations committee staffer suggested that the NIH might need a billion-dollar increase every year "just to stay even," and NIH officials suggested that they would need annual increases between 7% and 12% to match inflation and maintain their current programs.[74]

As the NIH budget stagnated, disease lobbying was ineffective because of the difficulty of tinkering with existing expenditures. Beginning with fiscal year 2005, diseases with lots of lobbying had no funding advantage (see Figure 5.2). The head of Research!America recognized this pattern, saying that after the budget doubling, "additional money wasn't there any more, and advocacy fell apart."[75]

In fact, the more mobilized diseases actually tended to get *less* money (see Figure 5.2). Of the seven diseases with the biggest drops in NIH funding in 2006, the year the budget was cut, all but one were targeted by large lobbying efforts and had received dramatic funding increases during the budget doubling (see Figure 5.3 for the case of diabetes and Alzheimer's disease). Having funneled money to these politically powerful diseases, NIH officials may have been pulling back out of a sense of balance.[76] In an

---

[71] Greenberg, *Science, Money, and Politics.*

[72] Murphy and Topel, "Introduction," 2.

[73] Alberts, "Overbuilding Research Capacity"; Boat, "Biomedical Research Funding," 170; Couzin and Miller, "Boom and Bust"; Greenberg, *Science, Money, and Politics*; Insel, Volkow, and Li, "Research Funding"; Nurse, "US Biomedical Research Under Siege"; Sarewitz, *Frontiers of Illusion*; Stephan, *How Economics Shapes Science*; Teitelbaum, *Falling Behind?*; Teitelbaum, "Structural Disequilibria in Biomedical Research"; Zerhouni, "NIH in the Post-Doubling Era," 1088.

[74] Malakoff, "NIH Prays for a Soft Landing," 1993; Marshall, "Plan to Reduce," 953.

[75] Mary Woolley, quoted in Kastor, *National Institutes of Health*, 157.

[76] In a similar example from a few decades earlier, the National Cancer Act of 1971 provided a major budget boost for the National Cancer Institute (NCI). Since several other institutes saw budget

interview, one NIH official told me about his frustration with an earmark for a highly mobilized disease:

> I go to Center reviews, and the experts from the field are saying "this is very unlikely to yield substantive results," and Congress is telling me to fund it. And that hurts because I have in my back pocket a hundred good grants that I can't fund.

Such an official would be likely to support funding cuts for such diseases in subsequent years.

In 2009, President Barack Obama entered office in the midst of a severe recession and immediately began work on an $800-billion economic stimulus package. Obama needed Senator Arlen Specter's vote to avoid a filibuster, and Specter made his support contingent on recouping the NIH's inflation-adjusted losses since the end of the budget doubling.[77] The stimulus legislation achieved this goal with an extra $10.4 billion for the NIH, split over two years, amounting to a 17% budget increase for FY 2009 (see Figure 5.1).[78]

But repeating history again, the budget's takeoff was followed by a hard landing. Republicans took control of the House in the 2010 election, promising to cut funding for all federal agencies.[79] Officially, NIH appropriations were cut by less than 1%.[80] But this calculation excludes the previous year's stimulus funding. The NIH actually received 17.8% less in 2011 than in 2010 (see Figure 5.1). Scientists had complained about a hard landing after the budget doubling, when the NIH budget merely failed to keep up with inflation. This was a much harder crash.[81]

Meanwhile, fiscal fights led to another law designed to force budget cuts. The Budget Control Act of 2011 (BCA) ordered Congress to reduce discretionary spending by $1 trillion by 2021. In 2013, the BCA required 5%

cuts in the early 1970s, some senators argued that the War on Cancer had moved money away from other diseases. Spingarn, *Heartbeat*, 89. But over the next decade and a half, the NCI's budget sometimes decreased in current dollars and other institutes gained ground. Consequently, the proportion of NIH funding going to the NCI dropped steadily. Ginzberg and Dutka, *Financing of Biomedical Research*, 27.

[77] Kaiser, "NIH Hopes Stimulus Isn't a Roller-Coaster Ride"; Kintisch, "Science Wins"; Wilson, "Bruised by Stimulus Battle."
[78] Mervis, "Science and the Stimulus," 1176.
[79] Wayne, "GOP Budget Cuts."
[80] *Nature*, "NIH Spared Budget Slash"; Raloff, "2012 Budget."
[81] Collins and Kaiser, "Francis Collins," 1090.

across-the-board cuts for much of the federal budget, including the NIH.[82] In the NIH's "darkest year," grant success rates declined to their lowest level ever.[83] Another budget stalemate, including a government shutdown, was resolved with the Bipartisan Budget Act of 2013, which raised the BCA caps enough to ease sequestration.[84] The NIH budget increased modestly from 2013 to 2016. This pattern continued for fiscal years 2017 and 2018, with Congress rejecting President Trump's proposed budget cuts for the NIH but without major funding increases.[85]

Turning to the quantitative data, we see again that lobbying directs the flow of new money but is hard-pressed to siphon funds from existing programs. Just as they had during the previous decade's budget doubling and subsequent stagnation, diseases with more lobbying expenditures got significantly larger funding increases during the stimulus (see Figure 5.2). But these diseases then received significantly *less* money in 2011 (when the stimulus ended) and 2013 (when the BCA led to budget cuts) (see Figure 5.2). For example, diabetes and Alzheimer's, both targeted by major lobbying campaigns, each got major chunks of the stimulus money but saw declines in the subsequent years (see Figure 5.3).

Across the decades, the competition between diseases rarely became a zero-sum game because policymakers tended to reward lobbying only when there was extra money to go around. The general pattern was not that big increases for one disease were taken from other diseases. Instead, the good years were good for everyone—but especially good for highly mobilized diseases.

Conclusion

Since beneficiaries invariably protest budget cuts, it's difficult for policymakers to set priorities by moving money around. It's much easier to reward favored causes when new money becomes available. Congressional allies consistently steered money to the NIH, at the expense either of other domestic spending or of budget balancing. But the NIH's largest gains came

---

[82] Mole, "Science Slowdown," 14; Mullin, "Congressional Budget Deal"; *Nature*, "NIH Budget Blues."

[83] Lowrey, "Budget Battles"; *Washington Post* Editorial Board, "NIH Research Is Ailing."

[84] Morello et al., "Budget Offers Recovery Hope."

[85] Pear, "Congress Rejects Trump Proposals."

from the federal budget surplus and economic stimulus package—money that wasn't visibly being taken from any other program. Zooming in reveals the same pattern within the NIH budget. Disease lobbying primarily paid off during boom times—the budget doubling of 1999–2003 and the economic stimulus of 2009–2010—when money could flow to favored diseases without budget cuts for other diseases. When we discuss how political opportunities help social movements succeed, we need to consider *budgetary* opportunities, recognizing that advocacy organizations are most influential in times of expansion.[86]

This fact meant that funding increases for one disease rarely come from another disease's budget. Instead of competing in a zero-sum game, diseases tend to lift each other up. After disease campaigns help the NIH secure budget increases, officials have substantial flexibility in how they spend and account for that money, "for example classifying a basic biology project as 'breast cancer research.'"[87] This "creative accounting" can allow officials to use money earmarked for politically popular diseases for other health priorities.[88] Additionally, one disease's political successes can set a precedent for other diseases. At a 1971 hearing about the War on Cancer, when an American Heart Association representative worried that heart disease research was being shortchanged, Senator Ted Kennedy replied, "There are those who say if you can't get a raise yourself, the best thing that can happen is for the fellow next to you to get a raise."[89] And, in fact, the National Heart, Blood Vessel, Lung, and Blood Act passed the following year.[90] Moreover, since it's politically difficult to cut budgets, money that's added to the NIH budget tends to stay there, year after year. This money can later flow to other diseases. Similar priorities do not invariably compete with one another; in contrast, gains tend to spill over across related causes.[91]

---

[86] Kamlet and Mowery, "Budgetary Base"; Rubin, *Politics of Public Budgeting*, 30, 154. This argument parallels Zald and McCarthy's hypothesis that "under conditions of the declining availability of marginal resources, direct competition and conflict between SMOs with similar goals can be expected to increase" because "where there are limited numbers of institutional funders, competition appears to be zero-sum." Zald and McCarthy, "Social Movement Industries," 5, 8. But in this case, instead of competing for money from donors to fund their own operations, social movement organizations (SMOs) are competing for federal funds to target their problems.

[87] Rubin, *Politics of Public Budgeting*, 14.

[88] Anderson, "Opponents of Earmarks," 4.

[89] US Senate, "Conquest of Cancer Act," 232; see discussion in Studer and Chubin, *Cancer Mission*, 77.

[90] Studer and Chubin, *Cancer Mission*, 102.

[91] Hilgartner and Bosk, "Rise and Fall of Social Problems," 68; Jones and Baumgartner, *Politics of Attention*, 259; Kingdon, *Agendas, Alternatives, and Public Policies*, 201–2.

At some point, government spending priorities must compete, either with each other or with the goals of keeping taxes and deficits low.[92] Every game becomes zero-sum if you expand the boundaries wide enough.[93] But stating that a game is zero-sum is meaningless without defining the boundaries of the competition. During the fiscal year, disease competition is zero-sum within the NIH budget, with grant applicants competing for funding within a preset budget. But at appropriations time, the NIH budget can increase or decrease, changing the size of the pie. The NIH budget itself competes with various other priorities, depending on political institutions and strategic action.

The "fiscalization of lawmaking" has made trade-offs more explicit and fiscal constraints more influential.[94] Laws like GRH, BEA, and BCA created constraints that sought to force trade-offs between the NIH and other domestic spending.[95] These constraints meant that funding increases for popular diseases occasionally came at the expense of other domestic spending. However, as the creation of the DOD-CDMRP shows, policymakers can maneuver around these rules, expanding the boundaries of the competition to benefit a favored cause. As one budget official explained, "there's always room in the budget if you are willing to raise taxes or if you are willing to cut other programs. The budget constraint isn't so much there, as it is a question of how you handle the budgetary implications."[96] Whether advocacy becomes a zero-sum game depends on how advocates and policymakers construct the boundaries of the competition.

And so instead of asking whether particular priorities always compete in a zero-sum game, we should ask how and why particular trade-offs are made.[97] For instance, social scientists have asked for decades whether

[92] Eichenberg, "Do We Yet Know Who Pays for Defense?"; Kamlet and Mowery, "Executive and Congressional Budgetary Priorities."

[93] This chapter focuses on budgets and asks when funding battles become zero-sum. A related research tradition asks whether social problems invariably compete for attention in zero-sum games, with attention measured by media coverage, public concern, or the policy agenda. Hilgartner and Bosk, "Rise and Fall of Social Problems"; Kingdon, *Agendas, Alternatives, and Public Policies.*

[94] Nelson, *Making an Issue of Child Abuse*, 123, 135; Pierson, "Deficit and Domestic Reform," 127. Steuerle argues that the early 1980s marked a shift from the "easy financing era" to the "fiscal straightjacket era." Previously, expanding government revenues meant that legislation "appeared to involve only winners." In the latter period, the fiscal situation and prior policy commitments mean that "legislation appears mainly to identify losers." Steuerle, "Financing the American State," 422, 431.

[95] As Jones and Baumgartner note, these "general fiscal targets or constraints . . . are top-down propagators of interdependencies" between policy priorities. Jones and Baumgartner, *Politics of Attention*, 143; see also Padgett, "Hierarchy and Ecological Control."

[96] Kingdon, *Agendas, Alternatives, and Public Policies*, 114.

[97] We should neither assume that policies are always independent (an assumption implicit in common statistical methods used to predict policy outcomes) nor assume that they are always

countries tend to make trade-offs between military and welfare spending.[98] But there's no reason to believe that every country will make the same trade-offs every year—some might finance military expansion by cutting welfare spending, while others raise taxes or run deficits.[99] Some programs are thought of as connected because they benefit the same group of people (e.g., the elderly, rural residents), leading to the expectation of trade-offs between them.[100] Political structures can also determine which trade-offs will be made. Since housing and defense are on different subcommittees, "budgeters do not ask, Do you want to house the homeless or buy the navy a new helicopter?"[101] Trade-offs between various types of scientific research may be more common in countries with a central scientific ministry, while the decentralized US system places the competition within single agencies' budgets or between research and other government priorities.[102]

Critics worried that the NIH budget would never grow if advocates only asked for funding increases for particular diseases. But, in fact, the height of disease advocacy coincided with the doubling of the NIH budget, and some congressional staffers and experts attributed the budget increases in part to the cacophony of disease constituencies. A chorus of advocates demanding help for their particular diseases may have been *more* effective than a rational, technocratic request for a larger NIH budget. After a century of disease campaigns, we shouldn't be surprised that a campaign to fight breast cancer is more politically powerful than a technocratic campaign to fund more biomedical research. While some social scientists have argued that smaller, specialized, or identity-based movements are less likely to achieve broad goals,[103] these findings support researchers who argue that

---

interdependent. Jones and Baumgartner, *Politics of Attention*. Hayes argues that it's easier "to keep the legislative stakes non-zero-sum" when policies have concentrated benefits and diffuse costs, so that "material rewards for the participants [can be] drawn almost entirely from the inattentive in the form of higher taxes or higher prices." Hayes, *Lobbyists and Legislators*, 99.

[98] Domke, Eichenberg, and Kelleher, "Illusion of Choice"; Gifford, "Why No Trade-off"; Huber and Stephens, *Development and Crisis*; Kamlet and Mowery, "Executive and Congressional Budgetary Priorities"; Pampel and Williamson, "Welfare Spending"; Russett, "Defense Expenditures and National Well-Being."

[99] Eichenberg, "Do We Yet Know Who Pays for Defense?," 234.

[100] Hilgartner and Bosk, "Rise and Fall of Social Problems," 73–74; Rubin, *Politics of Public Budgeting*, 126, 134, 159.

[101] Rubin, *Politics of Public Budgeting*, 135.

[102] Cook-Deegan and McGeary, "Jewel in the Federal Crown?"

[103] Collins, *Black Feminist Thought*; Gamson, "Hiroshima"; Gitlin, "From Universality to Difference"; Gitlin, *Twilight of Common Dreams*; Hobsbawm, "Identity Politics and the Left"; hooks, *Talking Back*; McAdam, *Political Process*; Mushaben, "Struggle Within"; Piore, *Beyond Individualism*; Putnam, *Bowling Alone*; Rorty, *Achieving Our Country*; Skocpol, *Diminished Democracy*; Turner, "Intersex Identities."

diversity, specialization, and identity politics can help movements survive and thrive.[104] Biomedical research advocates needn't have worried: when disease advocates came to Washington, they were good for the bottom line at the NIH.

When budget rules enforced a zero-sum competition between domestic discretionary programs, medical research to cure disease sometimes won out over more redistributive and politically controversial programs. This trade-off is shortsighted even if we consider health promotion the primary goal for public policy because programs from housing to education to poverty reduction can have dramatic impacts on health.[105] The outsize growth of medical research results in part from our propensity for disease campaigns.

But why did disease campaigns funnel so much of their energy into medical research funding in the first place? Medical research is not the only possible goal for disease campaigns—they might also focus on ensuring access to treatment, lobbying for patients' rights, or applying existing knowledge to prevent disease. The next chapter explains why disease campaigns tend to prioritize research and awareness and why they often neglect prevention and treatment access.

---

[104] Armstrong, *Forging Gay Identities*; Bernstein, "Celebration and Suppression"; Bernstein, "Identity Politics"; Berry, *New Liberalism*; Bickford, "Anti-Anti-Identity Politics"; Ghaziani and Baldassarri, "Cultural Anchors"; Haines, "Black Radicalization"; Levitsky, "Niche Activism"; Minkoff, *Organizing for Equality*; Minkoff, "Sequencing of Social Movements"; Minkoff, Aisenbrey, and Agnone, "Organizational Diversity"; Polletta, "Strategy and Identity."

[105] Pollack et al., "Social and Economic Policies as Health Policy," 387.

6

Publicity Over Prevention, Cures Over Care

In 1904, organizers of the first national disease association described broad goals including research, awareness, prevention, and treatment access.[1] The following century of disease campaigns tended to prioritize some of these goals and neglect others. Disease organizations vary widely in the goals they pursue. But looking across hundreds of organizations over the decades reveals that when we fight one disease at a time, we tend to prioritize some goals over others. When organizations and laws focus on single diseases, they tend to promote awareness and lobby for research, paying less attention to prevention and treatment access. To understand why, we need to bring together theories about how individual organizations choose goals with theories of how fields of organizations develop over time.

Organizations face pressure to define an organizational identity and act consistently with it.[2] Since acting "out of character" threatens organizational legitimacy and survival,[3] organizations prioritize goals that align with their organizational identities and avoid issues that cross the boundaries of categories of organizations.[4] In the case of disease advocacy, many prevention efforts, including environmental protection and health behavior change, cross disease categories. So do most efforts to expand access to healthcare. Since these goals don't match up neatly with disease categories, pursuing them may threaten single-disease organizations' legitimacy with potential members and donors. The pressure to maintain a clear, disease-focused

---

[1] "(1) The study of tuberculosis in all its forms and relations. (2) The dissemination of knowledge about the causes, treatment, and prevention of tuberculosis. (3) The encouragement of the prevention and scientific treatment of tuberculosis." Knopf, *History of the National Tuberculosis Association*, 29.

[2] Albert and Whetten, "Organizational Identity"; Whetten, "Albert and Whetten Revisited."

[3] Whetten, "Albert and Whetten Revisited," 223, 227; see also Suchman, "Managing Legitimacy"; Walker and Stepick, "Valuing the Cause"; Zuckerman, "Categorical Imperative," 1398.

[4] Baumgartner and Jones, *Agendas and Instability*; Carpenter, "Setting the Advocacy Agenda," 115–16; Kingdon, *Agendas, Alternatives, and Public Policies*; Wilson, *Political Organizations*.

organizational identity discourages some organizations from prioritizing these broader goals.

In addition to maintaining a consistent organizational identity, organizations must consider their ability to attract resources and members. Since visible successes motivate participants and encourage donations, advocates respond to political opportunities and try to choose achievable goals.[5] Organizations also select goals that will appeal to donors and corporate funders.[6] Both sets of incentives often push organizations to prioritize uncontroversial goals.[7] In the case of disease advocacy, corporate influence and the lure of short-term success discouraged a focus on environmental hazards and encouraged a focus on awareness, an actionable goal that aligns well with corporate interests. Meanwhile, the need for political "wins" pushed organizations to prioritize research over treatment access.

For individual organizations, choosing narrow goals that maximize identity consistency, resources, and political opportunities can be a sensible short-term strategy.[8] But over time, these effects accumulate beyond the boundaries of individual organizations. Organizations model themselves after one another, eventually creating taken-for-granted ideas about what it's possible or sensible to ask for.[9] This means that short-term strategic calculations influence the development of organizational fields over the long term, making some goals seem more legitimate than others. Over time, disease advocates institutionalized a model for what a disease advocacy organization should look like: it promotes awareness and lobbies for

---

[5] Diani, "Linking Mobilization Frames"; Einwohner, "Practices, Opportunity"; Ferree, "Resonance and Radicalism"; Gamson and Meyer, "Framing Political Opportunity"; Gordon, *Dead on Arrival*; Gould, *Moving Politics*, 3; Jenkins, "Nonprofit Organizations and Political Advocacy," 319; Kingdon, *Agendas, Alternatives, and Public Policies*, 38; Klandermans, "Social Construction of Protest," 78–86; McAdam, *Political Process*; McCarthy and Zald, "Resource Mobilization and Social Movements," 1228–29; Meyer, "Protest and Political Opportunities," 127–28, 139; Meyer and Staggenborg, "Movements, Countermovements," 1651; Steinberg, "Talk and Back Talk"; Tarrow, *Power in Movement*; Zald and Ash, "Social Movement Organizations," 333.

[6] Campbell, "Where Do We Stand?," 41; McCarthy and Zald, "Resource Mobilization and Social Movements"; Zald and Ash, "Social Movement Organizations."

[7] Diani, "Linking Mobilization Frames"; Einwohner, "Practices, Opportunity"; Ferree, "Resonance and Radicalism"; Jenkins, "Nonprofit Organizations and Political Advocacy," 319; Kingdon, *Agendas, Alternatives, and Public Policies*; Klandermans, "Social Construction of Protest," 78–86; McAdam, *Political Process*; McCarthy and Zald, "Resource Mobilization and Social Movements," 1228–29; Meyer, "Protest and Political Opportunities"; Tarrow, *Power in Movement*.

[8] Halpin, Fraussen, and Nownes, "Balancing Act."

[9] Clemens, "Organizational Repertoires and Institutional Change"; Clemens, *People's Lobby*; DiMaggio and Powell, "Iron Cage Revisited"; Ferree, "Resonance and Radicalism," 307; Gamson and Meyer, "Framing Political Opportunity"; Lake and Wong, "Politics of Networks"; Steinberg, "Talk and Back Talk," 746–50; Walker, *Grassroots for Hire*, 48.

government research funding. And so single-disease campaigns tend to push health policy and health charity toward awareness and research.

These choices help maintain consensus around disease campaigns but also prevent them from achieving their maximum potential to improve our health. Research is sometimes framed as a benefit to current patients, but given the slow pace of medical research, current patients might be better served by improved access to existing treatments and services. Meanwhile, awareness campaigns promote the idea that earlier diagnosis and more medical treatment are always better. This way of thinking can encourage overtreatment, in which people who face very small risks of disease are exposed to larger risks from medical treatment itself.[10] Overblown awareness campaigns can actually make us *less* healthy.

Disease campaigns could do more to improve Americans' health and well-being if they shifted some of their attention from research and awareness to prevention and treatment access. But this statement does not imply that the existing focus on research and awareness *causes* less attention to be paid to prevention and treatment. The previous chapter showed that diseases do not compete for research funding in a zero-sum game. This chapter explains that goals do not displace each other, either. At a societal level, we pay more attention to prevention and treatment than we would if there were no disease campaigns. While various pressures push individual organizations to adopt limited goals, these choices foster consensus and help the field grow in ways that also favor transformative campaigns and broader goals.

Limited Goals

Examining *Encyclopedia* listings, congressional testimony, and laws reveals that disease campaigns tend to prioritize awareness and research while downplaying prevention and treatment access.[11] The divergences are starkest among organizations and laws that target single diseases. These differences are statistically significant in multivariate models (see Appendix, Table A.4).

---

[10] Brownlee, *Overtreated*; Welch, Schwartz, and Woloshin, *Overdiagnosed*.
[11] See Appendix for a discussion of the data sources for this chapter.

Relative to other goals, disease campaigns underemphasize prevention, defined here as attempts to stop people from coming down with a disease. These efforts, also known as "primary prevention," include steps that individuals can take to prevent disease (e.g., diet, exercise, safe sex), measures societies can take to prevent disease (e.g., limiting pollution, encouraging food companies to use healthier ingredients), and vaccines.[12] For most of the last six decades, fewer than a quarter of disease advocacy organizations mentioned disease prevention at all in their *Encyclopedia* listings or congressional testimony (see Figure 6.1). The tighter the focus on a single disease, the less likely organizations are to prioritize prevention. When organizations focus on multiple diseases (e.g., an organization targeting both breast cancer and cervical cancer) and broader categories (e.g., mental illness or cancer in general), 28% adopt prevention goals, compared to only 15% of single-disease organizations (see Figure 6.2).[13]

Likewise, a minority of disease campaigns focus on access to treatment[14] (see Figure 6.1). In multivariate models, single-disease organizations are significantly less likely to prioritize treatment (see Appendix, Table A.4). Similarly, the more tightly a law focuses on a disease, the less likely it is to refer to treatment access. A majority of non-disease-specific health laws focus on treatment access—for example, regulating health insurance or funding hospital construction. Single-disease laws related to treatment access, such as the National Sickle Cell Disease Control Act or the Ryan White CARE Act, are much rarer. Only 16% of single-disease laws have a treatment access component (see Figure 6.3).

---

[12] Over the decades, health professionals have expanded the definition of "prevention" beyond its colloquial meaning. "Primary prevention" means stopping someone from developing a disease, reducing the number of new cases. "Secondary prevention" means detecting and curing disease, perhaps before patients develop symptoms, reducing the number of people living with the disease. "Tertiary prevention" halts decline among people who already have a disease, reducing the amount of disability an illness causes. Cantor, "Introduction"; Fletcher and Fletcher, *Clinical Epidemiology*, 153; US Commission on Chronic Illness, *Chronic Illness*. Critics argue that these definitions have "blurred the distinctions between prevention and other measures such as screening or therapy" so that prevention has "lost its precise meaning and [become] a flexible concept." Goodman and Goodman, "Prevention," 26; Leopold, *Darker Ribbon*, 182; Welch, Schwartz, and Woloshin, *Overdiagnosed*, 197. Some view tertiary prevention as "an attempt by therapists to sponge off of the new enthusiasm for prevention." Cantor, "Introduction," 29. When I use the word "prevention" in this chapter, I am referring to primary prevention.

[13] The difference is marginally significant ($p < .1$) in multivariate analyses (see Appendix, Table A.4).

[14] I defined access to treatment as providing treatment, paying for treatment, and/or pushing for access to treatment. If a listing or statement focused only on research into new treatments, I coded it as treatment research, not treatment access.

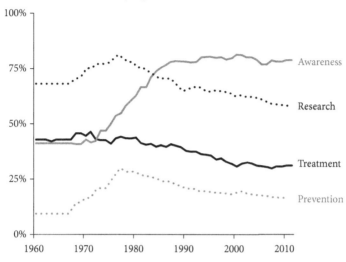

Encyclopedia Entries

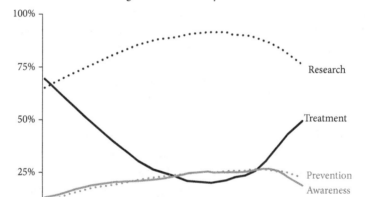

Congressional Testimony

Figure 6.1 Disease advocacy organizations' goals, 1960–2014

Percent of disease-related voluntary associations mentioning awareness, research, treatment access, and prevention in their *Encyclopedia of Associations* listings and in their testimony at Health and Human Services, Labor, and Education Appropriations Hearings (Labor, Health, Education and Welfare, pre-1980). Values sum to more than 100% because organizations can list multiple goals. Lowess smoother applied to bottom panel.

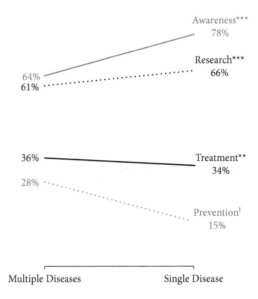

Figure 6.2 Single-disease organizations prioritize awareness, neglect prevention

Percent of multiple-disease and single-disease organizations mentioning treatment access, prevention, awareness, and research goals in their *Encyclopedia of Associations* entries. Values sum to more than 100% because entries can include multiple goals.

***p < .001, **p < .01, ᵗp < .1 indicate statistically significant differences between single- and multiple-disease organizations in multivariate models (details in Appendix).

Meanwhile, a majority of disease organizations emphasize research[15] in their *Encyclopedia* listings. Research is also the dominant request made of the government, the only goal espoused by a majority of disease advocates in congressional hearings (see Figure 6.1). Single-disease organizations are slightly more likely to include research in their *Encyclopedia* listings than organizations targeting multiple diseases or broader disease categories (66% versus 61%). This difference is statistically significant in multivariate analyses.

Over time, awareness has become a dominant goal for disease organizations. Fewer than half of 1960s-era disease organizations promoted awareness, but by the 1990s, more than three-quarters did so (see Figure 6.1).[16]

---

[15] My codes for research include references to research, study, development, or discovery things. I included basic and clinical research into treatment, services, screening, and prevention.

[16] I identified an awareness focus when organizations mentioned public education campaigns (workshops, seminars, classes, etc., for the public and/or medical professionals),

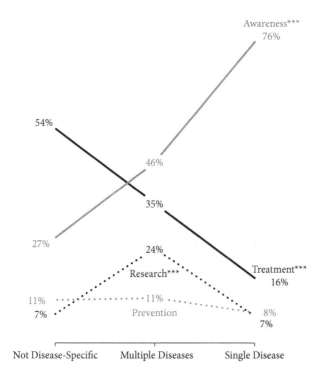

Figure 6.3 Disease-focused laws emphasize awareness more, treatment access less

Percent of non-disease-specific health laws, multiple-disease laws, and single-disease laws passed by Congress focusing on treatment access, prevention, awareness, and research. Values sum to more than 100% because laws can have multiple goals.

***p < .001 indicates statistically significant differences across specificity of disease focus (details in Appendix).

The tighter an organization's focus on a disease, the more it tends to focus on awareness. Among organizations focused on multiple diseases and broader categories of disease, 65% emphasized awareness in their *Encyclopedia* listings. Meanwhile, 79% of single-disease organizations did so (see Figure 6.2). We see the same pattern among laws passed by Congress: the more disease-focused a law, the more likely it is to be focused on awareness. When Congress passes health laws that are not disease-focused, only a

provision of information (including hotlines, brochures, pamphlets, educational materials), and explicit references to "awareness."

quarter promote awareness (e.g., laws instituting National Hospice Month or National Nursing Home Residents Day). Meanwhile, about half of multi-disease laws promote awareness, and fully three-quarters of single-disease laws do so (see Figure 6.3).

The more we organize our philanthropy and public policy around disease categories, the more resources we devote to awareness and research. And the more tightly these campaigns focus on single diseases, the less likely they are to emphasize prevention and treatment access. These patterns can be explained by the pressure to align goals with disease categories, corporate influence, and the pursuit of consensus.

Aligning Goals with Disease Categories

Advocacy organizations face pressure to find a specialized niche and to prioritize goals that align with their organizational identity.[17] Research and awareness line up neatly with disease categories. Since research money can be targeted to a particular disease, it's a more visible success for a disease advocacy group than, say, improvements in access to medical care overall. Meanwhile, many awareness campaigns call public attention to particular diseases. In contrast, prevention campaigns and pushes for treatment access sometimes face boundary problems.

Prevention Crosses Disease Categories

Most primary prevention efforts are not specific to any particular disease but instead target "upstream" factors that raise the risks of multiple diseases (e.g., smoking, environmental pollution, diet, and exercise).[18] This makes prevention less likely to get onto a single-disease organization's agenda. One health advocate I interviewed argued that "everyone wants to have

---

[17] Gamson, *Strategy of Social Protest*, 41–49; Hsu, Hannan, and Koçak, "Multiple Category Memberships"; Levitsky, "Niche Activism"; Olzak, "Effect of Category Spanning"; Walker and Stepick, "Valuing the Cause"; Zuckerman, "Categorical Imperative."

[18] McGinnis, Williams-Russo, and Knickman, "Policy Attention to Health Promotion," 84. Disease categories line up better with secondary and tertiary prevention. We can screen people for a particular cancer (e.g., using mammograms to detect breast cancer), detect it early, and offer treatment with the hope of slowing or halting the progression of the disease.

something to report back to their constituencies, who care about 'what have you done for diabetes.'" This pressure makes it "hard to get the advocacy groups to see the common ground" around prevention interventions like "clean air, nutrition, etc."

Prevention campaigns are an especially poor fit for organizations seeking to benefit current patients. In the early twentieth century, the charitable crusades saw their beneficiaries as potential *future* patients, and they embraced prevention methods from quarantining infected patients to funding vaccine research.[19] But disease advocacy is now fueled by patients' constituencies. As one advocate told me, "people are not afraid of diseases they don't already have," and "the people who aren't getting sick don't march on Washington."[20] Meanwhile, the patients who do mobilize have less to gain from preventing future cases. Organizations with patients as members are less likely to have prevention goals than other organizations (14% versus 21%), though this difference is not statistically significant when we account for whether the organizations focus on a single disease (see Appendix, Table A.4, models 1 and 2).

The trajectories of mainstream and environmental breast cancer activism illustrate the awkward fit between single-disease advocacy and primary prevention. Seeking to maintain its breast cancer focus, the mainstream movement increasingly avoided prevention. The National Breast Cancer Coalition's (NBCC's) original concerns about environmental causes "got pushed to the margins" as NBCC leaders worried that a broader environmental agenda would "dilute the focus on breast cancer as a single issue."[21] At one board meeting, the NBCC director reportedly said, "I'm all for clean air, but what does the Clean Air Act have to do with breast cancer?"[22] In contrast, prioritizing prevention led environmental breast cancer organizations to "think outside the organ," linking breast cancer to other environmental health issues.[23] Prevention goals push organizations to broaden their focus beyond a single disease, which not all organizations are willing to do.

---

[19] Oshinsky, *Polio*, 169; Sills, *Volunteers*; Teller, *Tuberculosis Movement*, 85. Contemporary organizations targeting infectious diseases retain this focus and are more likely than chronic disease organizations to emphasize prevention (see Appendix, Table A.4, Model 1).

[20] For a similar point, see McGinnis, Williams-Russo, and Knickman, "Policy Attention to Health Promotion," 85.

[21] McCormick, *No Family History*, 70; Cynthia Pearson, interviewed by Lerner, *Breast Cancer Wars*, 263.

[22] Fran Visco, paraphrased in the Women's Community Cancer Project Archives, "Report from the March Meeting."

[23] Janice Barlow, quoted in Ley, *From Pink to Green*, 201; see also 13, 39–40, 107–9, 164–76, 202; Klawiter, *Biopolitics of Breast Cancer*, 174, 205–6; McCormick et al., "Personal Is Scientific," 154.

Government policies organized around disease categories may also underemphasize prevention.[24] Most National Institutes of Health (NIH) institutes and centers focus on particular diseases and organs, raising concerns that "existing paradigms of categorical disease and organ-specific research do not adequately accommodate prevention research on modifiable risk factors that affect multiple diseases."[25] Since 1980, the NIH has established various committees and offices to encourage prevention research across institutes and centers.[26] Still, less than 5% of the NIH budget funds primary prevention studies,[27] and only about 2% of the National Cancer Institute's budget goes to prevention.[28]

In the world of public health, much prevention funding comes through categorical grants, many of which focus on particular diseases, creating "duplicative and inefficient" prevention efforts.[29] These separate programs are inefficient for patients with multiple chronic conditions and for conditions that share the same risk factors.[30] Attempting to address the problem, the Affordable Care Act established the Prevention and Public Health Fund, and the Centers for Disease Control and Prevention's recent Coordinated Chronic Disease Prevention program distributes coordinated prevention funding to state health departments.[31] These efforts resemble earlier decades' attempts to rationalize health funding by moving away from the disease campaign model. Lacking the political appeal of disease campaigns, these coordination projects remain a small proportion of the public health budget.

[24] This pattern is part of a larger trend of silo-like policies that may have trouble achieving broader goals. Christensen and Lægreid, "Whole-of-Government," 1060; Exworthy and Hunter, "Challenge of Joined-Up Government"; Nelson, *Making an Issue of Child Abuse*, 125, 135; Smith, "Institutional Filters," 88–90.

[25] Kalberer and Parkinson, "Workshop H," 566; see also Furberg, "Challenges to the Funding of Prevention Research," 599.

[26] Greenberg, *Science, Money, and Politics*, 420; Marshall, "Prevention Research," 1508; National Institutes of Health, "Research in Prevention"; National Institutes of Health, "History of the Office of Disease Prevention."

[27] While the NIH reports that it spends about one-fifth of its budget on prevention research, less than a quarter of that money targets primary prevention. Calitz et al., "Funding for Behavioral Interventions," 462.

[28] Bode and Dong, "Cancer Prevention Research," 508; see also Cuomo, *World Without Cancer*, 16.

[29] Institute of Medicine, "For the Public's Health," 54; see also Slonim et al., "Integration of Chronic Disease Programs," 1; Voetsch, Sequeira, and Chavez, "Chronic Disease Coordination," 1.

[30] Allen et al., "Benefits and Challenges."

[31] Institute of Medicine, "For the Public's Health," 107; Rigby, "National Prevention Council," 2150; Voetsch, Sequeira, and Chavez, "Chronic Disease Coordination," 1.

Access to Treatment Crosses Disease Categories

Most policies providing access to treatment also cross disease categories. Some scholars have asked if narrow constituencies, including disease patients' groups, invariably neglect the broader goal of universal access to healthcare.[32] Deborah Heath and colleagues ask whether a focus on genetic identities tends to "lead individuals to assert claims based on their specific, usually rare, conditions rather than for health care more broadly."[33] Beatrix Hoffman notes that when constituency-based social movements, from civil rights to the women's movement to AIDS, have focused on healthcare, they have tended to demand "specific changes on behalf of their particular group, such as racial desegregation of hospitals, access to abortion, and the release of experimental AIDS drugs."[34] But some did demand universal access to healthcare, especially when they realized that this was the only way to achieve their goals.[35] Steven Epstein argues that disease constituencies are not "necessarily isolated and particularistic"; they can also turn to "universalistic efforts to transform the meaning and practice of health and health care in the United States."[36]

Disease advocacy organizations have sometimes perceived a mismatch between broad treatment politics and their disease-specific goals. A founder of the National Tuberculosis Association wrote that in the early twentieth century, "the Association's directors felt no urge to support the incipient health insurance movement . . . because they viewed the Association as a body devoted to a specific program based on generally accepted principles."[37] When Congress debated several health insurance bills in the 1940s, the association "supported these in so far as they related definitely to tuberculosis" but "did not take any stand on compulsory health insurance in principle."[38]

When disease advocates promote healthcare access, they sometimes need to justify having the issue in their portfolio. When the NBCC supported

---

[32] Epstein, "Measuring Success," 269; Gordon, *Dead on Arrival*; Hoffman, "Health Care Reform"; King, *Pink Ribbons, Inc.*, 120; Levitsky and Banaszak-Holl, "Introduction," 3.

[33] Heath, Rapp, and Taussig, "Genetic Citizenship," 159.

[34] Hoffman, "Health Care Reform," 75; see also Hoffman, *Health Care for Some*, 143; Levitsky and Banaszak-Holl, "Introduction," 3.

[35] Hoffman, "Health Care Reform," 76, 79.

[36] Epstein, "Politics of Health Mobilization," 246.

[37] Shryock, *National Tuberculosis Association*, 98.

[38] Shryock, 266.

Clinton's healthcare plan, one member asked NBCC President Fran Vicso "what health care reform had to do with the mission of the National Breast Cancer Coalition." Visco argued that "to eradicate the breast cancer epidemic . . . we must make certain that no woman dies needlessly because she lacked access to appropriate screening or detection or to treatment.[39] In explaining why healthcare access is a breast cancer issue, Visco tried to head off the argument that treatment advocacy was inconsistent with her organization's identity. Other disease advocates avoid the hassle by focusing on policy goals that can be explicitly divided into disease categories.

The Lure of Success and the Pursuit of Consensus

The pressure to maintain a clear organizational identity is only part of the story. Advocacy organizations must also consider their ability to attract resources and participants. Since members and funders respond well to visible successes, advocates often focus on immediate, actionable goals and follow political opportunities.[40] Corporate funders and policymakers also tend to reward organizations that avoid radical challenges and controversial positions. These pressures shape the distribution of organizational goals through adaptation (organizations change their goals) and selection (radical organizations are less likely to survive).[41] They encourage disease advocacy organizations to launch awareness campaigns and lobby for research and avoid discussing environmental hazards or public funding of healthcare.

Raising Awareness, Neglecting Prevention: Quick Wins and Corporate Influence

Awareness campaigns provide important benefits to organizations. Every advocacy organization must convince donors, members, and policymakers that its problem is important; awareness campaigns help achieve this goal.[42]

---

[39] Kay Dickersin Papers, "Memo to NBCC State Coordinators."

[40] Campbell, "Where Do We Stand?," 41; McCarthy and Zald, "Resource Mobilization and Social Movements"; Zald and Ash, "Social Movement Organizations."

[41] Clemens and Minkoff, "Beyond the Iron Law," 164; McCarthy, Britt, and Wolfson, "Institutional Channeling."

[42] Benford and Snow, "Framing Processes and Social Movements," 615; McCarthy and Wolfson, "Resource Mobilization," 1072.

Additionally, American volunteers feel an imperative "to show that regular citizens really can make a difference," leading them to focus on problems and solutions that seem "do-able";[43] awareness campaigns meet this need by allowing for immediate action. In the mid-twentieth century, the American Cancer Society (ACS) turned to screening campaigns "to create opportunities for service among their many volunteers, which would also create a reservoir of emotional and human capital for the future."[44] Years later, one woman wrote on a breast cancer message board that "the only tangible thing we can do to prevent our sisters, friends and daughters from going through this terrible experience is to serve as a reminder to the women in our lives to 'get your mammograms', 'do your self-exams', 'be proactive'."[45]

Seeking to maximize public attention and donations, disease advocacy organizations have a financial stake in ensuring that the public believes that their diseases are terrible but curable.[46] This encourages them to launch awareness campaigns that may misstate scientific evidence. In the early days of the tuberculosis association, a founding member explained that education campaigns should create "an enlightened public opinion in which everyone is frightened just enough to act sensibly, and not enough to act foolishly; just enough to insure necessary public appropriations and private donations."[47] To encourage these beliefs, the organization concealed scientific uncertainty. One leader exhorted campaigners to "adopt our creed and doctrines and present them to the laity as though they were unanimously adopted and almost spontaneously created. Our controversies of orthodoxy and faith should be reserved for the inner chambers of our scientific and professional conferences."[48]

Public messages about cancer have been similarly motivated by the desire to maximize medical testing and public donations. From its birth, the ACS sought to find a "middle ground between too much hope and too much horror"[49] that would maximize donations; one ACS official noted that "the attitudes towards cancer which seem to be most closely associated with the

[43] Eliasoph, *Avoiding Politics*, 2, 21.

[44] Aronowitz, *Unnatural History*, 212.

[45] Quoted in Barker and Galardi, "Dead by 50," 1356.

[46] Aronowitz, *Unnatural History*, 211–29, 331; Leopold, *Darker Ribbon*, 171.

[47] Edward Devine 1905, quoted in Teller, *Tuberculosis Movement*, 56; see also Shryock, *National Tuberculosis Association*, 86–87.

[48] George Palmer, president of the Illinois State Association for the Prevention of Tuberculosis, 1915, quoted in Teller, *Tuberculosis Movement*, 57.

[49] Thomas Debevoise, quoted in Ross, *Crusade*, 24–25; see also Klawiter, *Biopolitics of Breast Cancer*, 67; Lerner, *Breast Cancer Wars*, 30, 42.

tendency to give to the campaign are the beliefs that today cancer is one of the most terrible diseases in the country but that we are making definite progress in getting it under control."[50] ACS publications sought to promote these donation-inspiring beliefs, even in the absence of scientific evidence.[51]

Once organizations begin raising awareness and promoting screening, multiple factors discourage them from changing course, including start-up costs, built-up knowledge, and the need to maintain a consistent organizational identity over time.[52] In the 1990s and 2000s, expert panels raised concerns that routine mammograms for women under 50 caused more harm than good—the few cancer deaths avoided did not outweigh all the unnecessary biopsies and disabling treatments. These recommendations were greeted with a chorus of criticism from breast cancer advocates.[53] Leading cancer organizations, including the ACS and the Komen Foundation, continue to recommend annual mammograms for women in their 40s or younger.[54] One ACS official explained, "we had made such strides, and the thought of going backward was very distressing."[55] Similarly, when the US Preventive Services Task Force warned that indiscriminate prostate specific antigen (PSA) testing does more harm than good, disease advocacy groups continued to recommend PSA screenings.[56]

The tenacity with which advocates hold on to screening campaigns may reflect corporate influence. When they encourage more people to be screened and treated, awareness campaigns increase profits for drug makers and the rest of the healthcare industry. Pharmaceutical companies fund patients' organizations that encourage people to seek diagnoses.[57]

---

[50] Quoted in Lerner, *Breast Cancer Wars*, 45.

[51] Aronowitz, "Do Not Delay"; Klawiter, *Biopolitics of Breast Cancer*, 67; Lerner, *Breast Cancer Wars*, 67.

[52] Pierson, "Not Just What, but When"; Whetten, "Albert and Whetten Revisited," 223.

[53] Grady, "Mammogram Advice"; Kolata, "Mammogram Debate"; Lerner, *Breast Cancer Wars*, 244–45; Orenstein, "Feel-Good War"; Sulik, *Pink Ribbon Blues*, 179.

[54] American Cancer Society, "History of ACS Recommendations"; Barbells for Boobs; Jørgensen and Gøtzsche, "Presentation on Websites"; Klawiter, *Biopolitics of Breast Cancer*, 145; Sulik, *Pink Ribbon Blues*, 207.

[55] Joann Schellenbach, quoted in Stolberg, "Confronting Cancer."

[56] American Cancer Society, "History of ACS Recommendations"; Harris, "Panel Advises."

[57] Angell, *Truth About the Drug Companies*, 30, 152; Batt, "A Community Fractured," 138; Brownlee, *Overtreated*, 183–95; Cox, "Forging Alliances"; Drinkard, "Drugmakers"; Harris, "Drug Makers"; Herxheimer, "Pharmaceutical Industry and Patients' Organisations"; Jones, "In Whose Interest?"; Lipton and Abrams, "EpiPen Maker"; Lofgren, "Pharmaceuticals and the Consumer Movement"; Mintzes, "Money from Drug Companies"; Moynihan and Cassels, *Selling Sickness*, 8–9, 63–69; O'Donovan, "Corporate Colonization of Health Activism?"; Rothman et al., "Health Advocacy Organizations"; Silverstein, "Prozac.Org."

The ACS has received donations from GE and DuPont, which make mammography machines and their film; these corporations profit when awareness campaigns encourage more screening.[58] Cancer advocates were quicker to cut back on screening recommendations when there wasn't money at stake, in the case of breast self-examination. Early ACS campaigns urged women to "examine their own breasts at least twice a week."[59] For decades, the ACS recommended monthly breast self-exams, beginning either in high school or at age 20. But amid growing evidence that the exams did little to detect breast cancer, in 2003, the ACS changed its recommendation for breast self-exams to "optional" and stopped recommending it at all in 2015.[60]

While awareness campaigns attract corporate sponsors, prevention campaigns often run up against corporate interests. Corporations that make their money from treating diseases stand to lose when diseases are prevented (unless the diseases are prevented with drugs). While medical and pharmaceutical corporations are unlikely to directly *oppose* disease prevention, they are not incentivized to promote it. Other industries' profits can also be threatened by disease prevention efforts, as when government regulations address environmental health hazards. Activists have criticized the ACS for taking donations from chemical companies and for putting manufacturers of toxic products on its board. They charge that these corporate links explain why the ACS rarely mentions environmental risks in its publications, why it opposed regulations on potentially toxic chemicals, and why it has "insisted on unequivocal proof that a substance causes cancer in humans before taking a position on public health hazards."[61] The Zeneca Group, which manufactures a blockbuster breast cancer drug and has been sued for dumping carcinogenic chemicals, created Breast Cancer Awareness Month.[62] Cancer prevention efforts hurt both its pharmaceutical and chemical businesses, but it profits when awareness campaigns lead more women to be diagnosed early and spend more years taking tamoxifen.[63] It holds the copyright for Breast Cancer Awareness Month and controls what's written

[58] Lerner, *Breast Cancer Wars*, 208; Paulsen, "Cancer Business."
[59] Little, *Civilization Against Cancer*, 87.
[60] American Cancer Society, "History of ACS Recommendations."
[61] Batt and Gross, "Cancer, Inc."
[62] Batt and Gross; Ehrenreich, "Welcome to Cancerland"; Paulsen, "Cancer Business"; Zones, "Profits from Pain."
[63] Klawiter, *Biopolitics of Breast Cancer*, 98–99; McCormick, *No Family History*, 36.

in promotional materials, which have generally "downplayed environmental causes of breast cancer and prevention."[64]

For disease advocacy organizations, corporate influence encourages a
focus on awareness and discourages broad prevention efforts. Organizations
with more corporate funding were somewhat less likely to mention prevention and more likely to mention awareness in their initial *Encyclopedia*
listings, though these patterns were not statistically significant.[65]

Avoiding Treatment, Seeking Research: Political Gains and the Avoidance of Controversy

While corporate influence encouraged disease organizations to promote
awareness and neglect prevention, the avoidance of political controversy
pushed them to deprioritize treatment access and lobby for research. Many
disease advocates care deeply about treatment access, but politics trained
them to focus on research as a politically palatable alternative.

During the 1960s and 1970s, when disease organizations testified before
Congress, about half of them mentioned treatment access. For example,
in 1979, the Cooley's Anemia Foundation recommended the creation of a
"a catastrophic or comprehensive national health insurance program" that
would "cover the medical and hospital costs of those now ill with the disease."[66] But in the 1980s, a changing political climate made it seem irrational to ask for healthcare provision. As one witness told the Reagan-era
Congress, "I have been told that it is perhaps very appropriate that I come
from the Mental Health Association, because anybody who comes to
Congress this year and asks for more money for health service programs
ought to have their head examined."[67]

Healthcare politics soon became even more divisive. In 1993, President
Clinton proposed a major federal intervention in healthcare. After attacks

---

[64] Ley, *From Pink to Green*, 39; see also Batt and Gross, "Cancer, Inc."; McCormick, *No Family History*, 36; Zones, "Profits from Pain," 144.

[65] See Appendix, Table A.4, models 2 and 4. We should not assume that corporate funding is causing organizations to change their goals since corporations tend to seek out organizations that already share their priorities. Moynihan and Cassels, *Selling Sickness*, 64–65; Walker, *Grassroots for Hire*, 10.

[66] US House of Representatives, "Appropriations for 1980, Part 8," 877.

[67] US House of Representatives, "Appropriations for 1985, Part 10," 573.

from Republicans and insurance companies, public opinion turned against the plan, and it was abandoned in 1994.[68] As the tide turned against Clinton's plan, disease organizations were significantly less likely to testify about treatment access (see Figure 6.1, bottom panel).[69] In 1993 and 1994, only 8% of disease advocates mentioned treatment provision in their congressional testimony, despite the fact that 36% of disease advocacy organizations had treatment goals in their *Encyclopedia* entries.

While government-funded medical treatment seemed like an unattainable goal, asking for research funding set advocates up for success. Medical research is a lavishly funded "distributive arena" in which benefits can be given out in small units, making it easier for lobbying to be effective.[70] And so as treatment access came to seem like a non-starter, disease advocates framed research as an uncontroversial alternative. In 1994, a Juvenile Diabetes Foundation representative testified, "In this the year of health care reform, it seems odd to me that we do not invest more in research, the one area which would have the most dramatic impact on our health care costs."[71] Throughout hearings in the 1990s, witnesses discussed problems with access to medical care but concluded by arguing for more research. The mother of a boy with epilepsy described the financial burden of repeated hospitalizations and special schooling. But she didn't ask the government to help with her medical bills or to improve public school services for students with special needs. Instead, she argued that "research alone holds the key to his future."[72] Likewise, a witness for the National Prostate Cancer Coalition discussed the difficulties she and her husband faced in securing adequate pain medications but translated this difficulty into a request for research funding, saying that

> eventually we dealt with hospice people who understood pain medication better than any other professionals that we dealt with through the entire course of Bill's illness. Even with all of these facts, spending for research continues to lag.[73]

[68] Quadagno, *One Nation, Uninsured*; Skocpol, *Boomerang*.
[69] The treatment testimony counts in this figure differ from those in Figure 1 in Best, "Disease Campaigns and the Decline of Treatment Advocacy" due to smoothing and due to the inclusion of all disease witnesses (not just those with treatment goals in the *Encyclopedia*).
[70] Lowi, "American Business."
[71] US House of Representatives, "Appropriations for 1995, Part 7," 173.
[72] US House of Representatives, "Appropriations for 2000, Part 7a," 360.
[73] US House of Representatives, "Appropriations for 2001, Part 7b," 493.

These witnesses testified movingly about the hardships they faced due to inadequate or unaffordable treatment and services. And yet none of them asked the government to help with these problems directly; instead, they asked only for medical research. This pattern suggests a tension between advocates' goals and the requests they felt they could reasonably make to Congress. Even among organizations that *didn't* mention research in their *Encyclopedia* listings, 81% mentioned it in their congressional testimony.[74] Witnesses seemed to take it for granted that research was the most reasonable thing for them to ask for.[75] A representative of the National Multiple Sclerosis Society began by saying, "We are talking today about funding for the National Institutes of Health, of course," suggesting that it was obvious that she would ask for research.[76]

Returning to the case of the NBCC reveals how political victories guide disease advocates to favor research over treatment access. Early on, the NBCC had three main task forces: research, access (to healthcare), and influence. By July 1991, the research task force had hit the ground running, with a range of specific projects and strong relationships with the Congressional Women's Caucus and NIH director Bernadine Healy. The access task force had fewer members and was tied to Clinton's doomed health plan.[77] The next year, when an NBCC document highlighted the organization's major accomplishments, the first six focused on research, and none were primarily about access to treatment.[78] Board members argued that the "BCC should continue its successful focus on increasing the funding of research" and that a "position paper should be slanted toward what the politicos want."[79] The NBCC never gave up on treatment access and prevention, but the allure of success pushed it to focus more and more on research funding.[80]

---

[74] In contrast, fewer than 20% of organizations without treatment, prevention, and awareness goals in their *Encyclopedia* listings mentioned these goals in Congress.

[75] Qualitative studies concur that disease advocacy organizations have increased their research focus over time. Aronowitz, *Unnatural History*, 214; Casamayou, *Politics of Breast Cancer*, 58; Couzin, "Advocating, the Clinical Way"; Dresser, *When Science Offers Salvation*; Hess, "Medical Modernisation"; Koay and Sharp, "Shaping Genomic Science"; Kolker, "Framing," 820; Ley, *From Pink to Green*, 126; Novas, "Political Economy of Hope"; Panofsky, "Generating Sociability"; Pinto, Martin, and Chenhall, "Rare Disease Research"; Rabeharisoa, "Struggle Against Neuromuscular Diseases"; Strickland, *Politics, Science, and Dread Disease*, 37.

[76] US House of Representatives, "Appropriations for 2000, Part 7a," 1377.

[77] Kay Dickersin Papers, "Working Board Meeting." The NBCC found more success with research funding than with efforts to promote treatment access, genetic discrimination, and a patients' bill of rights. King, *Pink Ribbons, Inc.*, 78.

[78] Kay Dickersin Papers, "History, Goals, Accomplishments."

[79] Kay Dickersin Papers, "Meeting Minutes"; "National Breast Cancer Coalition Meeting."

[80] Kaufert argues that the NBCC needed goals that could unite a membership that ranged from mainstream to feminist to environmental breast cancer organizations. All the member organizations

The removal of treatment provision from congressional testimony may have been a short-term political calculation. Disease advocates focused on achievable goals, and some of them later returned to their other priorities. As the years passed since the Clinton plan controversy, witnesses gradually became more willing to discuss access to medical treatment. In the early 2000s, government testimony again resembled organizations' *Encyclopedia* entries, with similar percentages of witnesses and listings mentioning treatment access (see Figure 6.1).

However, these short-term political calculations reshaped the field of disease advocacy. After removing treatment requests from their testimony, some organizations also removed them from their *Encyclopedia* listings. Organizations were significantly more likely to remove treatment access from their missions during the years immediately following congressional testimony (see Figure 6.4).[81] Among organizations that ever listed treatment goals, one in ten eventually dropped them. Speaking to Congress didn't inspire organizations to drop research, prevention, or awareness from their missions—on the contrary, they tended to *add* all those goals (see Figure 6.4).[82] The dispiriting effect of testimony was limited to treatment provision.

Social movement organizations sometimes do well to "forego the (slim) chance for immediate gains in favor of concentrated efforts to cultivate political opportunities for subsequent action." But for this "strategic restraint" to pay off in terms of later opportunities, it must not lead movements to fundamentally redefine their goals.[83] In 1970, 45% of disease advocates had treatment missions. By 2000, that number had declined to 31%, and it did not rebound (see Figure 6.1). The political climate in the 1980s and 1990s encouraged organizations to redefine what it meant to be a disease advocacy organization—a definition that discouraged treatment access goals.

could agree on the need for research, helping to keep the coalition together. Kaufert, "Women, Resistance," 299.

[81] This pattern is discussed further in Best, "Disease Campaigns and the Decline of Treatment Advocacy."

[82] Event history analyses show that these differences are statistically significant (see Appendix, Tables A.5 and A.6).

[83] Downey, "Elaborating Consensus," 351.

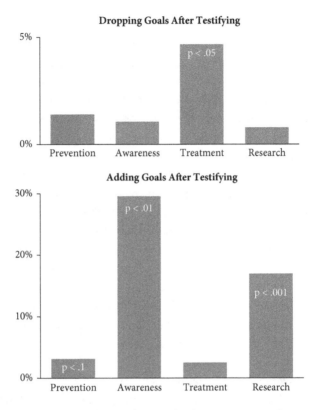

Figure 6.4 Organizations change their goals after congressional testimony

Percent of organizations with a given goal that dropped it from their *Encyclopedia of Associations* listings, and percent without a given goal that added it, in the five years after congressional testimony. *p* values indicate statistically significant increases in the rate of goal changes during the five years following testimony (see Appendix Tables A.6 and A.7).

Imperfect Goals

These trends are not universal; there are many disease advocacy organizations lobbying for access to treatment, challenging environmental hazards, and working to prevent disease. But over time, the field of disease advocacy organizations has increasingly centered around promoting awareness and lobbying for government research funding. Does this agenda best serve the interests of patients and the general public?

Does Research Serve Patients' Interests?

The United States spends more on medical research than any other nation.[84] Our research focus is also high in proportional terms: the United States devotes 5.6% of healthcare spending to research, a much higher proportion than any other country.[85] Our overall science budget is heavily skewed toward biomedical research, with two-thirds of university research and development funding going to the life sciences.[86] These investments in medical research have been spurred onward by disease campaigns. But does research best serve the interests of disease campaigns' constituents?

Many advocates argue that research, even basic biological research, will proceed quickly enough to benefit *today's* patients, not just future generations. The sister of a man with schizophrenia testified that she "can't overemphasize the importance of all three research efforts—basic neuroscience research, clinical research and service systems research. With[out] all three, my brother wouldn't get the help he needs."[87] A Parkinson's disease patient reported that scientists had promised her "Joan, this is going to be in time for you."[88] The mother of three sons with dystonia predicted that a cure would come that "will not only help my sons . . . but . . . the hundreds of thousands of others as well who suffer with this disease."[89] In 1994, disease advocates told Congress that we were on "the edge of important discoveries" for Alzheimer's, "at the precipice of major breakthroughs in osteoporosis research," and "on the brink of multiple new breakthroughs" for schizophrenia.[90] In 1999, they reported that "more treatments and a cure are in the near horizon" for dystonia; that "scientists stand ready right now to deliver, what I call, rescue" for Parkinson's disease; that "we are very close to the finish line" for retinitis pigmentosa, for which "sightsaving treatments would be available today if we could only fund the research opportunities that exist."[91] As of 2019, despite substantial investments in research, none of these conditions have been cured.

---

[84] Greenberg, *Science, Money, and Politics*, 23; *Nature Medicine*, "Windfall for Biomedical Science," 115.

[85] Moses et al., "Financial Anatomy of Biomedical Research," 1340.

[86] Stephan, *How Economics Shapes Science*, 237.

[87] US House of Representatives, "Appropriations for 1995, Part 7," 1190.

[88] US House of Representatives, 214.

[89] US House of Representatives, "Appropriations for 2000, Part 7a," 771.

[90] US House of Representatives, "Appropriations for 1995, Part 7," 117, 769, 1189.

[91] US House of Representatives, "Appropriations for 2000, Part 7a," 771, 212, 349.

In reality, healthcare breakthroughs are expensive and inefficient.[92] It often takes decades to develop a new drug or treatment.[93] Once a drug has been developed, it takes an average of seven to ten years to be approved.[94] Most drugs never make it to this point, failing at some point in the process.[95] There are exceptions to the rule. For example, after pressure from AIDS activists, AZT went from its first clinical tests to Food and Drug Administration approval in under two years.[96] But AZT had already been synthesized twenty years before as a possible cancer drug, so it cannot serve as an example of the speedy development of a new drug.[97] For most diseases, patients should not expect advances to come soon enough to help them, and research advocacy is better understood as a philanthropic effort to help future generations.

Rebecca Dresser calls the faith that research will help current patients the "collective therapeutic misconception."[98] At an individual level, the therapeutic misconception refers to patients thinking of clinical trials as a way to get access to cutting-edge treatments, missing the fact that the trials are primarily designed to advance knowledge.[99] At a collective level, advocates assume that research will benefit the current generation of patients, when in all likelihood treatments are decades away. The collective therapeutic misconception may lead to bad decisions by individuals; an NIH panel warned that overly optimistic "patients, their families, and health providers may make unwise decisions regarding treatment alternatives, holding out for cures that they mistakenly believe are 'just around the corner.' "[100] It can also lead organizations to overprioritize research when their members would be

---

[92] Stergiopoulos and Getz, "Development Pathway."

[93] For instance, it took at least 20 years to develop bone marrow transplantation and cholesterol-lowering statin drugs. Li, *Triumph of the Heart*; Orkin and Motulsky, "Report and Recommendations"; Steinberg and Gotto, "Preventing Coronary Artery Disease"; Tobert, "Lovastatin and Beyond."

[94] Kaitin, "Drug Development Process"; PhRMA, "Biopharmaceutical Research & Development." Others estimate that the entire process usually takes about 15 years for drugs that are ultimately approved. Rowberg, "Pharmaceutical Research and Development."

[95] Booth and Zemmel, "Prospects for Productivity," 451; Kaitin, "Drug Development Process," 358.

[96] Broder, "Development of Antiretroviral Therapy"; Cimons, "Sale of AZT."

[97] *New York Times*, "AZT's Inhuman Cost."

[98] Dresser, *When Science Offers Salvation*, 9.

[99] Appelbaum et al., "False Hopes and Best Data"; Lidz et al., "Therapeutic Misconception."

[100] Orkin and Motulsky, "Report and Recommendations," 13. Scientific researchers are sometimes the source of this misconception. In the case of stem cell research, scientists seeking funding gave journalists lists of diseases that might someday be cured by stem cell research. Reading these lists, "patients came to recognize themselves as . . . the projected users of stem cell technologies" even though the research was at a basic stage. Langstrup, "Interpellating Patients," 173.

better served by improved access to treatment or services.[101] Dresser points out the irony that "research funding is depicted as a way to help people currently burdened by poor health, while an appreciable number of those same people have trouble obtaining the basic, established treatments and services that could extend and improve their lives."[102]

Patients sometimes push back, arguing that treatment and services would do more for them than research. In the late 1960s, the American Diabetes Association's lay members opposed the organization's increased focus on research because they were primarily focused on the day-to-day problems they faced in managing the disease.[103] In an interview with researchers, a contemporary disease advocate described conflicts between organization leaders' focus on research and members' concerns about insurance reimbursement.[104] When the Cystic Fibrosis Foundation promoted gene therapy research, one patient argued that "their search for a cure will not help me or many of my friends with CF," and another stated that "the Foundation's almost total neglect in aiding PWCF [people with cystic fibrosis] in our day-to-day lives is criminal."[105] Surprisingly, organizations with patients as members were significantly *less* likely to prioritize treatment access (32% versus 42%; see Appendix, Table A.4, model 5).[106] But patients may lack power, even when they are nominally members. A study of rare disease organizations found that in organizations that focused primarily on supporting research, members often had little say in decision-making.[107] Medical research yields important health benefits but often only for future generations of patients.

[101] Silberman, *Neurotribes*; Stockdale, "Waiting for the Cure," 589–90. Some disease organizations recognize this problem. Pinto, Martin, and Chenhall, "Chasing Cures," 13–15.

[102] Dresser, *When Science Offers Salvation*, 9. Of course, not all patients have trouble obtaining access to medical treatment. Access to treatment is of greater concern for low-income and/or uninsured patients, while research (if it comes quickly enough to benefit any current patients) will benefit the richest patients first. Sarewitz, *Frontiers of Illusion*, 149. Like all advocacy groups, disease organizations tend to focus disproportionate attention on the concerns of their most advantaged members. Strolovitch, *Affirmative Advocacy*.

[103] American Diabetes Association, *Journey & and the Dream*, 131.

[104] Keller and Packel, "Going for the Cure," 353.

[105] Stockdale, "Waiting for the Cure," 589.

[106] These organizations were more likely than others to focus on providing mutual support (49% versus 17%; $p < .001$); these support groups may have avoided discussions of treatment access in order to focus on things patients can accomplish among themselves.

[107] Pinto, Martin, and Chenhall, "Chasing Cures," 15.

Does Awareness Make Us Healthier?

Americans are exposed to a staggering number of disease awareness campaigns. Walks and ribbons represent dozens of diseases.[108] Pink ribbons promoting breast cancer awareness decorate everything from sneakers to buckets of fried chicken.[109] October is simultaneously ADHD Awareness Month, AIDS Awareness Month, Breast Cancer Awareness Month, Down Syndrome Awareness Month, Rett Syndrome Awareness Month, and Selective Mutism Awareness Month.[110]

In certain circumstances—if there are good treatments available, if early detection improves outcomes, or if behavioral changes can prevent a disease—disease awareness saves lives. Campaigns encouraging cervical cancer screening and discouraging smoking have saved thousands of lives. But more and earlier medical treatment isn't always a good thing. All medical interventions come with risks and side effects. For people with no symptoms and low risks, like those with slow-growing cancers, benign abnormalities, or mildly elevated blood pressure, the harms of treatment can outweigh the benefits. Early detection and aggressive diagnosing of risks can literally make us sicker by exposing us to risky, harmful, and unneeded medical care.[111] In the "popularity paradox" of screening, the people who are most harmed—who undergo difficult, disabling, and disfiguring treatments for cancers that would never have harmed them—believe that screening saved their lives, detecting cancer while it could still be "cured." They become ready-made constituents for disease advocacy organizations.[112]

In addition to direct effects on health, awareness campaigns have intangible effects on patients, some positive and some negative. Being able to talk about a diagnosis and joining a community of survivors can make patients feel less alone. But awareness campaigns may make non-patients unnecessarily fearful.[113] By most objective measures, Americans today are healthier

---

[108] Charity Walks Blog, "Charity Walk Events"; Awareness Depot.

[109] Sulik, *Pink Ribbon Blues*.

[110] Lohmann, "2016 Awareness Calendar."

[111] Brownlee, *Overtreated*, 144–66, 265; Furtado et al., "Whole-Body CT Screening"; Welch, Schwartz, and Woloshin, *Overdiagnosed*, 11, 32–43, 50–65, 131, 142, 178, 190.

[112] Aronowitz, *Risky Medicine*, 39; Barker and Galardi, "Dead by 50," 1357; Brownlee, *Overtreated*, 206; Klawiter, *Biopolitics of Breast Cancer*, 86; Orenstein, "Feel-Good War"; Raffle and Gray, *Screening*; Ransohoff, Collins, and Fowler, "Prostate Cancer Screening"; Welch, Schwartz, and Woloshin, *Overdiagnosed*, 183–84, 194.

[113] Klawiter, *Biopolitics of Breast Cancer*; Orenstein, "Feel-Good War"; Welch, Schwartz, and Woloshin, *Overdiagnosed*.

than previous generations. But when survey-takers ask, we report feeling *less* healthy: we've been diagnosed with more conditions, and we worry about the ones we might develop.[114] Awareness campaigns can also pressure patients to adopt particular roles and identities. After her breast cancer diagnosis, Barbara Ehrenreich described a climate in which "cheerfulness is more or less mandatory, dissent a kind of treason."[115] Another patient wrote of feeling expected "to exude the upbeat attitude of the survivors on television commercials, donning pink ribbons and walking marathons, declaring a new lease on life."[116] The relentless optimism can be especially difficult for patients with terminal cancer.[117] The myth that early diagnosis makes everything curable can also create stigma and self-blame.[118] While disease awareness can sometimes improve our health, more awareness is not always a good thing.

Do Goals Crowd Each Other Out?

Disease campaigns could better improve our health if they devoted more attention to prevention and treatment access. But saying that they *overemphasize* research and awareness does not mean that pursuing these goals is *harmful*. While too much disease awareness sometimes makes us less healthy, the main concern about funding too much research and campaigning for too much awareness is that they would *crowd out* other goals. Does adopting research and awareness goals cause organizations to drop prevention and treatment access from their agendas? Does the prominence of single-disease campaigns mean we have less prevention and treatment advocacy at a societal level? And does the dominant idea that the way to fight a disease is through research and awareness make it more difficult for other approaches to gain traction?

Within organizations, awareness and research do not crowd out other goals. Instead, organizations that have awareness and/or research goals in their *Encyclopedia* listings are significantly *more* likely to prioritize

---

[114] Brownlee, *Overtreated*, 199; Welch, Schwartz, and Woloshin, *Overdiagnosed*, 8–9, 89, 198.

[115] Ehrenreich, "Welcome to Cancerland," 50; see also Jain, "Be Prepared"; Sulik, *Pink Ribbon Blues*, 231–67.

[116] Sczudlo, "Positivity Is Bullshit."

[117] Quoted in Orenstein, "Feel-Good War."

[118] Gardner, *Early Detection*; Phelan et al., "Stigma."

treatment access and/or prevention as well.[119] Goals might still displace each other if organizations need to choose where to spend limited resources. But if awareness and research goals help organizations attract funding, goals might not compete for resources, either.

A given single-disease organization is less likely to prioritize prevention and treatment access than a given multi-disease organization. But as the previous chapters showed, the appeal of single-disease campaigns allowed their numbers to expand dramatically. Looking at raw numbers of organizations, rather than percentages, reveals that larger numbers of single-disease than multi-disease organizations pursue prevention and treatment access (see Figure 6.5). Targeting a single disease pushes individual organizations away from prioritizing prevention and treatment access, but the growth of the field—itself made possible by the appeal of narrowly targeted campaigns—means we see more total attention to these important goals. We're less likely to prioritize prevention and treatment access when we fight one disease at a time than when we launch general public health campaigns. But fighting one disease at a time attracts more money and attention to health promotion, some of which flows to prevention and treatment access.

At a societal level, does the dominance of research and awareness make it more difficult to imagine other ways of responding to disease? Some critics argue that mainstream breast cancer advocacy "displace[s]" or "diminishes" other ways of addressing the disease.[120] Barron Lerner asks, "is all of this attention to breast cancer screening and treatment distracting American society from pursuing a more productive goal—primary prevention of the disease by eliminating environmental and other toxins?"[121] Patricia Strach argues that the dominance of mainstream breast cancer advocacy means that advocates promoting alternative approaches are "faced with an overwhelming task: destabilizing the issue understanding [and] dismantling the monopoly" and that environmental breast cancer activists would fare better if breast cancer were completely "off the American agenda."[122] Similarly,

---

[119] $\chi^2(1) = 23.3, p < .001; \chi^2(1) = 165.8, p < .001; \chi^2(1) = 261.8, p < .001; \chi^2(1) = 321.1, p < .001$, respectively. These results confirm Downey's finding that organizations tended to combine awareness efforts with other goals and "were acutely aware of the danger of letting education become an end in itself." Downey, "Elaborating Consensus," 344, 347.

[120] King, Pink Ribbons, Inc., 59; Strach, Hiding Politics in Plain Sight, 50.

[121] Lerner, Breast Cancer Wars, 13; see also Strach, Hiding Politics in Plain Sight, 41, 173, 178–79; Orenstein, "Feel-Good War."

[122] Strach, Hiding Politics in Plain Sight, 178–79; see also 39. Strach suggests that it would be preferable if breast cancer were off the agenda because advocates might be able to start fresh after "a major disaster or bombshell research report that puts the issue on the front page." Strach, 178. But a disaster

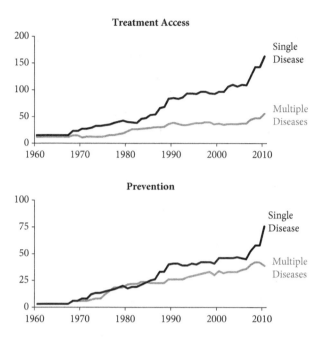

Figure 6.5 Single- and multiple-disease organizations with treatment access and prevention goals, 1960–2010

Number of single-disease and multiple-disease voluntary associations mentioning treatment access (top panel) and prevention (bottom panel) in their *Encyclopedia of Associations* listings.

Samantha King and Gayle Sulik both argue that small, radical breast cancer organizations would be more successful if they didn't have to compete with large, mainstream breast cancer advocacy organizations for funds and attention.[123] These arguments imply that the environmental breast cancer movement would be more influential if the mainstream breast cancer movement did not exist. But, in fact, environmental breast cancer organizations can attract more media attention during Breast Cancer Awareness Month, as when Breast Cancer Action launched a campaign criticizing corporations that use pink ribbons while marketing carcinogenic chemicals.[124] Activists

---

or bombshell with non-mainstream advocates taking control over its interpretation seems less likely to occur than a successful reframing of an issue already on the agenda.

[123] King, *Pink Ribbons, Inc.*, 58; Sulik, *Pink Ribbon Blues*, 54.
[124] King, *Pink Ribbons, Inc.*, 24–28.

promoting prevention and treatment access may be helped by the visibility of mainstream disease campaigns, even if they are outnumbered by them.[125] Instead of a zero-sum competition between goals, we see resources and attention spilling over from awareness and research to prevention and treatment.

And so, while disease campaigns disproportionately focus on research and awareness, important subsets of the field emphasize prevention and treatment access. Feminist and environmental breast cancer activists have often been harsh critics of the "screening orthodoxy" and have brought attention to environmental carcinogens.[126] AIDS activists have fought for universal healthcare and embraced a social justice agenda, fighting against poverty and inequality.[127] Recently, some large, mainstream disease advocacy organizations have begun questioning the orthodoxy of early detection and lobbying for treatment access and disease prevention. In 2002, the NBCC broke with other breast cancer organizations when it stopped unilaterally recommending routine mammograms for younger women.[128] The ACS's new chief medical officer has shown an unprecedented willingness to question screening, saying that "the advantages to screening have been exaggerated" and "we are actually hurting people with overtreatment."[129] Some mainstream organizations have also become more willing to push for access to medical care. In the run-up to the 2008 presidential election, the ACS spent its entire advertising budget publicizing the fact that many Americans lacked health insurance. The ACS also collaborated with the American Heart Association, the American Diabetes Association, and the Alzheimer's Association to promote access to "quality, affordable health care with transparent costs."[130] These organizations are fighting against the tide, and their efforts are encouraging.

---

[125] Klawiter, *Biopolitics of Breast Cancer*, 224.

[126] Klawiter, 210; see also Epstein, "Measuring Success"; Epstein, "Politics of Health Mobilization"; Ley, *From Pink to Green*; McCormick, *No Family History*; McCormick et al., "Personal Is Scientific"; Moffett, "Moving Beyond the Ribbon," 288.

[127] Brier, *Infectious Ideas*, 156–84; Duggan, *Twilight of Equality?*, 68; Hoffman, "Health Care Reform," 82; Hoffman, *Health Care for Some*, 176–80.

[128] National Breast Cancer Coalition, "Mammography"; Stolberg, "Confronting Cancer."

[129] Brawley, "Quotation of the Day"; Otis Brawley, quoted in Parker-Pope, "Plenty of Blame."

[130] Sack, "Cancer Society."

Conclusion

Contemporary disease advocacy organizations often claim to represent the interests of patients and their families. But what are those interests? Even people who are active enough to participate in associations may not have a defined set of political goals. For instance, when sociologist Sandra Levitsky asked a woman caring for a relative with Alzheimer's if she had ever contacted an elected official, she responded, "I really should. It's just that I don't know what to ask for. You know, find a cure for Alzheimer's? . . . Help us take care of our parents who have Alzheimer's? I don't know what to ask for."[131] Since patients' and caregivers' interests are not predefined, disease advocacy organizations play a key role in shaping their political agendas.[132] Disease advocates tend to focus on lobbying for research funding and promoting awareness, underemphasizing the collective risks that predispose us to multiple diseases and the inequalities we face in access to treatment. The resulting health campaigns often fail to meet patients' needs, subsidize corporate interests, and may actually be making us sicker.

Measuring goals across organizations and over time reveals how advocacy organizations decide which goals to pursue. Disease advocates' goals have been shaped by the need to match their goals to disease categories and by the pursuit of consensus, corporate support, and short-term gains. Avoiding controversy, disease advocates sometimes turn away from the goals that would do most to improve our health.

This chapter has identified troubling tendencies of disease campaigns, but this is not to say that we'd be better off without them. Narrow specialization may discourage *individual organizations* from pursuing broad goals. But the appeal of specialized campaigns encourages the proliferation of organizations, some of which buck these trends. Mainstream organizations promoting awareness and research do not crowd out more radical organizations promoting prevention and treatment access. And so instead of rejecting disease campaigns, we should recognize and encourage promising countertrends. Some scholars criticize consensus politics and narrowly targeted campaigns, arguing that they displace more contentious activism

---

[131] Levitsky, *Caring for Our Own*, 153.
[132] Advocacy organizations' prioritization of issues "sifts and filters salient voices and perspectives on public policy *before* they become manifest in advocacy work." Halpin, Fraussen, and Nownes, "Balancing Act," 216.

and advocacy for broadly shared goals.[133] This chapter suggests that while various pressures push individual organizations to prioritize narrow goals and pursue consensus, these choices help the advocacy field grow, making room for potentially transformative campaigns as well.

[133] Eliasoph, *Avoiding Politics*; Eliasoph, *Making Volunteers*; Ferree, "Resonance and Radicalism"; Gitlin, *Twilight of Common Dreams*; Gitlin, "From Universality to Difference"; Michels, *Political Parties*; Lofland, *Polite Protesters*; Lofland, "Consensus Movements"; Piven and Cloward, *Poor People's Movements*.

Conclusion

Picking Fights

In the 1930s, the president of the organization that would become the American Cancer Society hoped that the cancer campaign would reduce social conflict:

> At a time when our country is inclined to develop class, race or creed consciousness or hatreds the menace of a common enemy and the inspiration of fighting it together may have a sorely needed and deeply significant religious and moral force.[1]

He hoped that fighting the "common enemy" of cancer would discourage Americans from fighting each other.[2] Across the decades, Americans have indeed come together to fight diseases. Knowing that no one will be offended by a request for money to fight a disease, millions have volunteered their time and donated their money. Politicians from both parties have united to fund medical research; "major-disease research" is a quintessential example of the "high-salience, low-conflict areas" that "offer the strongest incentives to congressional involvement."[3] In the 1980s, the conservative Heritage Foundation singled out the National Institutes of Health (NIH) as "virtually the only domestic agency of government whose work was so important, so efficiently carried out, and of such high benefit-to-cost ratio, that no cuts should be made in it."[4] Politicians use medical research funding as a "tactical retreat to least common denominator politics."[5]

Social scientists tend to focus on contentious politics, and so studies of agenda setting and advocacy often overlook disease campaigns

---

[1] Clarence Little, quoted in *Time* Magazine, "Cancer Army."
[2] Little, *Civilization Against Cancer*, 115, 138.
[3] Price, "Policy Making in Congressional Committees," 548.
[4] Strickland, *NIH Grants Programs*, 90.
[5] Malakoff, "Clinton's Science Legacy," 2236.

entirely, while medical sociologists focus on the most radical and contentious among them. When we ignore consensus politics, we overlook campaigns that attract vast resources, inspire mass participation, build up institutions, and transform fields. Rather than normalizing things that are considered banal or ordinary, scholars should study mainstream and "boring" organizations and experiences, asking how taken-for-granted activities distribute resources, privilege some groups over others, and transform society.

This book has revealed the powerful effects of consensus campaigns. Bringing Americans together, disease campaigns have attracted huge sums of money to fight terrible diseases. Awareness and screening campaigns have yielded major declines in diseases such as cervical and colon cancer. Disease campaigns have amplified patients' voices. Consumer groups are often described as too heterogeneous and fragmented to mobilize effectively.[6] And yet recent decades have seen dramatic growth in patients' involvement in decision-making, policymaking, and research priority setting, brought about in large part by disease campaigns.[7] They have spurred medical breakthroughs from the polio vaccine to AZT and led the United States to develop a world-leading biomedical research establishment.[8] Consensus campaigns may be especially well suited for attracting resources and building lasting institutions.

Across the decades, disease campaigns have concentrated attention and resources on a few diseases and neglected others. The same criticisms recently leveled at breast cancer advocacy and the amyotrophic lateral sclerosis ice bucket challenge once targeted the tuberculosis and polio campaigns. Public participation in disease campaigns produces an "irrational" distribution of funds, in that we overinvest in fighting some diseases and underinvest in others.

But repeated efforts over a century to rationalize the disease funding system have failed; people just don't get as excited about contributing to public health campaigns or funding basic science. In private charity and in the federal budget, we're not choosing between the same amount of money, distributed irrationally or rationally. We're choosing between a large

---

[6] Alford, *Health Care Politics*, 15, 218; Wood, *Patient Power?*, 7.

[7] Epstein, "Measuring Success."

[8] Greenberg, *Science, Money, and Politics*, 74; *Nature Medicine*, "Windfall for Biomedical Science," 115.

amount of money distributed irrationally and a small amount of money distributed rationally. The former is probably better.

In addition to focusing on a few diseases, the campaigns focus on a few goals—generally those that are the least controversial and the least redistributive. Disease campaigners tend to emphasize the goals that are least challenging to inequality and corporate interests—promoting awareness and supporting research—while neglecting primary prevention and treatment access. Investing in medical research without equalizing access to care creates profound inequalities, a problem that has been recognized for decades. In 1967, NIH Director Shannon wrote that

> progress in our medical capability has been substantial. The benefits of this progress, however, are not universally available. . . . The solution lies not in medical science but in medical economics and sociology.[9]

Three decades later, NIH Director Varmus similarly worried that investments in medical research were outpacing access to healthcare:

> We have a problem in this country in that there is nothing people place a higher value on than a healthy life, but . . . we're going to cut a very significant portion of our population out of the benefits of certain kinds of approaches to health that were paid for by public money and ought to be publicly accessible.[10]

When disease campaigns encourage us to invest in medical research without ensuring access to care, they exacerbate these inequalities. As Daniel Callahan notes, "medical research for the benefit of affluent countries raises their already high quality of life to one that is still higher."[11] When we allocate resources to the things we can agree on, we often end up helping the rich the most.

When disease campaigns prioritize research, they also help institutionalize massive public subsidies to pharmaceutical companies. The rise of disease advocacy has coincided with a dramatic expansion of the pharmaceutical industry. Since the 1980s, a series of policy changes—extending

[9] Shannon, "Advancement of Medical Research," 105.
[10] Harold Varmus, quoted in McManus, "Varmus Counsels Successor."
[11] Callahan, *What Price Better Health?*, 262.

patent protections, easing the commercialization of publicly funded research, outlawing the importation of drugs from other countries, and forbidding Medicare to negotiate drug prices—allowed pharma's profits to skyrocket.[12] This powerful industry has increasingly collaborated with disease organizations. Patient advocacy groups and pharmaceutical companies often had a confrontational relationship in the 1960s and 1970s. But beginning in the 1980s, they were increasingly likely to find common ground.[13] There is variation in the extent to which disease advocacy organizations accept pharmaceutical funding,[14] but even in the absence of direct influence, patients' groups generally pursue a pharma-friendly agenda, pushing for publicly funded research and access to expensive drugs.[15]

Sometimes, disease campaigns are explicit alternatives to addressing inequality. In the early 1990s, supporting breast cancer research was a politically attractive option for members of Congress seeking to "demonstrate a commitment to women's issues" while avoiding controversy.[16] The Nixon administration, seeking a "safe" black issue, favored funding for sickle cell disease research.[17] Medical research into particular diseases may not meet these communities' primary needs—or even their primary health needs.

But at other times, we provide services through disease categories that are not otherwise available. In the early twentieth century, institutions for treating tuberculosis provided food and shelter that decreased the burdens on poor families (if those families happened to include a tuberculosis patient).[18] Health reform was a popular goal for progressives "because sanitary improvement alleviated the conditions of poverty without restructuring society."[19] Today, AIDS patients can access drug treatment, housing vouchers, case managers, and bus passes through the Ryan White CARE Act. The director of one AIDS organization argued that "we are basically an

[12] Angell, *Truth About the Drug Companies.*

[13] Batt, "A Community Fractured," 139; Cox, "Forging Alliances," 9; Lofgren, "Pharmaceuticals and the Consumer Movement," 232.

[14] Baggott, Allsop, and Jones, *Speaking for Patients and Carers*; O'Donovan, "Corporate Colonization of Health Activism?"; Rose et al., "Patient Advocacy Organizations."

[15] Batt, "A Community Fractured"; Jones, "In Whose Interest?"; Rothman et al., "Health Advocacy Organizations." Walker notes that corporations don't need to co-opt the charities they sponsor to achieve their goals. They can, instead, strategically select organizations that align with corporate interests and provide the funding to allow these organizations to become more influential. Walker, *Grassroots for Hire,* 10.

[16] Kedrowski and Sarow, *Cancer Activism,* 145.

[17] Spingarn, *Heartbeat,* 78–79.

[18] Bates, "Quid Pro Quo," 244–45.

[19] Porter, *Health, Civilization, and the State,* 156; see also Fee, "Public Health and the State," 234.

anti-poverty agency for people with AIDS."[20] But to minimize controversy, the law must not *appear* to be an anti-poverty program; one AIDS advocate defended the act by saying that "the Ryan White CARE Act is not a welfare program, and it is not an entitlement."[21] Charles Rosenberg notes that "a poor or homeless person becomes visible to the health-care system when diagnosed with an acute ailment but then returns to invisibility once that episode has been managed. It is almost as though the disease, not its victim, justifies treatment."[22] Similarly, Kristin Barker calls Gulf War syndrome an "attempt to have the suffering and sacrifice of combat service recognized medically when it has been denied politically."[23] She argues that

> harsh cutbacks in recent decades have created a climate in which one of the only ways to make a worthy claim on the ever-less-generous welfare state is to do so on the basis of a medical diagnosis. Demands on the state by citizens, workers, or even mothers are less politically viable, driving more and more individuals to frame their needs and demands as medical.[24]

Targeting social welfare programs to particular disease categories reflects a larger trend in American politics toward narrow categorical programs.[25] Barbara Nelson argues that "in the absence of cultural support for even minor redistributive efforts . . . the resulting segmented demands for social intervention" are met through "interest group politics, where many social problems are constructed as self-contained and essentially noneconomic."[26] We end up with narrowly targeted policies and we "hope that the whole of all categorical social programs will be greater than the sum of their parts. This is rarely so."[27]

The shortcomings of disease campaigns reveal why charity cannot replace political solutions to social problems. For over a century, conservatives have argued that government aid is harmful, while charity is uplifting for

---

[20] Quoted in Chambré, *Fighting for Our Lives*, 199, see also 106; see also Watkins-Hayes, *Remaking a Life*.

[21] Mark Barnes, AIDS Action Council, quoted in Siplon, *AIDS and the Policy Struggle*, 95.

[22] Rosenberg, *Our Present Complaint*, 31.

[23] Barker, *Fibromyalgia Story*, 195.

[24] Barker, 195.

[25] Baumgartner and Jones, *Politics of Information*, 3; Weir, "Ideas and the Politics of Bounded Innovation," 193.

[26] Nelson, *Making an Issue of Child Abuse*, 135.

[27] Nelson, 125.

volunteers, donors, and recipients. These beliefs have led to efforts to curtail public spending and let the voluntary sector pick up the slack.[28] At the beginning of the Great Depression, President Hoover argued that public relief programs would "break down this sense of responsibility of individual generosity to individual and mutual self-help," "[impair] something infinitely valuable in the life of the American people," and "[strike] at the roots of self-government."[29] Half a century later, President Reagan claimed that "the truth is that we've let government take away many of the things we once considered were really ours to do voluntarily."[30] His administration sought to limit the size of government and let nonprofits meet social needs.[31] The following decade, President Bush envisioned a sea of donors and volunteers—"a thousand points of light"—who could replace the federal safety net.[32] It's not just conservative politicians; many American citizens have long believed that our communities flourish through voluntary service to help our neighbors.[33] In the 2000s, majorities of Americans told surveytakers that "the government is trying to do too many things that should be left to individuals and businesses" and that "religious, charitable and community organizations can do a better job than government of providing services to people in need."[34] Disease campaigns played a role in convincing Americans to believe that voluntary efforts are a key way to solve collective problems: the experience of buying Christmas Seals, donating dimes, and wearing ribbons trained Americans "to view philanthropy as both a quintessential part of being American and another means of achieving major objectives."[35] The problem with viewing voluntarism as a replacement for a

---

[28] Berlant, *Queen of America*, 7; Clemens, "In the Shadow of the New Deal"; Eliasoph, *Avoiding Politics*, 13, 50, 58; Grønbjerg and Smith, "Nonprofit Organizations and Public Policies," 140; O'Connell, "Voluntary Activity"; Salamon and Abramson, *Federal Budget and the Nonprofit Sector*, 21; Zunz, *Philanthropy in America*, 233. These arguments, which view public spending and private charity as opposing each other, have coexisted with a long-standing system of public subsidies to private charities and the use of nonprofits to administer government programs. Clemens, "In the Shadow of the New Deal," 79, 82, 105–7; Grønbjerg and Smith, "Nonprofit Organizations and Public Policies," 146–47, 167; Salamon, *Resilient Sector*, 39, 53–54; Salamon and Abramson, *Federal Budget and the Nonprofit Sector*, 35.

[29] Herbert Hoover, 1931, quoted in Clemens, "In the Shadow of the New Deal," 88.

[30] Ronald Reagan, quoted in Salamon and Abramson, *Federal Budget and the Nonprofit Sector*, 22.

[31] King, *Pink Ribbons, Inc.*, xxvii, 5, 67; Salamon, *Resilient Sector*, 17; Salamon and Abramson, *Federal Budget and the Nonprofit Sector*, 2.

[32] Berlant, *Queen of America*, 7.

[33] Bellah et al., *Habits of the Heart*, 199.

[34] Fischer, *Made in America*, 58, 269; Kaiser Family Foundation, "Americans Distrust Government"; Saad, "Support for Active Government."

[35] Zunz, *Philanthropy in America*, 3.

public safety net is that charity flows toward a few specialized causes, favors valorized and advantaged groups, and avoids controversial goals.[36] Private charity can be an enormous force for good in American society, but it tends to prioritize things like disease campaigns—narrow, corporate-friendly, uncontroversial causes.

But while the narrow campaigns we can agree on may not be the most efficient way to improve our collective well-being, this book has shown that they do not crowd out broader attempts to solve social problems. To understand the aggregate effects of specialized, consensus campaigns, we need to consider how things would be different in their absence. Stigmatized diseases don't tend to have as much advocacy as other diseases, but they would have even less if there were no disease campaigns. Disease campaigns may not lobby for basic research or for the NIH as a whole, but they can still help achieve funding increases. Only a minority of single-disease organizations push for prevention and treatment access, but without them, we would pay even less attention to these important goals. Studying large fields of organizations over decades reveals that consensus politics do not automatically displace controversy and that specialized campaigns do not doom broader goals.[37]

We sometimes assume that caring about one problem will use up time, resources, or even empathy that would otherwise be available for other problems. Some scholars have argued that the public only has the mental or emotional capacity to care about a handful of issues at once. But this finding may be an artifact of how they measure public concern: by asking respondents to name the single most important problem facing America and counting how many issues are selected by at least 10% of the population.[38] In fact, individuals who care about one problem may be *more* likely to care about another. As Bernard-Henri Levy notes, we shouldn't assume

---

[36] O'Connell, "Voluntary Activity," 488.

[37] Downey, "Elaborating Consensus," 338; McCarthy and Wolfson, "Consensus Movements."

[38] McCombs, *Setting the Agenda*; Shaw and McCombs, *Emergence of Political Issues*; McCombs and Shaw, "Agenda-Setting Function"; Funkhouser, "Issues of the Sixties"; Zhu, "Issue Competition"; McCombs and Zhu, "Capacity, Diversity, and Volatility." A survey question forcing respondents to choose a single most important problem enforces a zero-sum competition that may not exist in reality. The 10% threshold is also an artificial limitation. Even if there were nine problems that all Americans believed were important targets for policy, we would not expect each problem to be selected as the "most important" by 10% of the public (with almost no one selecting another issue). Researchers have claimed that problems must be named by a "critical mass" of 10% of the public in order to take off (see McCombs, *Setting the Agenda*; McCombs and Zhu, "Capacity, Diversity, and Volatility"). They cite Neuman, "Threshold of Public Attention," for this claim, but it neither appears in Neuman's article nor follows from his data.

"that the capacity for empathy and the capacity for indignation is limited" because "the brain doesn't work like this—you can care about the Holocaust *and* slavery. The more you are concerned by one, the more you are likely to be concerned by the other."[39] Other scholars suggest that policy priorities invariably compete with each other because media and policy arenas have a limited "carrying capacity."[40] But the number of bills and amendments introduced in Congress and the number of laws passed vary dramatically over time.[41] So does the density of media coverage of social problems.[42] And political responses to one problem can spill over to another.[43] Some critics contend that identity politics displace attention to class struggle.[44] But identifying with a smaller group does not necessarily preclude commitments to broader goals, and identity-based movements can address class issues.[45] While social movements sometimes compete, they can also benefit each other.[46] When we build effective political institutions and lasting bureaucracies, we increase our ability to address multiple problems.

Zero-sum models assume that we're already as empathetic as human nature allows, that we're donating and volunteering as much as we possibly could, and that our policies devote the maximum possible amount of public resources toward improving society. If this were true, then devoting so much charitable and political attention to disease campaigns would come at a terrible cost, draining resources from other problems that most Americans think of as more important. But it seems likelier that we're not operating anywhere near capacity—that we could be much more sympathetic, attentive, and giving if we learned how. Disease campaigns, while not the optimal place to devote our efforts, can help train us to come together to solve social problems.

---

[39] Bernard-Henri Levy, quoted in Reiss, "Laugh Riots," 49.

[40] Hilgartner and Bosk, "Rise and Fall of Social Problems"; Kingdon, *Agendas, Alternatives, and Public Policies*.

[41] Binder, "Going Nowhere"; Heinz et al., *Hollow Core*, 390.

[42] Best, "Situation or Social Problem."

[43] Skrentny, *Minority Rights Revolution*.

[44] Gitlin, *Twilight of Common Dreams*; Piore, *Beyond Individualism*; Rorty, *Achieving Our Country*; Waters, "Succession in the Stratification System"; Weakliem, "Race versus Class?"

[45] Bickford, "Anti-Anti-Identity Politics"; Bernstein, "Celebration and Suppression"; Bernstein, "Identity Politics"; Polletta, "Strategy and Identity."

[46] McAdam, "'Initiator' and 'Spin-off' Movements"; Meyer and Whittier, "Social Movement Spillover"; Minkoff, *Organizing for Equality*; Olzak and Ryo, "Organizational Diversity"; Soule and King, "Competition and Resource Partitioning"; Tarrow, *Struggle, Politics, and Reform*.

Data and Methods

Understanding the emergence and effects of disease campaigns requires data on large fields of organizations over long time periods. Studies of advocacy organizations often rely on interviews or surveys of advocates.[1] But survey data are not well suited to studying changing fields of organizations over time. First, surveys must wrestle with the problem that not everyone is willing to respond to them, raising concerns that the eventual sample may differ from the population of interest. One study found that the average response rate for surveys of nonprofits is 42%.[2] Second, respondents often lack accurate information about the past, making surveys an inappropriate data source for historical information about organizational activities, finances, and goals. Third, survey data are not ideal for studying populations of organizations over time. Researchers sometimes try to track the growth of advocacy fields over time using survey questions about the founding dates of existing organizations. But since they only include surviving organizations, these studies overestimate increases in the number of organizations over time (since defunct organizations are excluded) and provide biased information about the types of organizations that existed in the past (since we only know about the most hardy organizations).[3]

Other studies rely on newspaper coverage of protest activity to track advocacy over time. When studying the past, newspaper coverage is preferable to surveys, and it may be the best choice for studying protest events over time. But journalistic standards and values create biases in which events make it into the newspaper.[4] Focusing on protest also excludes much of the activity of consensus movements.

---

[1] Berry, *New Liberalism*; Heinz et al., *Hollow Core*; Schlozman and Tierney, *Organized Interests and American Democracy*; Strolovitch, *Affirmative Advocacy*; Walker, *Mobilizing Interest Groups*.

[2] Hager et al., "Response Rates," 257.

[3] Walker, McCarthy, and Baumgartner, "Replacing Members with Managers?," 1286.

[4] For a review, see Earl et al., "Newspaper Data."

Table A.1 Main Data Sources

Data	Years Available
Associations	1961–2014
Congressional witnesses	1959–2013
Nonprofits	1989–2011
Corporate giving	1985–2015
Senate lobbying disclosures	1999–2014
Mortality	1979–2014
Disability-adjusted life years	1990–2013
Research funding	1987–2015
Health laws	1948–2011

Taking these concerns into account, I sought out records and documents that could provide insight into disease advocacy over decades.[5] Since each type of record comes with its own biases,[6] I combined multiple data sources whenever possible, collecting comprehensive information on advocacy and public policy targeting a wide range of diseases. First, I'll describe the quantitative data, which are organized in three units of analysis: organizations, diseases, and years. Table A.1 summarizes the main data sources. Next, I'll describe the qualitative data.

Data on Organizations

For some questions, I use organizations as the unit of analysis. For example, Chapter 6 asks when and why disease advocacy organizations emphasized prevention, awareness, treatment access, and/or research. Can these goals be explained by the extent to which the organization focuses on a single disease? By the type of disease? By the organization's finances and funding? To answer questions at the organization level, I created a file with information on 1,744 unique disease organizations from 1960 to 2014.

The first decision to make was which types of organizations to include. Previous studies of health campaigns have defined the field in various ways.

---

[5] Other researchers have also used written records to study advocacy organizations over time, for example, Baumgartner and Jones, *Agendas and Instability*; Tichenor and Harris, "Interest Group Politics."

[6] Andrews et al., "Sampling Social Movement Organizations."

Some included all social movements related to health.[7] Others focused on groups for patients, caregivers, and/or health consumers.[8] It can be difficult, though, to draw boundaries between organizations that are "truly" patient-led and those that are not. For example, one study of "patients' associations" found multiple organizations that "claimed or appeared to be patient-centered but [were] in practice profession-led."[9] This complexity would not surprise scholars of advocacy organizations, who realize that membership is a "slippery concept"; it's difficult to draw a clean line between membership and non-membership organizations.[10] In practice, many studies that set out to study health movements or patients' associations are actually studying disease advocacy because most existing health activism is organized around disease categories. For example, one study of "health consumer groups" is almost entirely focused on disease organizations.[11]

Since my overriding subject is disease campaigns, I exclude organizations that do not focus on diseases. But within that group, I include as many types of organizations as possible. I include professional associations when they are organized around a disease category (e.g., the American Association of Diabetes Educators) but not when they are organized around a broader medical specialty (e.g., the American College of Cardiology). I include groups that might traditionally have been called social movements or interest groups, recognizing that these groups exist on a spectrum and cannot be neatly separated into categories.[12] I include groups with members and groups with no members. I include groups with varying levels of control given to patients, health professionals, and corporate interests. I include groups that lobby the government and those with no political involvement. Whenever possible, I collect data on these variables to get a fuller picture of the field of disease-related organizations.

I combined multiple data sources to get as comprehensive a picture as possible. I collected data on disease advocacy organizations from the *Encyclopedia of Associations*, witnesses at congressional hearings, Internal Revenue Service (IRS) data on nonprofits, directories of corporate grants,

---

[7] Brown et al., "Embodied Health Movements"; Epstein, "Patient Groups and Health Movements."

[8] Baggott, Allsop, and Jones, *Speaking for Patients and Carers*; Keller and Packel, "Going for the Cure"; Landzelius, "Patient Organization Movements"; Wood, *Patient Power?*

[9] Wood, *Patient Power?*, 23.

[10] Andrews and Edwards, "Advocacy Organizations," 485.

[11] Baggott, Allsop, and Jones, *Speaking for Patients and Carers*, 4.

[12] Andrews and Edwards, "Advocacy Organizations"; Burstein, "Interest Organizations"; Burstein, "Social Movements and Public Policy"; Gamson, *Strategy of Social Protest*, 138; McAdam, Tarrow, and Tilly, *Dynamics of Contention*; Tarrow, "Foreword."

and disclosures of federal lobbying. These data sources have complementary strengths. To the extent to which they have overlapping weaknesses, they all tend to emphasize larger, national organizations.

Associations

The *Encyclopedia of Associations* provides comparable data about advocacy organizations across half a century. Since the 1950s, its publishers have identified as many national voluntary associations as possible and surveyed them about their goals and activities. Since 1974, they have published the results every year. The *Encyclopedia* is extremely consistent over time, published in the same format each year with listings of the same length, meaning that it provides an unusually good data source for tracing changes over time.[13]

The *Encyclopedia* has excellent coverage of large national organizations and is thus ideal for studying the types of organizations most likely to influence public policy. The editors attempt to include all national voluntary associations, meaning that the barriers to entry are purposefully kept low. However, their coverage is not perfect. Small, radical, and unstable organizations are underrepresented in the *Encyclopedia*.[14] Additionally, I only coded the volumes describing national organizations, which exclude local organizations. This decision limits the scope of my data but retains the organizations that are most likely to lobby the federal government.

For 1961 through 2014, I identified all organizations in the *Encyclopedia's* health category that were related to diseases.[15] The number of disease associations grew from 63 in 1961 to 707 in 2014. Overall, there were 924 unique organizations.[16] When the listing included a founding date, I used it to calculate the organization's age. Since the age distribution has a long tail, I use its natural

[13] Bevan et al., "Understanding Selection Bias," 1758; Johnson and Frickel, "Ecological Threat," 321–22; Walker, McCarthy, and Baumgartner, "Replacing Members with Managers?"

[14] Andrews et al., "Sampling Social Movement Organizations"; Bevan et al., "Understanding Selection Bias"; Martin, Baumgartner, and McCarthy, "Measuring Association Populations"; Minkoff, "Macro-Organizational Analysis"; Walker, McCarthy, and Baumgartner, "Replacing Members with Managers?"

[15] I began by examining all the health listings in the 1961, 1970, 1980, 1990, 2000, and 2010 volumes. When disease organizations appeared or disappeared, I examined the intervening volumes to identify when the change occurred. This strategy made coding more efficient, but has the downside of excluding organizations that only appeared in the *Encyclopedia* for a few years that did not overlap with the start of a decade.

[16] The total number of organizations exceeds the 2014 tally because some organizations became defunct.

logarithm in statistical analyses. I also created three membership variables, respectively equal to 1 if the organization mentioned having a) patients and their families, b) healthcare professionals, and c) medical researchers as members.

Since organizational representatives write their own descriptions, they can express a broad range of goals in their own words. This makes the *Encyclopedia* a good source of information about organizational goals. With the help of two graduate research assistants, I coded the *Encyclopedia* listings to see how organizations described their goals.[17] Missions change slowly, so we started by coding every 10 years, identified changes, and then looked at intervening years to see when changes occurred. For a few years in which the *Encyclopedia* was not published or we could not track down copies, including much of the 1960s, we assigned the most recent available year's goals.

The coding scheme included a broad range of goals, each coded as 1 if the listing mentioned the goal at least once.[18] For the analyses in Chapter 6, I focus on four goals: prevention, awareness, treatment access, and research. First, I ask whether the listing mentions prevention, defined as attempts to stop people from coming down with a disease. These efforts include steps that individuals can take to prevent disease (e.g., diet, exercise, safe sex), measures societies can take to prevent disease (e.g., limiting pollution, encouraging food companies to use healthier ingredients), and vaccines. Second, I coded for references to awareness, including public education campaigns, training for the public and/or medical professionals, provision of information (including hotlines, brochures, pamphlets, educational materials), and explicit references to "awareness." Third, I coded for treatment provision, including discussions of providing treatment, paying for treatment, and/or pushing for access to treatment. Fourth, I coded for research, including references to research, study, development, and finding or discovering things. I included basic and clinical research into treatment, services, screening, and prevention. These codes are not mutually exclusive; organizations could pursue all four goals at once, and an individual activity could relate to more than one goal.[19]

---

[17] During five weeks of coder training, the research assistants and I each coded the same *Encyclopedia* entries and then met to resolve disagreements and improve the coding scheme. We continued this process until we achieved levels of intercoder agreement exceeding 90%.

[18] I initially classified goals as related to treatment, services, screening, prevention, education, information, support, and/or manpower (human capital investments in the research or healthcare field). For each of these categories, I distinguished between a focus on research and a focus on provision.

[19] Since the "treatment access" code focuses specifically on *access* to treatment, it excludes mentions of research seeking new treatments.

Nonprofits

When social scientists study advocacy, they tend to focus on voluntary associations. They often overlook the nonprofit sector, which includes many more organizations that may differ in important ways.[20] To capture these organizations, I collected tax data on disease-focused nonprofits. Each year, most nonprofits with budgets exceeding a modest threshold must file Form 990 with the IRS.[21] These forms become publicly available and include substantial financial information. Compared to the *Encyclopedia* data, these tax data tend to include many more organizations.[22] Including them in the data adds information on disease charities that would not be classified by the *Encyclopedia* editors as voluntary associations.

Like any organizational data source, the IRS data have biases; they paint an incomplete picture of the nonprofit sector.[23] More radical and political organizations are less likely to register as tax-exempt organizations.[24] Thus, like the *Encyclopedia* data, the IRS data tend to underrepresent radical disease organizations, focusing on larger and more mainstream ones.

Previous researchers have raised concerns about using tax data to make comparisons over time, noting that the IRS 990 registry "has clearly grown increasingly comprehensive" over time.[25] I corrected one major source of this incongruity. Organizations with budgets below $25,000 (before

---

[20] Berry and Arons, *A Voice for Nonprofits*, 26.

[21] Organizations are included in the tax data if they are 1) a registered 501(c) organization; 2) have a budget of over $25,000 a year (before 2010) or $50,000 (2010 and later); and 3) are not in a number of excluded categories, such as churches, that are irrelevant for the current study.

[22] Andrews et al., "Sampling Social Movement Organizations," 237.

[23] For example, only about 10% of Indiana nonprofits filed financial information with the IRS. Gronbjerg, "Evaluating Nonprofit Databases." Most of the reasons for this discrepancy are not problems for my study. First, many of the nonprofits not represented in the IRS data are absent because they have revenues below $25,000; since excluded nonprofits tend to be very small, the IRS data likely capture most nonprofit revenues. Second, some discrepancies at the local level occur when nonprofits file their tax forms using the address of a headquarters organization. Nonprofits operating in Indiana with headquarters in other states would show up as discrepancies in these data but would not pose a problem for my national aggregations of the data. Third, the types of nonprofits least likely to appear in the IRS data (preschools and religiously affiliated nonprofits) are not included in this study. Thus, while there are serious concerns about using the IRS data to measure the nonprofit sector in local communities, these problems are much less severe when studying disease nonprofits at the national level.

[24] Andrews and Edwards, "Advocacy Organizations"; Bevan et al., "Understanding Selection Bias," 1760; Boris and Mosher-Williams, "Nonprofit Advocacy Organizations," 489; Brulle et al., "Measuring Social Movement Organization Populations"; Gronbjerg, "Using NTEE"; Grønbjerg and Clerkin, "Indiana's Nonprofit Sector"; Walker, McCarthy, and Baumgartner, "Replacing Members with Managers?"

[25] Bevan et al., "Understanding Selection Bias," 1760.

2010) or $50,000 (beginning in tax year 2010) do not file 990 forms.[26] Since the IRS did not adjust this cutoff for inflation until 2010, I drop all organizations with budgets below $25,000 in 1987 dollars to avoid inflating the number of organizations in later years. Another important step in making the data comparable over time is dropping years with incomplete data. Compilations of 990 forms include considerably fewer organizations in the first and last two years of coverage, perhaps because many nonprofits file their taxes late after receiving extensions. I therefore excluded these years from analyses of the nonprofit data.

The National Center for Charitable Statistics (NCCS), a program of the Urban Institute, compiles data from 990 forms. From the NCCS, I purchased two longitudinal data sets covering the years 1989–2011: the Core Trend File PC (501[c][3] public charities) and Core Trend File PF (private foundations). I also purchased the NCCS's annual Core Other files, which cover other tax-exempt organizations including 501(c)(4) social welfare organizations and trade unions. Together, these files yielded over 860,000 unique nonprofits, with data for up to 23 years, for a total of over 7.5 million lines of data.

The next task was to identify disease-focused nonprofits, code them by disease, and link them to data on the same organizations from other sources. The NCCS has developed a system for classifying nonprofits called the National Taxonomy of Exempt Entities (NTEE). The NTEE codes include a few disease categories, but these codes were insufficient for identifying disease organizations.[27] Time and resource constraints precluded a manual examination of all 860,000 nonprofits. I therefore undertook a several-step process to identify disease organizations. First, I searched for disease organizations I had identified through other data sources (the *Encyclopedia*, congressional testimony, Lilly disclosures, and the Taft directory). I searched for portions of the organizations' names, rather than the entire names, to allow for misspellings in the NCCS data. I manually examined each match and linked organizations by name.

---

[26] IRS, "Exempt Organizations Annual Reporting Requirements."

[27] I sought information about nonprofits targeting any disease, but the NTEE codes only include a handful of specific diseases (e.g., arthritis, epilepsy, asthma, Down's syndrome, cancer). Additionally, many organizations are misclassified, likely due to NCCS's use of keyword searches without human review. Gray, "A Puzzlement"; Gronbjerg, "Using NTEE"; Turner, Nygren, and Bowen, "NTEE Classification System." For example, organizations with "heart" in their names (e.g., Sacred Heart Catholic School) are classified as "Diseases of Specific Organs—Heart and Circulatory System." Likewise, organizations with "hand" in their names (e.g., Helping Hand Ministry) are classified as "Nerve, Muscle, and Bone Diseases—Arthritis."

Next, I focused on the five NTEE major categories most likely to include disease advocacy organizations: "Health—General & Rehabilitative"; "Mental Health, Crisis Intervention"; "Disease, Disorders, Medical Disciplines"; "Medical Research"; and "Human Services."[28] Among the 185,000 nonprofits in these categories, I searched for the diseases listed in Table A.2, again using substrings because of misspellings. I manually examined each match and coded organizations for the diseases they represented.

Finally, I focused on the top two categories for disease organizations: "Disease, Disorders, Medical Disciplines" and "Medical Research." For the 34,000 organizations in these categories, I manually examined each listing not already identified through organization or disease-name searches. I was able to code disease affiliations (or lack thereof) from the names of approximately three-quarters of the organizations. Web searches using Google and Guidestar (an online database of nonprofits) allowed me to identify all but 349 of the original 34,000. This manual coding ensured that I captured disease affiliations even for organizations without disease mentions in their names. It also allowed me to include organizations targeting diseases other than those listed in Table A.2. All in all, I identified 39,000 disease nonprofits, observed for up to 23 years, for a total of approximately 300,000 lines of data.[29]

Having identified disease nonprofits, I used the NCCS data to create three organization-level variables. As an indicator of organizational size, I include a variable for total revenues. Next, as an indicator of a focus on service provision, I include a variable for program service revenue, including government fees and contracts.[30] Finally, I include a variable for lobbying expenditures.[31] Each of these variables is collected for each year the nonprofit appears in

[28] While there are many problems with the more detailed NTEE codes, the broad codes classify organizations relatively validly. Gronbjerg, "Using NTEE," 311.

[29] This is a substantially larger data set than I used for my previous study of disease advocacy (Best, "Disease Politics and Medical Research Funding"). For that earlier article, I only used the Core PC file, meaning that the data only included 501(c)(3) charities and not other tax-exempt categories. I also had a shorter time range (1989–2007). Finally, for that data set I only examined the top two NTEE categories ("Disease, Disorders, Medical Disciplines" and "Medical Research"). The current data set is more comprehensive.

[30] The IRS data provide quite accurate information about organizations' finances. Froelich, Knoepfle, and Pollak, "Financial Measures"; Yetman, Yetman, and Badertscher, "Reliability of Nonprofit Disclosures."

[31] There's a common misconception that nonprofits are not allowed to lobby the government. In fact, they can lobby, but this lobbying must not constitute a "substantial part" of their activities. Uncertainty over what constitutes "substantial" lobbying does, however, dissuade many nonprofits from political activity. Berry and Arons, A Voice for Nonprofits; Internal Revenue Service, "Lobbying."

Table A.2 Disease Categories

Single diseases

ADD, ADHD	Glaucoma	Pancreatic cancer
Alpha-1	Headache	Parkinson's disease
ALS	Hemochromatosis	Pelvic inflammatory disease
Alzheimer's disease	Hemophilia	Peptic ulcer
Arthritis	Hepatitis	Phenylketonuria
Asthma	HIV/AIDS	Pneumonia
Atherosclerosis	Hodgkin's disease	Polio
Autism	Huntington's disease	Prader-Willi syndrome
Brain cancer	Hydrocephalus	Prostate cancer
Breast cancer	Hypertension	Psoriasis
Celiac disease	Influenza	Rett syndrome
Cerebral palsy	Interstitial cystitis	Reye's syndrome
Cervical cancer	Leprosy	Schizophrenia
Charcot-Marie-Tooth disease	Leukemia	Scleroderma
Inflammatory bowel disease	Liver cancer	Scoliosis
Chronic fatigue syndrome	Lung cancer	Septicemia
Chronic liver disease	Lupus	Sickle cell anemia
Craniofacial abnormality	Lyme disease	Skin cancer
Colorectal cancer	Lymphoma (non-Hodgkin's)	Spina bifida
COPD	Malaria	Spinal muscular atrophy
Cystic fibrosis	Marfan syndrome	Stroke
Depression	Multiple sclerosis	Stuttering
Diabetes	Muscular dystrophy	Sudden infant death syndrome
Down syndrome	Myasthenia gravis	Tay-Sachs
Dyslexia	Myeloma	Thalassemia
Dystonia	Neurofibromatosis	Tinnitus
Eczema	Niemann-Pick disease	Tourette's syndrome
Epidermolysis bullosa	Osteogenesis imperfecta	Tuberculosis
Epilepsy	Osteoporosis	Tuberous sclerosis
Fibromyalgia	Ovarian cancer	Uterine cancer
Fragile X/Martin-Bell	Paget's disease	

Broader disease categories

Cancer (general)	Heart disease	Lung (general)
Cardiovascular disease	Kidney disease	Mental illness (general)
Heart and lung disease	Liver (general)	

the data. Organizations that appeared only in the NCCS data, but no other source, have too little information to be used in organization-level analyses but become part of the disease- and year-level files.

Policy Advocacy

I also collected data on disease advocates' policy advocacy. I gleaned information about formal lobbying from the tax data and the Senate Lobbying Disclosure Act database, and I also collected data about the participation of disease advocacy organizations in congressional hearings.

As noted, the tax data include a measure of lobbying expenditures. Unfortunately, this variable is only useable through 2006.[32] I wanted more recent lobbying data and information on lobbying by organizations that were not registered nonprofits. The Lobbying Disclosure Act of 1995 required that firms report their lobbying activity twice a year.[33] The Senate maintains a searchable database of lobbying disclosures, beginning in 1999.[34] For each year from 1999 through 2014, I searched the database for all disease organizations identified in the *Encyclopedia* or IRS data, along with any from the congressional testimony data.[35]

Congressional testimony yields additional information about disease advocacy organizations' political claims-making thanks to a lucky quirk of a House of Representatives subcommittee. In most congressional hearings, committee chairs exert strong influence over witness lists.[36] But for decades, the committee overseeing appropriations for Labor, Health and

[32] The IRS removed the lobbying field for tax year 2008. Durnford, "IRS Documentation." The NCCS lobbying data were incomplete for 2007.

[33] Firms are only required to file reports if they spent at least $20,500 on lobbying in a six-month period. The covered lobbying activities do not include activities directed at the general public, including grass-roots lobbying or media campaigns, or activity that was already part of the public record, such as litigation or testimony at hearings. Activities are also not defined as lobbying if the target is not a relatively high government official; for instance, communication with the director of the NIH would count as lobbying but not communication with any other NIH staff member. The lobbying disclosure act focuses on only professional lobbyists, excluding employees or contractors who spend less than 20% of their time lobbying. Baumgartner and Leech, "Interest Niches and Policy Bandwagons," 1194, 1207; US Senate, "Lobbying Disclosure Act"; US House of Representatives, "Lobbying Disclosure Act."

[34] US Senate, "Lobbying Disclosure Act Database."

[35] The IRS and Senate lobbying data differ somewhat. The organizations included do not overlap completely since not all disease organizations that report lobbying to the Senate are nonprofits. Meanwhile, the same organizations may define lobbying differently for tax purposes and Senate reporting.

[36] Leyden, "Resources and Testimony."

Human Services, and Education[37] held unusually open hearings. Like other committees, they heard from the leaders of the relevant federal agencies and invited experts. But unlike most committees, including their Senate counterpart, this committee reserved significant time for testimony from "interested individuals," many of whom testified without invitations from congressional representatives.[38] A former committee staffer I interviewed explained that since this portion of the hearings was designed for public input, for the most part, people who requested slots received them. As the number of disease advocates ballooned, the committee implemented a lottery system; in 1999, one-third of the disease advocates who asked to testify received slots.[39] According to another staffer, the lottery became even more selective in the 2000s, but selection was still random. Random selection is a favorite of social scientists because it doesn't introduce any bias: the witnesses who testified don't differ in any systematic way from those who wanted to testify but didn't. From a data standpoint, this is extraordinary luck. This is the congressional committee that patients' groups interact with more than any other,[40] and it covers a vast swath of federal health spending, comprising multiple federal agencies with very different missions, including the National Institutes of Health (NIH).[41] And over the decades, it has offered advocates the same opportunity to state their concerns, even providing a representative sample of the advocates who wanted to testify. The testimony was transcribed and published by the federal government. Witnesses were given more time to speak in the 1960s, but in the 1970s through 2000s, the length of the oral testimony was quite consistent, with advocates given about five minutes to talk.[42] While other ways advocates

---

[37] Prior to 1980, the committee oversaw labor, health, education, and welfare.

[38] Stolberg, "Patients Lobby." In the earlier years of the data (the 1960s and 1970s), witnesses were more likely to be invited and managed by Congress. Policymakers called on key advocates "to produce expert witnesses" or invited their own witnesses for "window dressing." Strickland, *Politics, Science, and Dread Disease*, 138, 146–47, 152–53, 203; see also Drew, "Health Syndicate," 79; Kingdon, *Agendas, Alternatives, and Public Policies*, 36.

[39] Stolberg, "Patients Lobby."

[40] Keller and Packel, "Going for the Cure."

[41] This subcommittee does not cover appropriations for all federal health policy. Many new policies would require authorizing legislation, making it less likely that witnesses at appropriations hearings would discuss these policies (though some use advocates still do). The Food and Drug Administration is funded through the agriculture appropriations bill and is not discussed at these hearings. Neither are entitlement programs such as Medicare and Medicaid. Despite these limitations, the appropriations bill covers a vast swath of federal health spending—all of health and human services, comprising multiple federal agencies with very different missions—and provides advocates with the chance to talk about a broad range of issues.

[42] I analyze oral testimony, excluding longer written commentary.

interact with policymakers, including private meetings, may leave little trace, congressional testimony creates a decades-long written record of the participation and political desires of a representative sample of the disease advocates who sought to influence this major committee.

This testimony may not have been particularly influential; I interviewed several congressional staffers and advocates who noted that few committee members asked questions of the witnesses, and some viewed the process as a waste of time. But whether or not the advocates successfully influenced policymakers, the public testimony phase of the House appropriations hearings provides an unusually good opportunity to collect data on disease advocates' requests of the government over decades. While the *Encyclopedia* is commonly used by sociologists and political scientists, fewer scholars have collected data on congressional witnesses.[43] They are an underutilized source of data on which organized interests seek to influence policies and what goals they pursue. Of course, witness testimony excludes organizations without political goals and oversamples organizations with a Washington presence, reinforcing the importance of combining multiple data sources.

For each year from 1960 through 2015, research assistants and I read witness lists for the sections of the hearings reserved for "Other Interested Individuals and Organizations"[44] and identified all witnesses representing disease-related organizations or identified only as disease patients. We also classified all other witnesses at the hearings; this coding is discussed below (see Data on Years). For subsamples of witnesses, I also coded the content of their testimony. This coding proceeded in several phases with different coding teams. Each team included me and at least one graduate or undergraduate research assistant. Depending on availability of time and resources, some of these coding projects covered more years than others.

For the first phase of coding, I focused on every fifth year from 1959 through 2004 and randomly selected approximately 20 witnesses within each year. The proportion sampled per year ranged from 30% to 100%. This sampling strategy ensured that the samples are representative within years, while also yielding enough witnesses per year to allow me to examine trends over time. This procedure yielded witnesses representing 110 organizations testifying a total of 174 times. Two undergraduate research assistants and

[43] Burstein, *Public Opinion, Advocacy, and Policy*, 141.

[44] Over the years, these participants have also been called "interested organizations, and individuals" and "other individuals and organizations."

I coded how the witnesses made the case that their diseases deserved more attention—whether they emphasized health burden (e.g., mortality or prevalence), economic costs, and/or scientific potential.[45]

The next phase of content coding included a larger sample of witnesses and a different set of codes. For this phase, I selected 28 years between 1959 and 2010.[46] I included all disease witnesses who testified during the sampled years, for a total of 678 witnesses representing 235 organizations.[47] With one graduate research assistant, I coded whether each witness mentioned being a disease patient. With another research assistant, I coded the goals witnesses embraced and the requests they made of the government, using the same categories as the *Encyclopedia* coding: prevention, awareness, treatment access, and research.[48]

Corporate Donations

I also collected data on corporate funding of disease advocacy organizations using the *Taft Corporate Giving Directory* (*CGD*) for 1995, 2005, and 2015. Each year, the *CGD* compiles information on approximately 1,000 of the "top corporate charitable giving programs in the United States."[49] As a source of data on corporate giving, the *CGD* has several strengths. First, according to Taft's projections, the corporate giving programs included in the *CGD* gave out a majority of all corporate charitable donations that year.[50] Second, the editors gather data from various sources, including IRS forms, mail and telephone surveys, and analyses of corporate annual reports and proxy statements. Third, the data include both direct giving programs and

[45] Intercoder agreement percentages for these variables exceeded 90%. The initial coding scheme was more extensive, but most other variables failed to achieve adequate intercoder agreement.

[46] I selected years strategically to cover the entire time period while providing more detail during more recent years. We coded testimony in the following years: 1959, 1962, 1964, 1967, 1969, 1971, 1974, 1977, 1979, 1982, 1984, 1986, 1989, 1993, 1994, 1997, every year from 1999 through 2010, and 2013. Since these years were not randomly selected, the sample of witnesses is not representative of all witnesses who testified during these four decades. However, since we coded all witnesses within each year, the data are representative of claims made within years and provide unbiased measures of changes over time.

[47] In a previously published article, I focused only on organizations that appeared in the *Encyclopedia*, yielding a smaller number of witnesses. Best, "Disease Campaigns and the Decline of Treatment Advocacy."

[48] This same research assistant and I carried out the *Encyclopedia* coding, helping to ensure continuity in goals coding across the two data sources. Intercoder agreement rates exceeded 90%.

[49] Taft Group, *Corporate Giving Directory*, 2005, xiii.

[50] Taft Group, *Corporate Giving Directory*, 1995, vii.

corporate foundations. However, the *CGD* data also have some weaknesses. They do not include every corporate giving program. When they go beyond publicly available data, they are dependent on the information the corporations are willing to provide. Additionally, the *CGD* does not list every grant each corporation gave. I code disease organizations from the "recent grant" listings. The 1990 edition reported that these listings are "a sampling of recently awarded grants, usually 30"—this sample surely excludes many donations to disease associations. The editors report that "the list represents a cross-section of recipient organizations that follows the corporation's charitable priorities, with an emphasis on documenting the corporation's larger grants."[51] If the main bias is in favor of larger grants, then the organizations that received the most corporate dollars reported in the *CGD* are likely to be the organizations that received the most corporate dollars overall.

For each disease organization, I summed all donations reported in the *CGD* in each year. I imputed linear trends in corporate donations in intervening years. I also include a dummy variable for whether any of the organization's reported funding came from pharmaceutical or biotech companies.

I also collected data on grants that the pharmaceutical company Eli Lilly made to disease organizations. Since 2009, Lilly has published disclosures of its charitable giving. From 2009 through 2015, I read each year's disclosures and identified all disease-focused organizations. I then summed all grants to each organization in a given year.

Matching Organizations Across Data Sources

I gave each organization a unique identifier and used its name to match organizations across various data sources. Some organizations changed their names over time. I identified some name changes from *Encyclopedia* listings indicating organizations' previous names. I identified other name changes through my reading of the secondary literature and congressional testimony. In these cases, I was able to ensure continuity in my data by using the same organizational ID number over the years.

---

[51] Taft Group, *Corporate Giving Directory*, 1990, xiii.

All the organizations in the data set target at least one disease, including those listed in Table A.2; other, rarer diseases; and multiple diseases. I created a variable to distinguish between single-disease organizations and those targeting multiple diseases or broader categories like cancer or lung disease. I also include information about the type of disease (e.g., infectious, cancer, mental illness, preventable); these classifications are discussed in the following section.

Data on Diseases

Most sociological studies use individuals or organizations as the unit of analysis. Some of my questions required a less traditional approach, using diseases as the unit of analysis. For the disease-level data set, each line of data refers to a particular disease in a particular year, denoting, for example, how many nonprofits targeted diabetes, how many people diabetes killed, and how much federal research funding diabetes received in a particular year. This data set allows me to answer questions about which problems get attention and which get ignored. Are some diseases targeted by disproportionate levels of advocacy and funding? Do mobilized diseases get bigger funding increases? Researchers are often accused of sampling on the dependent variable by only studying mobilized issues and/or influential movements.[52] Sampling diseases instead of movements allows me to include diseases targeted by no advocacy and disease movements with varying effectiveness, permitting stronger conclusions about the determinants of mobilization and political efficacy.

Selecting Diseases

There is no single objective way to identify and classify diseases.[53] It's also not always clear what counts as a disease, as opposed to a condition or a symptom. I adopted a relatively broad definition, seeking to include campaigns targeting contested illnesses, conditions, syndromes, and

---

[52] Burstein, "Interest Organizations," 54; Leech, "Lobbying and Influence," 540; Olzak, "Analysis of Events," 121.

[53] Bowker and Star, *Sorting Things Out.*

disorders. For the quantitative data, I excluded campaigns focused on a particular medical procedure (e.g., ostomy) or symptom/problem (e.g., infertility, blindness). I included campaigns focused on relatively broad categories (e.g., heart disease, cancer, mental illness) but didn't include these broader categories in most disease-level analyses.

I began with the diseases about which the NIH reported data on research funding, choosing the lowest level of aggregation (e.g., breast cancer but not cancer). I matched them with the *International Classification of Diseases* codes used for Centers for Disease Control and Prevention (CDC) mortality data (ICD-9 and ICD-10). Fifty-three diseases appeared in both data sets, including all of the 15 leading causes of death in the United States besides murder, suicide, and accidents. Next, I added diseases targeted by more than two *Encyclopedia* organizations and/or congressional witnesses. This procedure yielded data on 92 diseases from 1960 through 2015, for a total of 5,152 observations (see Table A.2).

Aggregating Organization-Level Data

To include data on the advocacy targeting each disease, I needed to aggregate the organizational data. For most organization-level variables, I added up totals for each disease in each year. Nonprofits' financial data required a slightly different procedure. The NCCS data include organizations classified by the IRS as "public charities" and as "private foundations," with the latter making up about 10% of 501(c)(3) organizations. Since most private foundations distribute funds to charities, summing the budgets of charities and foundations targeting the same disease would risk double-counting their financial data.[54] Therefore, I summed financial data separately for charities and foundations and used whichever was larger as the measure for that disease in that year.

Some organizations appear in the organization-level data set but do not contribute to the disease-level data because they target rare diseases I did not include in the disease sample (e.g., the Xeroderma Pigmentosum Society) or because they target multiple diseases (e.g., the American Digestive Disease Society). Other organizations—those that appeared in the

---

[54] National Center for Charitable Statistics, "Guide to Using NCCS Data."

nonprofit tax data but no other organizational data source—contribute to
the disease-level data even though they are not used in organization-level
analyses.

Aggregating the organizational data created a series of variables related to the amount of advocacy targeting a given disease in a given
year: the number of associations, the number of nonprofits, nonprofits'
total lobbying, total Senate lobbying disclosures, number of congressional
witnesses,[55] total corporate donations from Taft, and total Lilly donations.
For instance, in 2010, 16 associations and 110 nonprofits targeted diabetes, and diabetes organizations disclosed over $2 million of lobbying
expenditures. For some analyses, I standardized these variables within
years (that is, I subtracted the mean and divided by the standard deviation so that instead of being expressed in dollars or numbers of organizations, the variables represent the number of standard deviations above or
below average). I used these standardized variables to create two indexes.
The *lobbying index* combines both sources of lobbying data. For 1999–
2006, it is the mean of two standardized variables: lobbying reported by
nonprofits and lobbying disclosed under the Senate Lobbying Disclosure
Act. Before 1999, only the nonprofit lobbying data are available, and after
2006, only the Senate data are available. For those years, the lobbying
index is equal to the single available standardized lobbying variable. In
order to have a single measure of advocacy to compare mobilization
across diseases for Chapter 3, I also created an *advocacy index*, which is
the mean of five standardized variables: number of nonprofits, number
of voluntary associations, number of organizations testifying before
Congress, and both measures of lobbying. Since both indexes are means
of standardized variables, values of zero indicate average levels. In 2010,
diabetes had a score of 6.9 on the lobbying index and 2.6 on the advocacy
index, indicating its higher than average levels of advocacy, compared to
other diseases that year.

---

[55] More precisely but less concisely, this is the number of organizations that sent at least one witness to testify at the House appropriations hearing. In an earlier article, I used counts of the number
of individual people testifying in each category. Best, "Disease Politics and Medical Research
Funding." Here, I sum organizations and not witnesses because some organizations send several
people to represent the organization, but they still only have one five-minute time slot, and often
only one speaks.

Disease Characteristics

I also sought measures of the health burden each disease inflicted in each year. I collected mortality data from the CDC,[56] matching my disease categories to ICD-9 codes for 1979–1998 and ICD-10 codes for 1999–2014. Some of my diseases are split across multiple ICD codes; in those cases, I added mortality totals, being careful never to double-count deaths by adding subcategories to supercategories. For some rare diseases, the CDC data were not specific enough (for instance, Niemann-Pick disease is included under E75.2, other sphingolipidosis). In these cases, mortality data are missing. I have mortality data for 74 of the 92 single diseases in my sample. In addition to providing data on total mortality, the CDC classifies deaths by race and gender. For each disease in each year, I created variables for the total number of deaths and the percent black and female fatalities. I also created dummy variables equal to 1 if over 95% of fatalities are women (breast, cervical, ovarian, and uterine cancers; pelvic inflammatory disease) or blacks (sickle cell anemia).

Measuring the burden of disease using mortality underemphasizes the burden of non-fatal conditions. Since the 1980s, researchers have sought to create measures that incorporate both mortality and morbidity into a single metric. The most widely used version is disability-adjusted life years (DALYs).[57] The Global Burden of Disease Study calculates DALYs for almost 300 causes in almost 200 countries.[58] I downloaded US DALY data for 1990, 1995, 2000, 2005, 2010, and 2013.[59] Staff from the Institute for Health Metrics and Evaluation provided data on pneumonia and influenza that were missing from the downloadable data files. I imputed linear trends for the intervening years. DALY data are available for 48 of the 92 single diseases in my sample.

I also tracked several other characteristics of diseases. I created variables equal to 1 if the disease was a cancer, an infectious disease, a mental illness, a childhood disease, a contested illness, and/or a sexually transmitted disease. I also used preventability scores from Phelan and colleagues, ranging from 1 (least preventable) to 5 (most preventable).[60] Preventability scores were available for 29 of the diseases in my study.

---

[56] Centers for Disease Control and Prevention, "Compressed Mortality File."

[57] Ashmore, Mulkay, and Pinch, *Health and Efficiency*, 89–105; Daniels, "Four Unsolved Rationing Problems"; Gold, Stevenson, and Fryback, "HALYS and QALYS and DALYS."

[58] Murray et al., "Disability-Adjusted Life Years."

[59] Institute for Health Metrics and Evaluation, "2015 Data."

[60] Phelan et al., "'Fundamental Causes.'"

Policy Responses

I also collected data on public policy responses to the diseases. First, I focused on medical research funding from the NIH, the primary public funder of medical research in the United States. With guidance and assistance from the NIH Office of Budget, I filed a Freedom of Information Act request for historical information on NIH research funding. The Office of Budget then shared an Excel spreadsheet with funding data for dozens of diseases and conditions back to 1987. I also compiled data on funding for leukemia, skin cancer, and pancreatic cancer (which were not tracked in the Budget Office data) from National Cancer Institute Fact Books.[61]

It's not completely straightforward to compile data on NIH funding to diseases since some grants address multiple conditions. Before 2007, different institutes coded such grants differently—some institutes prorated multidisease grants (assigning some of the funds to one disease and some to another), while others double-counted them. Since 2007, all institutes have used NIH's Research, Condition, and Disease Classification (RCDC) system, which double-counts these grants—for instance, if a grant targets diabetes and hypertension, 100% of the funding is counted for diabetes and 100% for hypertension (see Chapter 4).[62] Due to this double-counting (universal since 2007 and implemented by some institutes before then), I never sum NIH funding across disease categories.

In statistical analyses looking at the effects of advocacy on funding to diseases, the dependent variable is funding changes—that is, I'm asking if diseases targeted by lobbying tended to have larger funding increases (Chapter 5). The introduction of a new coding system could have created the illusion of large changes the year the new system was rolled out. Helpfully, for the first year of RCDC's implementation, the NIH provided data using both the old and new methods. Therefore, I could calculate funding changes for all years: I calculated funding changes from 2006 to 2007 using the old method's value for 2007 and from 2007 to 2008 using the new method's value for 2007.

The Department of Defense Congressionally Directed Medical Research Program (DOD-CDMRP) also distributes a significant amount of medical research funding (see Chapter 5). I compiled DOD-CDMRP funding data from the program's annual reports.[63] The more recent publications

[61] National Cancer Institute, "NCI Budget Fact Book Archive."
[62] National Institutes of Health, "August Crosswalk"; Studwell, "NIH Launches New System."
[63] Department of Defense, "Annual Reports."

list total appropriations and actual research grants, which often differ by approximately 10%. Only appropriations data are provided for the program's first seven years, so I rely on appropriations data for all years for consistency.

In some cases, it makes sense to sum the NIH and DOD funding together for a more complete measure of federal research funding to diseases. I do so when looking at the effects of lobbying in Chapter 5. When focusing specifically on NIH politics in Chapter 4, I look at NIH funding separately. Since NIH funding dwarfs DOD funding for almost all diseases but breast cancer, which I already exclude from most statistical analyses, including DOD funding in the totals makes no substantive changes in the results.

In addition to data on medical research funding, I compiled data on federal laws passed by Congress. As part of the Comparative Agendas Project, Baumgartner and Jones have classified every public law passed since 1948 into various categories.[64] For each law they classified as health-related, I coded whether it focused on prevention, awareness, treatment access, and/or research. I also classified each law as targeting a single disease, targeting multiple diseases, or not disease-specific. For single-disease laws, I coded which disease the law focused on. The disease-level data file includes annual counts of the total number of laws targeting each disease and counts of how many of those laws focused on prevention, awareness, treatment, and research.

Data on Years

Some of my questions concern changes over time in the entire field of disease politics. For example, in Chapter 4, I ask what percent of congressional witnesses represented disease organizations and health institutions and how these percentages changed over time. To answer these questions, I use the year as the unit of analysis.

---

[64] These data on federal laws were originally collected by Frank R. Baumgartner and Bryan D. Jones, with the support of National Science Foundation grant numbers SBR 9320922 and 0111611, and are distributed through the Department of Government at the University of Texas at Austin. Neither the National Science Foundation nor the original collectors of the data bear any responsibility for the analysis reported here.

To build the year data set, I began by aggregating the organization- and disease-level data up to the annual level. This file therefore includes annual totals for disease campaigns targeting multiple and single diseases: numbers of associations, nonprofits, and congressional witnesses; their total budgets and lobbying expenditures; how many of them made which claims in the *Encyclopedia* and congressional testimony; how many health laws were passed by level of disease specificity; etc.

Nonprofit organizations that a) did not appear in any other organization-level data source and b) target multiple diseases or diseases not listed in Table A.2 were not included in either the organization- or disease-level data set. These organizations *are* included in the year file's counts of disease nonprofits and sums of their financial variables. Another addition to the year-level data is information on the total NIH budget and the budgets for each NIH institute since 1938.

The year file also includes additional data about congressional witnesses. For every fifth year from 1965 to 1985 and every year from 1989 to 2007,[65] I downloaded lists of witnesses and their organizational affiliations from LexisNexis Congressional. With a team of seven undergraduate research assistants,[66] I classified the witnesses into 16 categories.[67] In Chapter 4, I use these data to look at the prevalence of witnesses representing health institutions (e.g., medical schools, hospitals, and medical research institutes) and disease advocacy organizations.[68] Since the overall number of witnesses changes from year to year, I look at these as a percentage of "outside" witnesses. The denominator is the number of witnesses testifying on the days reserved for "other interested persons" or "other interested individuals and organizations," excluding federal officials and members of Congress.

[65] I collected annual data beginning in 1989 to create independent variables for the statistical analyses.

[66] During each week of coder training, all research assistants coded the same hearing, and we then resolved disagreements and refined the coding scheme. After five weeks, intercoder agreement percentages ranged from 80% to 90%. We then finalized the codebook and began coding for data collection. Two research assistants coded each witness list.

[67] We classified witnesses as representatives of professional associations, places/programs, and private companies; advocates; federal officials; local officials; members of Congress; and individuals without organizational affiliations. Each category was split into health-related and non-health-related. I then coded whether witnesses classified as health advocates represented a disease or diseases.

[68] This count includes disease patients without organizational affiliations; these witnesses are not included in the organization-level data.

Inflation Adjusting

All financial variables are inflation-adjusted to 2013 dollars using the Current Population Index Research Series Using Current Methods (CPI-U-RS), which uses the Bureau of Labor Statistics' current methods to produce the best possible historical information about inflation.[69] The CPI-U-RS is available back to 1977; for earlier years, I use the Current Population Index (CPI).[70] When NIH reports budget data over time, it prefers to use the Biomedical Research and Development Price Index (BRDPI).[71] NIH officials argue that since the costs of biomedical research have increased faster than the rest of the economy, this adjustment better reflects changes in the NIH's purchasing power. I do not use the BRDPI because I'm less interested in the NIH's purchasing power than in how much of our societal resources we're devoting to medical research. Using the CPI-U-RS data allows me to inflation-adjust all financial data using the same ratios.

Qualitative Data

I complement these quantitative data sets with several sources of qualitative data that provide context and interpretive depth, reveal mechanisms for relationships between variables, and clarify details. The qualitative data also allow me to expand the study further back in time, to the first disease campaigns in the early twentieth century.

Congressional Hearings and *Encyclopedia* listings

I conducted a qualitative analysis of congressional testimony to explore how stigma shaped advocates' claims (Chapter 3), how advocates made the case that their diseases deserved more funds (Chapter 4), how members of Congress and NIH directors wrestled with ways to rank and compare diseases (Chapter 4), and how advocates described their goals (Chapter 6). I collected qualitative data from congressional hearings in

---

[69] Bureau of Labor Statistics, *Consumer Price Index Research Series*.
[70] Bureau of Labor Statistics, "CPI Inflation Calculator."
[71] Teitelbaum, *Falling Behind?*, 64, 232.

three ways. First, I read all the congressional testimony of organizations selected for the first phase of witness testimony coding (110 organizations testifying a total of 174 times). I noted emerging themes in how they described their diseases, how they justified their claims, and what they asked for.

Second, I used the quantitative data to identify additional witnesses for qualitative analysis. I sometimes identified witnesses who represented a broader trend (e.g., witnesses whose organizations discussed treatment access in the 1970s but did not in the 1980s or 1990s) and sometimes witnesses who were an exception to the rule (e.g., witnesses who mentioned treatment access in Congress in the mid-1990s, when few others did). I also read these organizations' *Encyclopedia* listings to compare their congressional testimony to their overall missions. Finally, I identified organizations that dropped treatment access goals from their *Encyclopedia* listings and read these listings to understand what types of changes were being made. I draw on a qualitative analysis of these organizations' testimony and *Encyclopedia* listings to illustrate trends from the quantitative data and to yield insights about mechanisms.

Third, with three graduate research assistants, I analyzed the NIH directors' testimony and discussions with Congress at the appropriations hearings for every fifth year from 1960 to 2010. These analyses focused on how the directors justified the NIH budget and how Congress held them responsible for the funding distribution.

Archives

I drew on two archives related to breast cancer advocacy. The first is the papers of Kay Dickersin, an epidemiology professor and breast cancer advocate who was a founding member and leader of the National Breast Cancer Coalition (NBCC).[72] The second is the records of the Women's Community Cancer Project, a feminist cancer organization that was also a founding organization of the NBCC.[73] I use these archives in Chapter 2 to discuss the

---

[72] Kay Dickersin Papers, 1976–2004. Schlesinger Library, Radcliffe Institute, Harvard University, Cambridge, MA.
[73] Women's Community Cancer Project Records, 1989–2003. Schlesinger Library, Radcliffe Institute, Harvard University, Cambridge, MA.

emergence of the breast cancer movement and in Chapter 6 to describe the NBCC's struggles to define its goals.

Interviews

I interviewed three former congressional staffers, three prominent health advocates, four NIH employees, and one patient advocacy consultant. I interviewed the NIH employees in person in 2008 and conducted the other interviews over the phone in later years. The interviews were granted exemption by the University of California, Berkeley's Office for the Protection of Human Subjects and the University of Michigan's Health Sciences and Behavioral Sciences Institutional Review Board on the condition that interviewees remain anonymous. Given their small numbers and public positions, I cannot provide details about how I selected these respondents without compromising their anonymity. This constraint limits the informativeness of the interview data, but the interviews still provide important context and illustration of key points.

Primary and Secondary Sources

When possible, I draw on written material from the time periods under study. For Chapters 1 and 2, I collected early and mid-twentieth-century studies of charity and philanthropy[74] and health voluntary associations.[75] I also drew on the *Social Work Yearbook*, which is "a record of organized efforts in the United States to deal with [social] problems" available from 1929 through 1957,[76] and official histories of disease advocacy organizations.[77] Some of these sources include quantitative or qualitative data (e.g., information about disease campaigns' budgets, donors, and

---

[74] American Association of Fund-Raising Counsel, "Giving USA"; Andrews, *Philanthropic Giving*; Cutlip, *Fund Raising*; Jenkins, *Philanthropy in America*; Lear, "Business of Giving"; Marts, *Generosity of Americans*.

[75] Breslow, *History of Cancer Control*; Carter, *Gentle Legions*; Cavins, *National Health Agencies*; Dublin, "Social Hygiene Movement"; Gunn and Platt, *Voluntary Health Agencies*; Hamlin, *Voluntary Health and Welfare Agencies*; Hiscock, "Opportunities of Voluntary Health Agencies"; Knopf, *History of the National Tuberculosis Association*; Lichtenstiger, "Philosophy and Significance"; Sills, *Volunteers*.

[76] Hall, *Social Work Year Book 1929*, 5.

[77] American Diabetes Association, *Journey & and the Dream*; Ross, *Crusade*; Knopf, *History of the National Tuberculosis Association*; Shryock, *National Tuberculosis Association*.

volunteers or interviews with organizations' participants and founders). These data provide insights about the scale and character of early and mid-twentieth-century disease advocacy for Chapters 1 and 2. The early and mid-twentieth-century studies also shed light on cultural reactions to disease campaigns by revealing how writers described disease campaigns in earlier time periods.

I also examined news coverage of disease campaigns and medical research politics in newspapers, magazines, scientific journals, and congressionally mandated reports from the Congressional Research Service and the Institute of Medicine. For example, Chapter 5 draws heavily on *Science* journalists' coverage of NIH budgeting. I also draw on existing studies of various disease movements and histories of charity, philanthropy, the NIH, and the CDC.

Details on Statistical Analyses

Analyses for Chapter 3

Chapter 3 asks which diseases are targeted by the most advocacy. For regression analyses, the dependent variable is the advocacy index, which includes information on lobbying, organizations, and congressional testimony. The analyses exclude HIV/AIDS and breast cancer, which are outliers in terms of their huge and successful advocacy campaigns. I use the Cochrane-Orcutt transformation to correct for first-order autocorrelation. I use robust standard errors to account for clustering by disease. Full results are presented in Table A.3.

I define diseases as female- or black-dominated if over 95% of deaths are women (breast, cervical, ovarian, and uterine cancers and pelvic inflammatory diseases) or blacks (sickle cell anemia). These models exclude breast cancer; if I include it, the female-dominated coefficient turns positive but is still non-significant. I also ran analyses using continuous variables for the percent of deaths that were black or female in a given year. In these analyses, I found a significant positive effect for percent black—that is, diseases that kill more black people tend to have more advocacy. But these results disappear when I exclude diabetes from the model, and as discussed in Chapter 3, much diabetes advocacy focuses on type 1 diabetes, which has a smaller proportion of black patients than type 2.

Table A.3 Which Diseases Have the Most Advocacy? (Chapter 3)

	1	2
Disease characteristics		
Highly preventable		-0.30*
		(0.13)
Infectious	-0.26***	-0.14
	-0.064	(0.14)
Mental illness[1]	-0.47***	
	(0.046)	
Patients' demographics		
Black-dominated[1]	-0.049	
	(0.047)	
Female-dominated	-0.19	-0.18
	(0.11)	(0.17)
Corporate funding (standardized)	0.21	0.20
	(0.13)	(0.15)
Mortality (thousands)	0.0011	0.00040
	(0.0018)	(0.0015)
Constant	0.0085	0.11
	(0.051)	(0.10)
Observations[1]	1,916	812
R^2	0.024	0.037

Cochrane-Orcutt regressions; dependent variable is advocacy index. Robust cluster standard errors in parentheses. Analyses exclude AIDS and breast cancer.

[1] Model 1 includes 72 diseases; model 2 includes only the 28 diseases for which preventability scores are available. Preventability scores were not available for any mental illnesses or black-dominated diseases, so these variables are omitted from model 2.

***$p < .001$, *$p < .05$ (two-tailed tests).

The analytic sample for model 1, determined by data availability, is 72 diseases from 1986 through 2014. Not all diseases are observed in all years. Model 2 includes preventability scores from Phelan et al..[78] The scores range from 1 (least preventable) to 5 (most preventable), and I classify diseases with scores of 4.5 or 5 as highly preventable. These scores were only available for 29 of the diseases in my study, limiting the analytic sample for model 2. Additionally, since Phelan et al. focus on the preventability of *mortality*,

[78] Phelan et al., " 'Fundamental Causes.' "

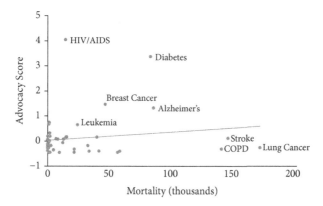

Figure A.1 Diseases' advocacy scores and mortality, 2005–2015

Alternate version of Figure 3.1, with mortality (deaths per year) rather than DALYs on the *x*-axis. The *y*-axis shows the advocacy score, an index of standardized measures of lobbying expenditures, organizations, and congressional testimony. Both variables are means for 2005–2015. COPD, chronic obstructive pulmonary disease.

they do not include conditions (like many mental illnesses) that do not cause many deaths.

While the statistical analyses for Chapter 3 cover the years from 1986 through 2014, one of the goals of Figures 3.1 and 3.2 is to provide descriptive information on contemporary disease advocacy. These figures therefore focus on the years 2005–2015. Figure 3.1 explores the relationship between the DALYs lost to a disease and the amount of advocacy targeting the disease. Figure A.1 is an alternate version of this graph, with mortality rather than DALYs on the *x*-axis.

Analyses for Chapter 4

Figure 4.4 explores the relationship between the amount of NIH funding diseases receive and the number of people they kill. Note that for most analyses, I predict funding *changes*. But since this chapter asks about the overall distribution of funds—the relationship between *total* funding and mortality—I use total funding, and not funding changes, as the dependent variable. For the years 1987–2015, I looked at the relationship between NIH funding and mortality for the same 29 diseases. These analyses are based on the diseases for which the NIH provided funding data and the CDC

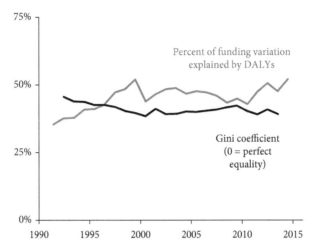

Figure A.2 Some equalization in DALYs per death over time

Alternate version of Figure 4.4, exploring the relationship between NIH funding and disability-adjusted life years (DALYs) lost instead of mortality. Gray line shows R^2 statistics from regressions of NIH funding to diseases on DALYs (lagged by one year). Black line shows the Gini coefficient, a measure of inequality in dollars per DALY. If NIH funding were distributed solely on the basis of DALYs, the Gini coefficient would equal zero. Both calculations are based on the same 22 diseases in each year.

collected mortality data in all years. I exclude AIDS and breast cancer, which were major outliers in terms of their funding successes. I also exclude larger disease categories (e.g., cancer in general, heart disease, kidney disease).

Within each year, I regressed NIH funding on mortality, lagged by one year. Figure 4.4 shows the R^2 values from these regressions. Figure A.2 is an alternate version of Figure 4.4, using DALYs instead of mortality. Since DALY data are available for fewer diseases, this figure only includes 22 diseases over a slightly shorter time period. Notably, we see much less change over time in the relationship between DALYs and funding, largely because there was less inequality in dollars per DALY at the start of the time period than there was in terms of dollars per death.

Analyses for Chapter 5

Chapter 5 summarizes the results of a series of regressions of funding changes on lobbying (see Figure 5.2). Each year, I ran a regression predicting

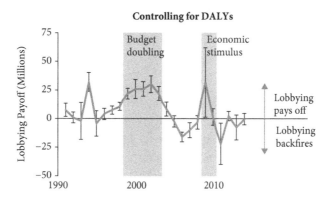

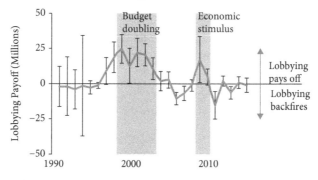

Figure A.3 Lobbying only sometimes pays

Alternate versions of Figure 5.2, controlling for DALYs instead of mortality, and excluding AIDS and breast cancer. Lobbying coefficients from regressions of NIH funding changes in millions, controlling for DALYs (top panel) and mortality (bottom panel), with 95% confidence intervals. Independent variables are lagged by one year.

changes in NIH and DOD funding for a disease. The key independent variable is the lobbying index. The regressions summarized in Figure 5.2 control for changes in mortality; findings were similar when controlling for changes in DALYs (see Figure A.3, top panel). Both independent variables are lagged by one year. Figure 5.2 includes AIDS and breast cancer, which are outliers in terms of the amount of advocacy and funding they received. Without these two diseases, the standard errors increase for most years, and the lobbying coefficient is no longer statistically significant in 1991 and 1994 (see Figure A.3, bottom panel).

Table A.4 Which Goals Did Disease Advocates Include in Their Initial *Encyclopedia* Entries? (Chapter 6)

	Prevention		Awareness		Treatment		Research	
	1	2	3	4	5	6	7	8
Single-disease organization	−0.39^t	−0.11	0.61***	−0.69	−0.44**	−0.46	0.70***	1.39***
	(0.22)	(0.62)	(0.18)	(0.51)	(0.17)	(0.42)	(0.17)	(0.42)
Infectious disease	1.12***	0.064	−0.23	0.26	−0.26	0.21	−0.59*	−1.70**
	(0.27)	(0.92)	(0.28)	(0.78)	(0.26)	(0.68)	(0.24)	(0.65)
Organization's age (ln)	−0.059	−0.23	−0.37***	−0.77*	0.12	0.52^t	−0.071	−0.17
	(0.13)	(0.40)	(0.11)	(0.33)	(0.10)	(0.29)	(0.098)	(0.28)
Membership								
Patients	0.38	1.29	0.74**	2.57**	−0.42*	−1.00	0.20	0.55
	(0.24)	(0.82)	(0.24)	(0.84)	(0.20)	(0.68)	(0.19)	(0.69)
Healthcare providers	−0.14	0.20	0.042	−1.68*	0.28	0.99	−0.12	−0.56
	(0.23)	(0.78)	(0.20)	(0.71)	(0.18)	(0.62)	(0.18)	(0.66)
Researchers[1]	0.88*		−0.43	1.80	−0.56	−1.75	1.35**	
	(0.39)		(0.38)	(1.40)	(0.39)	(1.29)	(0.44)	
Finances (in millions)								
Corporate funding		−0.38		7.07		4.53^t		3.38
		(2.07)		(7.32)		(2.34)		(3.12)
Total revenues		0.18***		0.024		−0.081*		0.043
		(0.049)		(0.036)		(0.035)		(0.030)
Program revenues		−0.54		−0.084		0.13		0.68
		(1.02)		(0.11)		(0.11)		(0.54)
Constant	−1.45***	−2.06^t	1.40***	3.32***	−0.53^t	−1.61*	−0.055	−0.38
	(0.37)	(1.07)	(0.32)	(0.98)	(0.29)	(0.80)	(0.28)	(0.75)
Observations	877	180	877	185	877	185	877	180

Logistic regressions; dependent variables are equal to 1 if the organization's first *Encyclopedia* entry mentioned prevention (models 1 and 2), awareness (models 3 and 4), treatment access (models 5 and 6), and research (models 7 and 8). Standard errors in parentheses.

[1] In models 2 and 8, zero organizations without researcher members mentioned the goal, so this variable is dropped and five observations are not used.

$^{***}p < .001$, $^{**}p < .01$, $^*p < .05$, $^t p < .1$ (two-tailed tests).

Analyses for Chapter 6

The first regression analyses in Chapter 6 ask whether organizations' initial *Encyclopedia* entries mentioned prevention, awareness, treatment access, and research goals. Each goal is explored in a separate logistic regression, with the dependent variable equal to 1 if the listing included the goal. These analyses use only one line of data per organization, from the year the organization first appeared in the *Encyclopedia*. Results are presented in Table A.4. Models 2, 4, 6, and 8 include financial information, which is only available for 501(c)(3) organizations after 1988, so these models draw on a smaller sample of organizations and years.

Figure 6.2 explores the relationship between level of disease focus (multiple diseases versus single disease) and goals included in organizations' *Encyclopedia* entries. Tests of statistical significance refer to the single-disease coefficients in models 1, 3, 5, and 7 (see Table A.4): these are two-tailed tests of differences between multiple- and single-disease organizations' goals, controlling for infectious diseases; organizational age; and patients, healthcare providers, and researchers as members. Figure 6.3 explores the relationship between level of disease focus (not disease-specific, multiple diseases, and single disease) and laws passed by Congress. Tests of statistical significance are $\chi^2(2)$ tests.

Figure 6.4 shows descriptive statistics indicating the percent of organizations that changed their goals within five years following congressional testimony. To see if organizations changed their goals significantly more frequently during these times, I conducted event history analyses: Weibull models predicting the hazard of dropping each goal (see Table A.5) and adding each goal (see Table A.6). The models for dropping goals limit the analytic sample to organizations that had the goal in the previous year; the models for adding goals limit the analytic sample to those that did not. Positive coefficients indicate an increased rate of either dropping or adding goals. All analyses use robust standard errors to account for clustering by disease. Tests of the proportional hazards assumption indicated that the membership coefficients varied over time; these variables are therefore interacted with organizational age.

Table A.5 Weibull Models of Dropping Goals (Chapter 6)

	Prevention 1	Awareness 2	Treatment 3	Research 4
Testified in the past 5 years	1.25	−0.45	1.42*	−0.46
	(1.06)	(0.86)	(0.65)	(1.07)
Single-disease organization	3.81	−0.092	−0.11	−0.45
	(2.46)	(1.12)	(0.83)	(0.97)
Infectious disease	4.10*	−16.6***	−0.22	2.04*
	(2.04)	(0.64)	(1.38)	(1.03)
Organization's age (ln)	3.72*	1.70*	0.67	0.17
	(1.80)	(0.67)	(0.50)	(0.55)
Membership				
Patients	26.2***	−2.53	−0.76	−16.9***
	(4.32)	(2.20)	(4.12)	(3.34)
Patients × ln(age)	−9.46***	0.79	0.84	0.24
	(1.64)	(0.75)	(1.66)	(1.10)
Healthcare professionals	8.39	5.35**	8.03*	−16.0***
	(5.60)	(1.81)	(4.01)	(3.81)
Healthcare professionals × ln(age)	−3.97ᵗ	−1.72**	−3.81*	0.085
	(2.28)	(0.55)	(1.65)	(1.17)
Researchers	−6.58	−18.6***	−26.5***	−17.2**
	(4.35)	(2.07)	(7.26)	(5.80)
Researchers × ln(age)	−2.00ᵗ	0.34	4.44ᵗ	1.26
	(1.16)	(0.61)	(2.46)	(1.63)
Finances				
Corporate funding	−427*	−0.52	0.72ᵗ	0.65*
	(183)	(0.72)	(0.38)	(0.29)
Total revenues	0.18*	0.00048	−0.015	−0.0012
	(0.076)	(0.0013)	(0.011)	(0.0018)
Program revenues	−0.052*	−0.0035	0.021ᵗ	0.0015
	(0.021)	(0.0042)	(0.013)	(0.0025)
Constant	−4,469*	−819***	−1,455***	−1,417***
	(2,092)	(189)	(245)	(213)
ln(p)	6.37***	4.67***	5.25***	5.23***
	(0.47)	(0.24)	(0.17)	(0.15)
Observations	743	2,843	1,440	2,717

Positive coefficients indicate a faster rate of dropping the relevant goal. Analytic samples include organizations that mentioned the relevant goal (prevention, awareness, treatment, or research) in their *Encyclopedia* entry. Robust standard errors in parentheses.

***$p < .001$, **$p < .01$, *$p < .05$, ᵗ$p < .1$.

Table A.6 Weibull Models of Adding Goals (Chapter 6)

	Prevention 5	Awareness 6	Treatment 7	Research 8
Testified in the past 5 years	2.08^t	1.86**	−0.64	3.84***
	(1.21)	(0.63)	(0.91)	(0.95)
Single-disease organization	1.65	0.75	0.51	1.69
	(2.47)	(0.78)	(0.84)	(1.32)
Infectious disease	1.79	−0.30	0.019	1.62
	(1.09)	(1.31)	(1.14)	(1.08)
Organization's age (ln)	−0.38	0.40	0.15	2.77*
	(0.77)	(0.59)	(0.46)	(1.08)
Membership				
Patients	5.62^t	17.2**	0.33	2.52
	(3.11)	(5.26)	(9.97)	(3.32)
Patients × ln(age)	−2.26*	−5.77**	−0.55	0.14
	(1.08)	(1.78)	(2.80)	(1.27)
Healthcare professionals	−20.1*	−0.96	0.13	11.1**
	(8.07)	(3.87)	(9.54)	(4.29)
Healthcare professionals × ln(age)	6.12**	−0.44	0.094	−4.78**
	(1.99)	(1.17)	(2.58)	(1.79)
Researchers	−2.52	−8.85*	4.77	0.35
	(11.3)	(3.87)	(6.75)	(5.56)
Researchers × ln(age)	0.27	2.83*	−1.49	1.73
	(2.96)	(1.22)	(1.96)	(2.28)
Finances				
Corporate funding	0.26	−2.43	−1.55	−23.6**
	(1.42)	(2.99)	(3.90)	(7.82)
Total revenues	−0.0092	−0.018	−0.031	0.13**
	(0.0083)	(0.037)	(0.045)	(0.042)
Program revenues	0.069***	−0.55	−0.16	−0.98
	(0.019)	(0.81)	(0.18)	(1.21)
Constant	−1,685*	−1,782***	−2,220**	−2,018*
	(845)	(382)	(732)	(817)
ln(p)	5.40***	5.45***	5.68***	5.57***
	(0.50)	(0.21)	(0.33)	(0.41)
Observations	2,727	599	2,023	762

Positive coefficients indicate a faster rate of adding the relevant goal. Analytic samples include organizations that did not mention the relevant goal (prevention, awareness, treatment, or research) in their *Encyclopedia* entry. Robust standard errors in parentheses.

$^{***}p < .001$, $^{**}p < .01$, $^*p < .05$, $^t p < .1$.

References

ACT UP. "ACT UP Capsule History." 2012. http://www.actupny.org/documents/capsule-home.html.

Agnew, Bruce. "Body-Count Budgeting: New Pressure to Shift Funding Among Diseases." *Journal of NIH Research* (1996): 21–22.

AIDS Project Los Angeles. "History of APLA." Accessed February 24, 2012. http://www.aplahealth.org/about/history.html.

AIDS Walk Los Angeles. "History." 2012. Accessed February 24, 2012. http://aidswalk.net/losangeles/about/history.

Albert, Stuart, and David A. Whetten. "Organizational Identity." *Research in Organizational Behavior* 7 (1985): 263–95.

Alberts, Bruce. "Overbuilding Research Capacity." *Science* 329 (2010): 1257.

Alford, Robert R. *Health Care Politics: Ideological and Interest Group Barriers to Reform.* Chicago: University of Chicago Press, 1975.

Allen, Peg, Sonia Sequeira, Leslie Best, Ellen Jones, Elizabeth A. Baker, and Ross C. Brownson. "Perceived Benefits and Challenges of Coordinated Approaches to Chronic Disease Prevention in State Health Departments." *Preventing Chronic Disease* 11 (2014): 130350.

ALS Association. "ALS Ice Bucket Challenge—FAQ." 2015. http://www.alsa.org/about-us/ice-bucket-challenge-faq.html.

ALS Association. "The ALS Association: What We Do." 2015. http://www.alsa.org/about-us/.

Amenta, Edwin, and Neal Caren. "The Legislative, Organizational, and Beneficiary Consequences of State-Oriented Challengers." In *The Blackwell Companion to Social Movements*, edited by David A. Snow, Sarah A. Soule, and Hanspeter Kriesi, 461–88. Oxford: Wiley-Blackwell, 2004.

Amenta, Edwin, Neal Caren, Elizabeth Chiarello, and Yang Su. "The Political Consequences of Social Movements." *Annual Review of Sociology* 36 (2010): 287–307.

Amenta, Edwin, and Michael P. Young. "Making an Impact: Conceptual and Methodological Implications of the Collective Goods Criterion." In *How Social Movements Matter*, edited by Marco Giugni, Doug McAdam, and Charles Tilly, 22–41. Minneapolis: University of Minnesota Press, 1999.

American Association of Fund-Raising Counsel. "Giving USA: A Compilation of Facts and Trends on American Philanthropy for the Year 1973." New York: American Association of Fund-Raising Counsel, 1974.

American Cancer Society. "History of ACS Recommendations for the Early Detection of Cancer in People Without Symptoms." 2015. http://www.cancer.org/healthy/findcancerearly/cancerscreeningguidelines/chronological-history-of-acs-recommendations.

American Diabetes Association. *The Journey & and the Dream: A History of the American Diabetes Association.* Arlington, VA: American Diabetes Association, 1990.

American Epilepsy Society. "History of AES." Accessed August 6, 2013. http://www.aesnet.org/go/about-aes/history.

Anderson, Christopher. "NSF Wins, NIH Loses in Clinton's 1994 Budget." *Science* 260 (1993): 24–25.

Anderson, Christopher. "Opponents of US Earmarks Propose Reviews to Temper Worst Elements of Growing Practice." *Nature* 360 (1992): 4–5.

Anderson, Robert N. "Coding and Classifying Causes of Death: Trends and International Differences." In *International Handbook of Adult Mortality*, edited by Richard G. Rogers and Eileen M. Crimmins, 467–89. Dordrecht, The Netherlands: Springer, 2011.

Andrews, Frank Emerson. *Philanthropic Giving*. New York: Russell Sage Foundation, 1950.

Andrews, Kenneth T., and Michael Biggs. "The Dynamics of Protest Diffusion: Movement Organizations, Social Networks, and News Media in the 1960 Sit-Ins." *American Sociological Review* 71, no. 5 (2006): 752–77.

Andrews, Kenneth T., and Bob Edwards. "Advocacy Organizations in the U.S. Political Process." *Annual Review of Sociology* 30 (2004): 479–506.

Andrews, Kenneth T., Bob Edwards, Akram Al-Turk, and Anne Kristen Hunter. "Sampling Social Movement Organizations." *Mobilization: An International Quarterly* 21, no. 2 (2016): 231–46.

Angell, Marcia. *The Truth About the Drug Companies: How They Deceive Us and What to Do About It*. New York: Random House, 2004.

Anglin, Mary K. "Working from the Inside Out: Implications of Breast Cancer Activism for Biomedical Policies and Practices." *Social Science and Medicine* 44, no. 9 (1997): 1403–15.

Anspach, Renee R. "From Stigma to Identity Politics: Political Activism Among the Physically Disabled and Former Mental Patients." *Social Science and Medicine* 13A (1979): 765–73.

Anspach, Renee R. "Notes on the Sociology of Medical Discourse: The Language of Case Presentation." *Journal of Health and Social Behavior* 29, no. 4 (1988): 357–75.

Appelbaum, Paul S., Loren H. Roth, Charles W. Lidz, Paul Benson, and William Winslade. "False Hopes and Best Data: Consent to Research and the Therapeutic Misconception." *Hastings Center Report* 17, no. 2 (1987): 20–24.

Archibald, Matthew E. *The Evolution of Self-Help: How a Health Movement Became an Institution*. New York: Palgrave Macmillan, 2007.

Armstrong, Elizabeth A. *Forging Gay Identities: Organizing Sexuality in San Francisco, 1950–1994*. Chicago: University of Chicago Press, 2002.

Armstrong, Elizabeth A., and Mary Bernstein. "Culture, Power, and Institutions: A Multi-Institutional Politics Approach to Social Movements." *Sociological Theory* 26, no. 1 (2008): 74–99.

Armstrong, Elizabeth M. *Conceiving Risk, Bearing Responsibility: Fetal Alcohol Syndrome & the Diagnosis of Moral Disorder*. Baltimore, MD: Johns Hopkins University Press, 2003.

Armstrong, Elizabeth M., Daniel P. Carpenter, and Marie Hojnacki. "Whose Deaths Matter? Mortality, Advocacy, and Attention to Disease in the Mass Media." *Journal of Health Politics, Policy, and Law* 31, no. 4 (2006): 729–72.

Arno, Peter, and Karyn L. Feiden. *Against the Odds: The Story of AIDS Drug Development, Politics and Profits*. New York: HarperCollins, 1992.

Aronowitz, Robert. *Risky Medicine: Our Quest to Cure Fear and Uncertainty.* Chicago: University of Chicago Press, 2015.

Aronowitz, Robert A. "Do Not Delay: Breast Cancer and Time, 1900–1970." *Milbank Quarterly* 79, no. 3 (2001): 355–86.

Aronowitz, Robert A. *Unnatural History: Breast Cancer and American Society.* Cambridge and New York: Cambridge University Press, 2007.

Ashmore, Malcolm, Michael Joseph Mulkay, and Trevor J. Pinch. *Health and Efficiency: A Sociology of Health Economics.* Milton Keynes, UK: Open University Press, 1989.

Awareness Depot. "By Cause Type." Accessed November 6, 2015. http://www.awarenessdepot.com/bycausetype.html.

Baggott, Rob, Judy Allsop, and Kathryn Jones. *Speaking for Patients and Carers: Health Consumer Groups and the Policy Process.* Houndmills, UK, and New York: Palgrave Macmillan, 2005.

Bakal, Carl. *Charity U.S.A.: An Investigation into the Hidden World of the Multi-Billion Dollar Charity Industry.* New York: Times Books, 1979.

Barbells for Boobs. Accessed July 6, 2016. http://www.barbellsforboobs.org/assets/5yrFundingt.pdf.

Barker, Kristin K., and Tasha R. Galardi. "Dead by 50: Lay Expertise and Breast Cancer Screening." *Social Science & Medicine* 72, no. 8 (2011): 1351–58.

Barker, Kristin. *The Fibromyalgia Story: Medical Authority and Women's Worlds of Pain.* Philadelphia: Temple University Press, 2005.

Barnartt, Sharon N., and Richard Scotch. *Disability Protests: Contentious Politics, 1970–1999.* Washington, DC: Gallaudet University Press, 2001.

Barrett, Deborah. "Illness Movements and the Classification of Pain and Fatigue." In *Emerging Illnesses and Society: Negotiating the Public Health Agenda*, edited by Randall M. Packard, Peter J. Brown, Ruth L. Berkelman, and Howard Frumkin, 139–70. Baltimore, MD: Johns Hopkins University Press, 2004.

Bastian, Hilda. "Speaking Up for Ourselves." *International Journal of Technological Assessment in Health Care* 14, no. 1 (1998): 3–23.

Bates, Barbara. "Quid Pro Quo in Chronic Illness: Tuberculosis in Pennsylvania, 1876–1926." In *Framing Disease: Studies in Cultural History*, edited by Charles E. Rosenberg and Janet Golden, 229–47. New Brunswick, NJ: Rutgers University Press, 1992.

Batt, Sharon. "A Community Fractured: Canada's Breast Cancer Movement, Pharmaceutical Company Funding, and Science-Related Advocacy." In *The Public Shaping of Medical Research: Patient Associations, Health Movements and Biomedicine*, edited by Peter Wehling, Willy Viehover, and Sophia Koenen, 132–50. London: Routledge, 2015.

Batt, Sharon, and Liza Gross. "Cancer, Inc." *Sierra Magazine* (1999). https://vault.sierraclub.org/sierra/199909/cancer.asp.

Batza, Katie. *Before AIDS: Gay Health Politics in the 1970s.* Philadelphia: University of Pennsylvania Press, 2018.

Baumgartner, Frank R., and Bryan D. Jones. *Agendas and Instability in American Politics.* Chicago: University of Chicago Press, 1993.

Baumgartner, Frank R., and Bryan D. Jones. *The Politics of Information: Problem Definition and the Course of Public Policy in America.* Chicago and London: University of Chicago Press, 2015.

Baumgartner, Frank R., Jeffrey M. Berry, Marie Hojnacki, Beth L. Leech, and David C. Kimball. *Lobbying and Policy Change: Who Wins, Who Loses, and Why.* Chicago: University of Chicago Press, 2009.

Baumgartner, Frank R., and Beth L. Leech. *Basic Interests: The Importance of Groups in Politics and in Political Science.* Princeton, NJ: Princeton University Press, 1998.

Baumgartner, Frank R., and Beth L. Leech. "Interest Niches and Policy Bandwagons: Patterns of Interest Group Involvement in National Politics." *Journal of Politics* 63, no. 4 (2001): 1191–1213.

Beard, Renée L. "Advocating Voice: Organisational, Historical and Social Milieux of the Alzheimer's Disease Movement." *Sociology of Health and Illness* 26, no. 6 (2004): 797–819.

Bearman, Peter S., and Kevin D. Everett. "The Structure of Social Protest, 1961–1983." *Social Networks* 15, no. 2 (1993): 171–200.

Belkin, Lisa. "Charity Begins at . . . the Marketing Meeting, the Gala Event, the Product Tie-In." *New York Times Magazine,* December 22, 1996.

Bell, Susan E. *DES Daughters: Embodied Knowledge, and the Transformation of Women's Health Politics in the Late Twentieth Century.* Philadelphia, PA: Temple University Press, 2009.

Bellafante, Ginia. "Alzheimer's, a Neglected Epidemic." *New York Times,* May 15, 2014.

Bellah, Robert N., Richard Madsen, William M. Sullivan, Ann Swidler, and Steven M. Tipton. *Habits of the Heart.* New York: HarperCollins, 1985.

Benford, Robert D., and David A. Snow. "Framing Processes and Social Movements: An Overview and Assessment." *Annual Review of Sociology* 26 (2000): 611–39.

Berlant, Lauren Gail. *The Queen of America Goes to Washington City: Essays on Sex and Citizenship.* Durham, NC: Duke University Press, 1997.

Bernstein, Mary. "The Analytic Dimensions of Identity: A Political Identity Framework." In *Identity Work in Social Movements,* edited by Jo Reger, Daniel J. Myers, and Rachel L. Einwohner. Minneapolis: University of Minnesota Press, 2008.

Bernstein, Mary. "Celebration and Suppression: The Strategic Uses of Identity by the Lesbian and Gay Movement." *American Journal of Sociology* 103, no. 3 (1997): 531–65.

Bernstein, Mary. "Identity Politics." *Annual Review of Sociology* 31 (2005): 47–74.

Berry, Jeffrey M. *The Interest Group Society.* Longman, 1997.

Berry, Jeffrey M. *The New Liberalism: The Rising Power of Citizen Groups.* Washington, DC: Brookings Institution Press, 1999.

Berry, Jeffrey M., and David F. Arons. *A Voice for Nonprofits.* Washington, DC: Brookings Institution Press, 2003.

Best, Joel. *Threatened Children: Rhetoric and Concern About Child-Victims.* Chicago: University of Chicago Press, 1990.

Best, Rachel. "Situation or Social Problem: The Influence of Events on Media Coverage of Homelessness." *Social Problems* 57, no. 1 (2010): 74–91.

Best, Rachel Kahn. "Disease Campaigns and the Decline of Treatment Advocacy." *Journal of Health Politics, Policy and Law* 42, no. 3 (2017): 425–57.

Best, Rachel Kahn. "Disease Politics and Medical Research Funding: Three Ways Advocacy Shapes Policy." *American Sociological Review* 77, no. 5 (2012): 780–803.

Bevan, Shaun, Frank R. Baumgartner, Erik W. Johnson, and John D. McCarthy. "Understanding Selection Bias, Time-Lags and Measurement Bias in Secondary Data Sources: Putting the Encyclopedia of Associations Database in Broader Context." *Social Science Research* 42, no. 6 (2013): 1750–64.

Bickford, Susan. "Anti-Anti-Identity Politics: Feminism, Democracy, and the Complexities of Citizenship." *Hypatia* 12, no. 4 (1997): 111–31.

Biggs, Michael, and Kenneth T. Andrews. "Protest Campaigns and Movement Success: Desegregating the U.S. South in the Early 1960s." *American Sociological Review* 80, no. 2 (2015): 416–43.

Binder, Sarah A. "Going Nowhere: A Gridlocked Congress?" *Brookings Review* 18, no. 1 (2000): 16–19.

Bishop, J. Michael, and Harold Varmus. "Editorial: Re-Aim Blame for NIH's Hard Times." *Science* 312, no. 5773 (2006): 499.

Bix, Amy Sue. "Disease Chasing Money and Power: Breast Cancer and AIDS Activism Challenging Authority." In *Health Care Policy in Contemporary America*, edited by Alan I. Marcus and Hamilton Cravens, 5–32. University Park: Pennsylvania State University Press, 1997.

Black, Mary E. "Self Help Groups and Professionals: What Is the Relationship?" *British Medical Journal* 296, no. 6635 (1988): 1485.

Blanchard, Ralph. "Community Chests." In *Social Work Year Book 1939*, edited by Russell H. Kurtz, 86–91. New York: Russell Sage Foundation, 1939.

Blendon, Robert J. "The Changing Role of Private Philanthropy in Health Affairs." In *Research Papers Sponsored by the Commission on Private Philanthropy and Public Needs*, Vol. 2, Part 1, edited by Commission on Private Philanthropy and Public Needs, 639–55. Washington, DC: Department of the Treasury, 1977.

Boat, Thomas F. "Biomedical Research Funding." *Journal of the American Medical Association* 303, no. 2 (2010): 170–71.

Bode, Ann M., and Zigang Dong. "Cancer Prevention Research—Then and Now." *Nature Reviews Cancer* 9, no. 7 (2009): 508–16.

Boehmer, Ulrike. *Personal & the Political: Women's Activism in Response to the Breast Cancer and AIDS Epidemics*. Albany: State University of New York Press, 2000.

Booth, Bruce, and Rodney Zemmel. "Prospects for Productivity." *Nature Reviews Drug Discovery* 3, no. 5 (2004): 451–56.

Booth, William. "No Longer Ignored, AIDS Funds Just Keep Growing." *Science* 242, no. 4880 (1988): 858–59.

Boris, Elizabeth, and Rachel Mosher-Williams. "Nonprofit Advocacy Organizations: Assessing the Definitions, Classifications, and Data." *Nonprofit and Voluntary Sector Quarterly* 27, no. 4 (1998): 488–506.

Borst, Homer W. "Community Chests and Councils." In *Social Work Year Book 1929*, edited by Fred S. Hall, 95–100. New York: Russell Sage Foundation, 1930.

Bowker, Geoffrey C., and Susan Leigh Star. *Sorting Things Out: Classification and Its Consequences*. Cambridge, MA: MIT Press, 1999.

Brawley, Otis. "Quotation of the Day." *New York Times*, October 21, 2009.

Brenner, Elsa. "Cast of Thousands Raises Money for Dozens of Worthy Causes." *New York Times*, May 23, 1999.

Breslow, Lester. *A History of Cancer Control in the United States, 1946–1971*. Washington, DC: National Cancer Institute, Division of Cancer Control and Rehabilitation, 1979.

Brier, Jennifer. *Infectious Ideas: U.S. Political Responses to the AIDS Crisis*. Chapel Hill: University of North Carolina Press, 2009.

Brinker, Nancy G. *Winning the Race: My Personal Story and Every Woman's Guide to Wellness*. Rev. ed. Irving, TX: Tapestry Press, 2001.

Britt, Lory, and David Heise. "From Shame to Pride in Identity Politics." In *Self, Identity, and Social Movements*, edited by Sheldon Stryker, Timothy J. Owens, and Robert W. White, 252–68. Minneapolos: University of Minnesota Press, 2000.

Broder, Samuel. "The Development of Antiretroviral Therapy and Its Impact on the HIV-1/AIDS Pandemic." *Antiviral Research* 85, no. 1 (2010): 1–18.

Brookmeyer, Ron, Sarah Gray, and Claudia Kawas. "Projections of Alzheimer's Disease in the United States and the Public Health Impact of Delaying Disease Onset." *American Journal of Public Health* 88, no. 9 (1998): 1337–42.

Brooks, Harvey. "The Problem of Research Priorities." *Daedalus* (1978): 171–90.

Brower, Vicki. "The Squeaky Wheel Gets the Grease." *EMBO Reports* 6, no. 11 (2005): 1014–17.

Brown, Hana E. "Race, Legality, and the Social Policy Consequences of Anti-Immigration Mobilization." *American Sociological Review* 78, no. 2 (2013): 290–314.

Brown, Phil. *Toxic Exposures: Contested Illnesses and the Environmental Health Movement*. New York: Columbia University Press, 2007.

Brown, Phil, Brian Mayer, Stephen Zavestoski, Theo Luebke, Joshua Mandelbaum, and Sabrina McCormick. "The Health Politics of Asthma: Environmental Justice and Collective Illness Experience in the United States." *Social Science & Medicine* 57, no. 3 (2003): 453–64.

Brown, Phil, Rachel Morello-Frosch, and Stephen Zavestoski, eds. *Contested Illnesses: Citizens, Science, and Health Social Movements*. Berkeley: University of California Press, 2011.

Brown, Phil, and Stephen Zavestoski. "Social Movements in Health: An Introduction." *Sociology of Health & Illness* 26, no. 6 (2004): 679–94.

Brown, Phil, Stephen Zavestoski, Sabrina McCormick, Meadow Linder, Joshua Mandelbaum, and Theo Luebke. "A Gulf of Difference: Disputes over Gulf War–Related Illnesses." *Journal of Health and Social Behavior* 42, no. 3 (2001): 235–57.

Brown, Phil, Stephen Zavestoski, Sabrina McCormick, Brian Mayer, Rachel Morello-Frosch, and Rebecca Gasior Altman. "Embodied Health Movements: New Approaches to Social Movements in Health." *Sociology of Health and Illness* 26, no. 1 (2004): 50–80.

Browne, William P. "Organized Interests and Their Issue Niches: A Search for Pluralism in a Policy Domain." *Journal of Politics* 52, no. 2 (1990): 477–509.

Brownlee, Shannon. *Overtreated: Why Too Much Medicine Is Making Us Sicker and Poorer*. New York: Bloomsbury, 2007.

Brulle, Robert J., and J. Craig Jenkins. "Foundations and the Environmental Movement: Priorities, Strategies, and Impact." In *Foundations for Social Change: Critical Perspectives on Philanthropy and Popular Movements*, edited by Daniel R. Faber and Deborah McCarthy, 151–73. Lanham, MD: Rowman & Littlefield, 2005.

Brulle, Robert, Liesel Turner, Jason Carmichael, and J. Jenkins. "Measuring Social Movement Organization Populations: A Comprehensive Census of US Environmental Movement Organizations." *Mobilization: An International Quarterly* 12, no. 3 (2007): 255–70.

Burd, Stephen. "Scientists Worry About Lawmakers' Approach to Breast-Cancer Research." *Chronicle of Higher Education* 39, no. 13 (1992): A23.

Bureau of Labor Statistics. *Consumer Price Index Research Series Using Current Methods*. Washington, DC: US Department of Labor, 2014.

Bureau of Labor Statistics. "CPI Inflation Calculator." Accessed July 5, 2018. https://www.bls.gov/data/inflation_calculator.htm.

Burstein, Paul. *American Public Opinion, Advocacy, and Policy in Congress: What the Public Wants and What It Gets*. New York: Cambridge University Press, 2014.

Burstein, Paul. "Interest Organizations, Political Parties, and the Study of Democratic Politics." In *Social Movements and American Political Institutions*, edited by Anne N. Costain and Andrew S. McFarland, 39–72. Lanham, MD: Rowman & Littlefield, 1998.

Burstein, Paul. "Social Movements and Public Policy." In *How Social Movements Matter*, edited by Marco Giugni, Doug Mcadam, and Charles Tilly, 3–21. Minneapolis: University of Minnesota Press, 1999.

Burstein, Paul, R. L. Einwohner, and J. A. Hollander. "The Success of Political Movements: A Bargaining Perspective." In *The Politics of Social Protest: Comparative Perspectives on States and Social Movements*, edited by J. Craig Jenkins and Bert Kandermans, 275–95. Minneapolis: University of Minnesota Press, 1995.

Burstein, Paul, and C. Elizabeth Hirsh. "Interest Organizations, Information, and Policy Innovation in the US Congress." *Sociological Forum* 22, no. 2 (2007): 174–99.

Bury, Michael. "The Sociology of Chronic Illness: A Review of Research and Prospects." *Sociology of Health and Illness* 13, no. 4 (1991): 451–68.

Cable, Sherry, Thomas E. Shriver, and Tamara L. Mix. "Risk Society and Contested Illness: The Case of Nuclear Weapons Workers." *American Sociological Review* 73, no. 3 (2008): 380–401.

Cain, Roy. "Community-Based AIDS Services: Formalization and Depoliticization." *International Journal of Health Services* 23, no. 4 (1993): 665–84.

Calitz, Chris, Keshia M. Pollack, Chris Millard, and Derek Yach. "National Institutes of Health Funding for Behavioral Interventions to Prevent Chronic Diseases." *American Journal of Preventive Medicine* 48, no. 4 (2015): 462–71.

Callahan, Daniel. "Shaping Biomedical Research Priorities: The Case of the National Institutes of Health." *Health Care Analysis* 7 (1999): 115–29.

Callahan, Daniel. *What Price Better Health? Hazards of the Research Imperative*. Berkeley: University of California Press, 2003.

Callon, Michel, and Vololona Rabeharisoa. "The Growing Engagement of Emergent Concerned Groups in Political and Economic Life: Lessons from the French Association of Neuromuscular Disease Patients." *Science, Technology, & Human Values* 33, no. 2 (2008): 230–61.

Campbell, Angus, Philip E. Converse, Warren E. Miller, and Donald E. Stokes. *Elections and the Political Order*. New York: Wiley, 1966.

Campbell, John L. "Ideas, Politics, and Public Policy." *Annual Review of Sociology*, no. 28 (2002): 21–38.

Campbell, John L. "Where Do We Stand? Common Mechanisms in Organizations and Social Movements Research." In *Social Movements and Organization Theory*, edited by Gerald F. Davis, Doug McAdam, W. Richard Scott, and Mayer N. Zald. New York: Cambridge University Press, 2005.

Cantor, David. "Introduction: Cancer Control and Prevention in the Twentieth Century." *Bulletin of the History of Medicine* 81, no. 1 (2007): 1–38.

Carpenter, Daniel. "Is Health Politics Different?" *Annual Review of Political Science* 15, no. 1 (2012): 287–311.

Carpenter, Daniel. *Reputation and Power: Organizational Image and Pharmaceutical Regulation at the FDA*. Princeton, NJ: Princeton University Press, 2010.

Carpenter, R. Charli. "Setting the Advocacy Agenda: Theorizing Issue Emergence and Nonemergence in Transnational Advocacy Networks." *International Studies Quarterly* 51, no. 1 (2007): 99–120.

Carter, Richard. *The Gentle Legions*. New York: Doubleday, 1961.

Casamayou, Maureen Hogan. *The Politics of Breast Cancer*. Washington, DC: Georgetown University Press, 2001.

Cavins, Harold M. *National Health Agencies: A Survey with Especial Reference to Voluntary Associations*. New York: Public Affairs Press, 1945.

Centers for Disease Control and Prevention. "Compressed Mortality File." 2016. https://wonder.cdc.gov/mortSQL.html.

Chambré, Susan Maizel. *Fighting for Our Lives: New York's AIDS Community and the Politics of Disease*. New Brunswick, NJ: Rutgers University Press, 2006.

Charity Walks Blog (blog). "Charity Walk Events." Accessed February 24, 2012. http://www.charitywalksblog.com/charity-walk-events/.

Charmaz, Kathy. *Good Days, Bad Days: The Self in Chronic Illness and Time*. New Brunswick, NJ: Rutgers University Press, 1993.

Chesler, Mark A., and Barbara K. Chesney. *Cancer and Self-Help: Bridging the Troubled Waters of Childhood Illness*. Madison: University of Wisconsin Press, 1995.

Christensen, Tom, and Per Lægreid. "The Whole-of-Government Approach to Public Sector Reform." *Public Administration Review* 67, no. 6 (2007): 1059–66.

Cimons, Marlene. "U.S. Approves Sale of AZT to AIDS Patients." *Los Angeles Times*, March 21, 1987.

Clarke, Adele E., Janet K. Shim, Laura Mamo, Jennifer Ruth Fosket, and Jennifer R. Fishman. "Biomedicalization: Technoscientific Transformations of Health, Illness, and U.S. Biomedicine." *American Sociological Review* 68, no. 2 (2003): 161–94.

Clemens, Elisabeth S. "In the Shadow of the New Deal: Reconfiguring the Roles of Government and Charity, 1928–1940." In *Politics and Partnerships: The Role of Voluntary Associations in America's Political Past and Present*, edited by Elisabeth S. Clemens and Doug Guthrie, 79–115. Chicago: University of Chicago Press, 2010.

Clemens, Elisabeth S. "Organizational Repertoires and Institutional Change: Women's Groups and the Transformation of U.S. Politics, 1890–1920." *American Journal of Sociology* 98, no. 4 (1993): 755–98.

Clemens, Elisabeth S. *The People's Lobby: Organizational Innovation and the Rise of Interest Group Politics in the United States, 1890–1925*. Chicago: University of Chicago Press, 1997.

Clemens, Elisabeth S., and James M. Cook. "Politics and Institutionalism: Explaining Durability and Change." *Annual Review of Sociology* 25 (1999): 441–66.

Clemens, Elisabeth S., and Debra C. Minkoff. "Beyond the Iron Law: Rethinking the Place of Organizations in Social Movement Research." In *The Blackwell Companion to Social Movements*, edited by David A. Snow, Sarah A. Soule, and Hanspeter Kriesi, 155–70. Oxford: Wiley-Blackwell, 2004.

Cloward, Richard A., and Frances Fox Piven. "Disruption and Organization: A Rejoinder." *Theory and Society* 13, no. 4 (1984): 587–99.

Cobb, Roger W., and Charles D. Elder. *Participation in American Politics: The Dynamics of Agenda-Building*. Baltimore, MD: Johns Hopkins University Press, 1983.

Cohen, Cathy J. *The Boundaries of Blackness: AIDS and the Breakdown of Black Politics*. Chicago: University of Chicago Press, 1999.

Cohen, Jon. "AIDS: A Justifiable Share." *Science* 276 (1997): 345.

Cohen, Jon. "Conflicting Agendas Shape NIH." *Science* 261 (1993): 1674–79.

Collins, Francis, and Jocelyn Kaiser. "Francis Collins: On Recruiting Varmus, Discovering Drugs, the Funding Cliff." *Science* 328 (2010): 1090–91.

Collins, Patricia Hill. *Black Feminist Thought*. New York and London: Routledge, 1991.

Congressional Budget Office. "Historical Budget Data." In *The Budget and Economic Outlook: 2014 to 2024*, 155–65. Washington, DC: Congressional Budget Office, 2014.

Conrad, Peter. "Medicalization and Social Control." *Annual Review of Sociology* 18 (1992): 209–32.

Conrad, Peter, and Deborah Potter. "From Hyperactive Children to ADHD Adults: Observations on the Expansion of Medical Categories." *Social Problems* 47, no. 4 (2000): 559–82.

Conrad, Peter, and Cheryl Stults. "The Internet and the Experience of Illness." In *Handbook of Medical Sociology*, edited by Chloe E. Bird, Peter Conrad, Allen M. Fremont, and Stefan Timmermans, 6th ed., 179–91. Nashville, TN: Vanderbilt University Press, 2010.

Cook-Deegan, Robert, and Michael McGeary. "The Jewel in the Federal Crown? History, Politics, and the National Institutes of Health." In *History and Health Policy in the United States: Putting the Past Back In*, edited by Rosemary Stevens, Charles E. Rosenberg, and Lawton R. Burns, 176–200. New Brunswick, NJ: Rutgers University Press, 2006.

Cooley's Anemia Foundation. "The Foundation's History." n.d. http://www.thalassemia.org/about-the-foundation/the-foundations-history/.

Couzin, Jennifer. "Advocating, the Clinical Way." *Science* 308 (2005): 940–42.

Couzin, Jennifer, and Greg Miller. "Boom and Bust." *Science* 316 (2007): 356–61.

Cowen, R. "Federal R&D Budget: Looking Good in '92." *Science News* 141, no. 6 (1992): 92.

Cowen, R., and J. Raloff. "Bush's '93 Budget Brightens Civilian R&D." *Science News* 141, no. 6 (1992): 86–92.

Cox, Teri P. "Forging Alliances." *Pharmaceutical Executive* (2002): 8–13.

craftsnscraps.com. "Awareness Ribbon Colors and Their Meanings." Accessed March 13, 2012. http://www.craftsnscraps.com/jewelry/ribbons.html.

Crawford, Mark. "Science and Congress: Outlook Uncertain." *Science* 247, no. 4941 (1990): 404–5.

Cress, David M., and David A. Snow. "The Outcomes of Homeless Mobilization: The Influence of Organization, Disruption, Political Mediation, and Framing." *American Journal of Sociology* 105, no. 4 (2000): 1063–1104.

Crohn's & Colitis Foundation. "About the Crohn's & Colitis Foundation." 2016. http://www.ccfa.org/about/.

Culliton, Barbara J. "A Battle over NIH Funds." *Science* 235, no. 4793 (1987): 1129–30.

Culliton, Barbara J. "AIDS Amendment Angers Cancer Institute." *Science* 226 (1984): 1056.

Culliton, Barbara J. "Congress Boosts NIH Budget 17.3%." *Science* 234 (1986): 808–9.

Culliton, Barbara J. "Congress Passes Generous NIH Budget." *Science* 222 (1983): 483–84.

Culliton, Barbara J. "House Battles over NIH Legislation." *Science* 221 (1983): 726–28.

Culliton, Barbara J. "NIH Budget Growth." *Science* 228 (1985): 1260.

Culliton, Barbara J. "NIH Faces $236-Million Budget Cut in FY 1986." *Science* 231 (1986): 444.

Culliton, Barbara J. "NIH to Award 2200 New Grants." *Science* 229 (1985): 947.

Culliton, Barbara J. "OMB Raid on NIH Budget Called 'Outrageous.'" *Science* 227 (1985): 1016–17.

Culliton, Barbara J. "Who Runs NIH?" *Science* 227 (1985): 1562–64.

Cuomo, Margaret I. *A World Without Cancer: The Making of a New Cure and the Real Promise of Prevention*. New York: Rodale, 2012.

Cutlip, Scott M. *Fund Raising in the United States: Its Role in America's Philanthropy*. New Brunswick, NJ: Rutgers University Press, 1965.

Daniels, Norman. "Four Unsolved Rationing Problems: A Challenge." *Hastings Center Report* 24, no. 4 (1994): 27–29.

Dastagir, Alia E. "'Largest-Ever' Climate-Change March Rolls Through NYC." *USA Today*, September 21, 2014.

David, Anne. *A Guide to Volunteer Services*. New York: Cornerstone Library, 1970.

Davis, Devra Lee. *The Secret History of the War on Cancer*. New York: BasicBooks, 2007.

Davis, Fred. *Passage Through Crisis: Polio Victims and Their Families*. Indianapolis: Bobbs-Merrill, 1963.

De Figueiredo, John M., and Brian S. Silverman. "How Does the Government (Want to) Fund Science?" In *Science and the University*, edited by Paula E. Stephan and Ronald G. Ehrenberg, 36–51. Madison: University of Wisconsin Press, 2007.

Department of Defense. *Annual Reports, Congressionally Directed Medical Research Program*. 2017. http://cdmrp.army.mil/pubs/annreports/annual_reports.

Department of Defense. "Funding History." 2013. http://cdmrp.army.mil/about/fundinghistory.

Diani, Mario. "Linking Mobilization Frames and Political Opportunities: Insights from Regional Populism in Italy." *American Sociological Review* 61, no. 6 (1996): 1053–69.

Diedrich, Lisa. *Indirect Action: Schizophrenia, Epilepsy, AIDS, and the Course of Health Activism*. Minneapolis: University of Minnesota Press, 2016.

DiMaggio, Paul J., and Walter W. Powell. "The Iron Cage Revisited: Institutional Isomorphism and Collective Rationality in Organizational Fields." *American Sociological Review* 48, no. 2 (1983): 147–60.

Dodge, Christopher D. "Doomed to Repeat: Why Sequestration and the Budget Control Act of 2011 Are Unlikely to Solve Our Solvency Woes." *New York University Journal of Legislation and Public Policy* 15 (2012): 835–80.

Domke, William K., Richard C. Eichenberg, and Catherine M. Kelleher. "The Illusion of Choice: Defense and Welfare in Advanced Industrial Democracies, 1948–1978." *American Political Science Review* 77, no. 1 (1983): 19–35.

Donovan, Mark C. *Taking Aim: Target Populations and the Wars on AIDS and Drugs*. Washington, DC: Georgetown University Press, 2001.

Downey, Dennis. "Elaborating Consensus: Strategic Orientations and Rationales in Wartime Intergroup Relations." *Mobilization: An International Quarterly* 11, no. 3 (2006): 337–56.

Dresser, Rebecca. "Public Advocacy and Allocation of Federal Funds for Biomedical Research." *Milbank Quarterly* 77, no. 2 (1999): 257–74.

Dresser, Rebecca. *When Science Offers Salvation: Patient Advocacy and Research Ethics*. New York: Oxford University Press, 2001.

Drew, Elizabeth Brenner. "The Health Syndicate: 'Washington's Noble Conspirators.'" *Atlantic*, December 1, 1967.

Drinkard, Jim. "Drugmakers Go Furthest to Sway Congress." *USA Today*, April 26, 2005.

Dublin, Louis I. "The Future of the Social Hygiene Movement in America." *Journal of Social Hygiene* 22, no. 2 (1936): 60–69.

Duggan, Lisa. *The Twilight of Equality? Neoliberalism, Cultural Politics, and the Attack on Democracy*. Boston: Beacon Press, 2003.

Dumit, Joseph. "Illnesses You Have to Fight to Get: Facts as Forces in Uncertain, Emergent Illnesses." *Social Science & Medicine* 62, no. 3 (2006): 577–90.

Durnford, Jon. "IRS Documentation—RTF Core File Layout and Mapping for 990 Redesign (Tax Year 2008 and Later)." National Center for Charitable Statistics, February 2011. Accessed February 28, 2017. http://nccsweb.urban.org/knowledgebase/detail.php?linkID=1221&category=13&xrefID=6528&close=0.

Earl, Jennifer, Andrew Martin, John D. McCarthy, and Sarah A. Soule. "The Use of Newspaper Data in the Study of Collective Action." *Annual Review of Sociology* 30 (2004): 65–80.

Eckstein, Harry. *Pressure Group Politics: The Case of the British Medical Association*. Palo Alto, CA: Stanford University Press, 1960.

Edgar, Harold, and David J. Rothman. "New Rules for New Drugs: The Challenge of AIDS to the Regulatory Process." In *A Disease of Society: Cultural and Institutional Responses to AIDS*, edited by Dorothy Nelkin, David P. Willis, and Scott Parris, 84–115. New York: Cambridge University Press, 1991.

Edwards, Bob, and John D. McCarthy. "Resources and Social Movement Mobilization." In *The Blackwell Companion to Social Movements*, edited by David A. Snow, Sarah A. Soule, and Hanspeter Kriesi, 116–52. Oxford: Wiley-Blackwell, 2004.

Ehrenreich, Barbara. "Welcome to Cancerland: A Mammogram Leads to a Cult of Pink Kitsch." *Harper's Magazine*, November 2001.

Eichenberg, Richard C. "Do We yet Know Who Pays for Defense? Conclusions and Synthesis." In *Defense, Welfare, and Growth*, edited by Steve Chan and Alex Mintz, 231–41. London and New York: Routledge, 1992.

Einwohner, Rachel L. "Practices, Opportunity, and Protest Effectiveness: Illustrations from Four Animal Rights Campaigns." *Social Problems* 46 (1999): 169.

Eliasoph, Nina. *Avoiding Politics: How Americans Produce Apathy in Everyday Life*. Cambridge and New York: Cambridge University Press, 1998.

Eliasoph, Nina. *Making Volunteers: Civic Life After Welfare's End*. Princeton, NJ: Princeton University Press, 2011.

EPSCoR/IDeA Foundation. "National Institutes of Health." November 30, 2015. http://www.epscorideafoundation.org/about/agencies/nih-idea.

Epstein, Steven. *Impure Science: AIDS, Activism, and the Politics of Knowledge*. Berkeley: University of California Press, 1996.

Epstein, Steven. *Inclusion: The Politics of Difference in Medical Research*. Chicago: University of Chicago Press, 2007.

Epstein, Steven. "Measuring Success: Scientific, Institutional, and Cultural Effects of Patient Advocacy." In *Patients as Policy Actors*, edited by Beatrix Hoffman, Nancy Tomes, Rachel Grob, and Mark Schlesinger, 257–77. New Brunswick, NJ: Rutgers University Press, 2011.

Epstein, Steven. "Patient Groups and Health Movements." In *Handbook of Science and Technology Studies*, edited by E. J. Hackett, O. Amsterdamska, M. Lynch, and J. Wajcman, 499–539. Cambridge, MA: MIT Press, 2008.

Epstein, Steven. "The Politics of Health Mobilization in the United States: The Promise and Pitfalls of 'Disease Constituencies.'" *Social Science & Medicine* 165 (2016): 246–54.

Espeland, Wendy Nelson, and Mitchell L. Stevens. "Commensuration as a Social Process." *Annual Review of Sociology* 24 (1998): 313–43.

Etheridge, Elizabeth W. *Sentinel for Health: A History of the Centers for Disease Control*. Berkeley: University of California Press, 1992.

Exworthy, Mark, and David J. Hunter. "The Challenge of Joined-Up Government in Tackling Health Inequalities." *International Journal of Public Administration* 34, no. 4 (2011): 201–12.

Fallows, James. "The Political Scientist." *New Yorker*, June 7, 1999.

Fee, Elizabeth. "Public Health and the State: The United States." In *The History of Public Health and the Modern State*, edited by Dorothy Porter, 224–75. Amsterdam, the Netherlands, and Atlanta, GA: Editions Rodopi, 1994.

Ferraro, Susan. "The Anguished Politics of Breast Cancer." *New York Times Magazine*, September 19, 1993.

Ferree, Myra Marx. "Resonance and Radicalism: Feminist Framing in the Abortion Debates of the United States and Germany." *American Journal of Sociology* 109, no. 2 (2003): 304–44.

Finer, Samuel Edward. "The Anonymous Empire." *Political Studies* 6, no. 1 (1958): 16–32.

Fischer, Claude S. *Made in America: A Social History of American Culture and Character.* Chicago: University of Chicago Press, 2010.

Fleischer, Doris Zames, and Frieda Zames. *Disability Rights Movement: From Charity to Confrontation.* Philadelphia: Temple University Press, 2001.

Fletcher, Robert, and Suzanne W. Fletcher. *Clinical Epidemiology: The Essentials.* Philadelphia: Lippincott Williams & Wilkins, 2013.

Flick, Ella M. E. *Beloved Crusader: Lawrence F. Flick, Physician.* Philadelphia: Dorrance & Company, 1944.

Foreman, Christopher H. "Grassroots Victim Organizations: Mobilizing for Personal and Public Health." In *Interest Group Politics*, edited by Allan. J. Cigler and Burdett. A. Loomis, 4th ed., 33–53. Washington, DC: Congressional Quarterly Press, 1995.

Fox, Patrick. "From Senility to Alzheimer's Disease: The Rise of the Alzheimer's Disease Movement." *Milbank Quarterly* 67, no. 1 (1989): 58–102.

Franklin, Daniel P. *Making Ends Meet: Congressional Budgeting in the Age of Deficits.* Washington, DC: Congressional Quarterly Press, 1993.

Freeman, Jo. "The Origins of the Women's Liberation Movement." *American Journal of Sociology* 78, no. 4 (1973): 792–811.

Frickel, Scott, and Kelly Moore. "Prospects and Challenges for a New Political Sociology of Science." In *The New Political Sociology of Science*, edited by Scott Frickel and Kelly Moore, 299–323. Madison: University of Wisconsin Press, 2006.

Friedman, Lawrence J. "Philanthropy in America: Historicism and Its Discontents." In *Charity, Philanthropy, and Civility in American History*, edited by Lawrence J. Friedman and Mark D. McGarvie, 1–21. Cambridge and New York: Cambridge University Press, 2003.

Frist, Bill. "Setting Biomedical Research Priorities at the National Institutes of Health." *FASEB Newsletter* (December 1997). http://www.faseb.org/portals/2/pdfs/opa/4x12x97.pdf.

Froelich, Karen A., Terry W. Knoepfle, and Thomas H. Pollak. "Financial Measures in Nonprofit Organization Research: Comparing IRS 990 Return and Audited Financial Statement Data." *Nonprofit and Voluntary Sector Quarterly* 29, no. 2 (2000): 232–54.

Fung, Archon. "Associations and Democracy: Between Theories, Hopes, and Realities." *Annual Review of Sociology* 29, no. 1 (2003): 515–39.

Funkhouser, G. Ray. "The Issues of the Sixties: An Exploratory Study in the Dynamics of Public Opinion." *Public Opinion Quarterly* 37, no. 1 (1973): 62–75.

Furberg, Curt D. "Challenges to the Funding of Prevention Research." *Preventive Medicine* 23, no. 5 (1994): 599–601.

Furtado, Claudia D., Diego A. Aguirre, Claude B. Sirlin, David Dang, Stephan K. Stamato, Patrick Lee, Farhad Sani, Michelle A. Brown, David L. Levin, and Giovanna Casola. "Whole-Body CT Screening: Spectrum of Findings and Recommendations in 1192 Patients." *Radiology* 237, no. 2 (2005): 385–94.

Gamson, Josh. "Silence, Death, and the Invisible Enemy: AIDS Activism and Social Movement 'Newness.'" *Social Problems* 36, no. 4 (1989): 351–67.

Gamson, Joshua, and Dawne Moon. "The Sociology of Sexualities: Queer and Beyond." *Annual Review of Sociology* 30, no. 1 (2004): 47–64.

Gamson, William A. "Hiroshima, the Holocaust, and the Politics of Exclusion." *American Sociological Review* 60, no. 1 (1995): 1–20.

Gamson, William A. "The Social Psychology of Collective Action." In *Frontiers in Social Movement Theory*, edited by Aldon D. Morris and Carol McClurg Mueller, 53–76. New Haven, CT: Yale University Press, 1992.

Gamson, William A. *The Strategy of Social Protest*. 2nd ed. Belmont, CA: Wadsworth, 1990.

Gamson, William A., and David S. Meyer. "Framing Political Opportunity." In *Comparative Perspectives on Social Movements: Political Opportunities, Mobilizing Structures, and Cultural Framings*, edited by Doug McAdam, John D. McCarthy, and Mayer N. Zald, 275–90. Cambridge and New York: Cambridge University Press, 1996.

Gardner, Kirsten E. *Early Detection: Women, Cancer, and Awareness Campaigns in the Twentieth-Century United States*. Chapel Hill: University of North Carolina Press, 2006.

Gerth, Jeff, and Sheryl Gay Stolberg. "Drug Firms Reap Profits on Tax-Backed Research." *New York Times*, April 23, 2000.

Ghaziani, Amin, and Delia Baldassarri. "Cultural Anchors and the Organization of Differences." *American Sociological Review* 76, no. 2 (2011): 179–206.

Gibbon, Sahra, and Carlos Novas. "Introduction: Biosocialities, Genetics and the Social Sciences." In *Biosocialities, Genetics and the Social Sciences: Making Biologies and Identities*, edited by Sahra Gibbon and Carlos Novas, 1–18. New York and London: Routledge, 2008.

Giddens, Anthony. *Modernity and Self-Identity: Self and Society in the Late Modern Age*. Cambridge: Polity Press, 1991.

Gifford, Brian. "Why No Trade-off Between 'Guns and Butter'? Armed Forces and Social Spending in the Advanced Industrial Democracies, 1960–1993." *American Journal of Sociology* 112, no. 2 (2006): 473–509.

Gilens, Martin. *Why Americans Hate Welfare*. Chicago: University of Chicago Press, 1999.

Gillum, Leslie A., Christopher Gouveia, E. Ray Dorsey, Mark Pletcher, Colin D. Mathers, Charles E. McCulloch, and S. Claiborne Johnston. "NIH Disease Funding Levels and Burden of Disease." *PLoS One* 6, no. 2 (2011): e16837.

Ginzberg, Eli, and Anna B. Dutka. *The Financing of Biomedical Research*. Baltimore, MD: Johns Hopkins University Press, 1989.

Gitlin, Todd. "From Universality to Difference: Notes on the Fragmentation of the New Left." In *Social Theory and the Politics of Identity*, edited by Craig Calhoun, 150–74. Cambridge, MA, and Oxford: Wiley-Blackwell, 1994.

Gitlin, Todd. *The Twilight of Common Dreams: Why America Is Wracked by Culture Wars*. New York: Holt Paperbacks, 1996.

Giugni, Marco. "How Social Movements Matter: Past Research, Present Problems, Future Developments." In *How Social Movements Matter*, edited by Marco Giugni, Doug Mcadam, and Charles Tilly, xiii–xxxiii. Minneapolis: University of Minnesota Press, 1999.

Giugni, Marco. *Social Protest and Policy Change: Ecology, Antinuclear, and Peace Movements in Comparative Perspective*. Lanham, MD: Rowman & Littlefield, 2004.

Gladwell, Malcolm. "Beyond HIV: The Legacies of Health Activism: Over a Decade, AIDS Battle Has Had Profound Impact on U.S. Regulation, Law and Society." *Washington Post*, October 15, 1992.

Globe and Mail. "AIDS Walk Aims to Raise $1.8 Million." August 22, 1983.

Goffman, Erving. *Stigma: Notes on the Management of Spoiled Identity*. New York: Simon and Schuster, 1986.

Gold, Marthe R., David Stevenson, and Dennis G. Fryback. "HALYS and QALYS and DALYS, Oh My: Similarities and Differences in Summary Measures of Population Health." *Annual Review of Public Health* 23, no. 1 (2002): 115–34.

Goldstone, Jack A. *States, Parties, and Social Movements*. New York: Cambridge University Press, 2003.

Goodman, Lenn E., and Madeleine J. Goodman. "Prevention—How Misuse of a Concept Undercuts Its Worth." *Hastings Center Report* 16, no. 2 (1986): 26–38.

Goodwin, Jeff, and James M. Jasper, eds. *Rethinking Social Movements: Structure, Meaning, and Emotion*. Lanham, MD: Rowman & Littlefield, 2004.

Gordon, Colin. *Dead on Arrival: The Politics of Health Care in Twentieth-Century America*. Princeton, NJ: Princeton University Press, 2003.

Gould, Deborah B. *Moving Politics: Emotion and ACT UP's Fight against AIDS*. Chicago: University of Chicago Press, 2009.

Grady, Denise. "Panel Reasserts Mammogram Advice That Triggered Breast Cancer Debate." *New York Times*, January 11, 2016.

Gray, Bradford H. "A Puzzlement: Health-Related Organisations in the Nonprofit Almanac." *Voluntas: International Journal of Voluntary and Nonprofit Organizations* 4, no. 2 (1993): 210–20.

Gray, Virginia, and David Lowery. "The Demography of Interest Organization Communities." *American Politics Research* 23, no. 1 (1995): 3–32.

Gray, Virginia, and David Lowery. *The Population Ecology of Interest Representation: Lobbying Communities in the American States*. Ann Arbor: University of Michigan Press, 1996.

Green, Jesse. "The Year of the Ribbon." *New York Times*, May 3, 1992.

Greenberg, Daniel S. *Science, Money, and Politics: Political Triumph and Ethical Erosion*. Chicago: University of Chicago Press, 2001.

Griffith, Dorsey. "Lung Cancer Patients Fight Societal Neglect." *Sacramento Bee*, December 5, 2005.

Grønbjerg, Kirsten A. "Evaluating Nonprofit Databases." *American Behavioral Scientist* 45, no. 11 (2002): 1741.

Grønbjerg, Kirsten A. "Using NTEE to Classify Non-Profit Organisations: An Assessment of Human Service and Regional Applications." *Voluntas: International Journal of Voluntary and Nonprofit Organizations* 5, no. 3 (1994): 301–28.

Grønbjerg, Kirsten A., and Richard M. Clerkin. "Examining the Landscape of Indiana's Nonprofit Sector: Does What You Know Depend on Where You Look?" *Nonprofit and Voluntary Sector Quarterly* 34, no. 2 (2005): 232–59.

Grønbjerg, Kirsten A., and Steven Rathgeb Smith. "Nonprofit Organizations and Public Policies in the Delivery of Human Services." In *Philanthropy and the Nonprofit Sector in a Changing America*, edited by Charles Clotfelter and Thomas Ehrlich, 139–71. Bloomington: Indiana University Press, 1999.

Gross, Cary P., Gerard F. Anderson, and Neil R. Powe. "The Relation Between Funding by the National Institutes of Health and the Burden of Disease." *New England Journal of Medicine* 340, no. 24 (1999): 1881–87.

Gross, Jane. "Turning Disease into Political Cause: First AIDS, and Now Breast Cancer." *New York Times*, January 7, 1991.

Gross, Robert A. "Giving in America: From Charity to Philanthropy." In *Charity, Philanthropy, and Civility in American History*, edited by Lawrence J. Friedman and Mark D. McGarvie, 29–48. New York and Cambridge: Cambridge University Press, 2003.

Guetzkow, Joshua. "Beyond Deservingness: Congressional Discourse on Poverty, 1964—1996." *Annals of the American Academy of Political and Social Science* 629, no. 1 (2010): 173–97.

Gunn, Selskar M., and Philip S. Platt. *Voluntary Health Agencies*. New York: Ronald Press Company, 1945.

Gurr, Ted Robert. *Why Men Rebel*. Princeton, NJ: Princeton University Press, 1970.

Gusfield, Joseph R. "Constructing the Ownership of Social Problems: Fun and Profit in the Welfare State." *Social Problems* 36, no. 5 (1989): 431–41.

Gusfield, Joseph R. *The Culture of Public Problems: Drinking-Driving and the Symbolic Order*. Chicago: University of Chicago Press, 1981.

Gussow, Zachary, and George S. Tracy. "The Role of Self-Help Clubs in Adaptation to Chronic Illness and Disability." *Social Science & Medicine* 10, no. 7-8 (1976): 407–14.

Guston, David H. *Between Politics and Science: Assuring the Integrity and Productivity of Research*. New York: Cambridge University Press, 2000.

Hacker, Jacob S., and Paul Pierson. "Winner-Take-All Politics: Public Policy, Political Organization, and the Precipitous Rise of Top Incomes in the United States." *Politics & Society* 38, no. 2 (2010): 152–204.

Hager, Mark A., Sarah Wilson, Thomas H. Pollak, and Patrick Michael Rooney. "Response Rates for Mail Surveys of Nonprofit Organizations: A Review and Empirical Test." *Nonprofit and Voluntary Sector Quarterly* 32, no. 2 (2003): 252–67.

Haines, Herbert H. "Black Radicalization and the Funding of Civil Rights: 1957–1970." *Social Problems* 32, no. 1 (1984): 31–43.

Haines, Herbert H. "Cognitive Claims-Making, Enclosure, and the Depoliticization of Social Problems." *Sociological Quarterly* 20, no. 1 (1979): 119–30.

Hall, Fred S., ed. *Social Work Year Book 1929*. New York: Russell Sage Foundation, 1930.

Hall, Peter Dobkin. "A Historical Overview of Philanthropy, Voluntary Associations, and Nonprofit Organizations in the United States, 1600–2000." In *The Nonprofit Sector: A Research Handbook*, edited by Walter W. Powell and Professor Richard Steinberg, 2nd ed., 32–65. New Haven, CT: Yale University Press, 2006.

Halpin, Darren. "Explaining Policy Bandwagons: Organized Interest Mobilization and Cascades of Attention." *Governance* 24, no. 2 (2011): 205–30.

Halpin, Darren R., Bert Fraussen, and Anthony J. Nownes. "The Balancing Act of Establishing a Policy Agenda: Conceptualizing and Measuring Drivers of Issue Prioritization Within Interest Groups." *Governance* 31, no. 2 (2018): 215–37.

Hamlin, Robert H. *Voluntary Health and Welfare Agencies in the United States: An Exploratory Study*. New York: Schoolmasters' Press, 1961.

Harden, Victoria Angela. *Inventing the NIH: Federal Biomedical Research Policy, 1887–1937*. Baltimore, MD: Johns Hopkins University Press, 1986.

Harris, Gardiner. "Drug Makers Are Advocacy Group's Biggest Donors." *New York Times*, October 22, 2009.

Harris, Gardiner. "U.S. Panel Advises Against Routine Prostate Test." *New York Times*, October 6, 2011.

Hart-Brinson, Peter. "New Ways of Bowling Together." *Contexts* 10, no. 4 (Fall 2011): 28–33.

Haveman, Heather A., Hayagreeva Rao, and Srikanth Paruchuri. "The Winds of Change: The Progressive Movement and the Bureaucratization of Thrift." *American Sociological Review* 72, no. 1 (2007): 117–42.

Havemann, Judith. "Crusading for Cash: Patient Groups Compete for Bigger Shares of NIH's Research Funding." *Washington Post*, December 15, 1998, Z10.

Hayes, Michael T. *Lobbyists and Legislators: A Theory of Political Markets*. New Brunswick, NJ: Rutgers University Press, 1981.

Heaney, Michael T., and Fabio Rojas. "Hybrid Activism: Social Movement Mobilization in a Multimovement Environment." *American Journal of Sociology* 119, no. 4 (2014): 1047–1103.

Heath, Deborah, Rayna Rapp, and Karen-Sue Taussig. "Genetic Citizenship." In *A Companion to the Anthropology of Politics*, edited by David Nugent and Joan. Vincent, 152–67. Malden, MA: Blackwell, 2004.

Heimer, Carol A. "Social Structure, Psychology, and the Estimation of Risk." *Annual Review of Sociology* 14, no. 1 (1988): 491–517.

Heinz, John P., Edward O. Laumann, Robert L. Nelson, and Robert H. Salisbury. *The Hollow Core: Private Interests in National Policy Making*. Cambridge, MA: Harvard University Press, 1993.

Hemminki, Elina, Hanna K. Toiviainen, and Lauri Vuorenkoski. "Co-Operation Between Patient Organisations and the Drug Industry in Finland." *Social Science & Medicine* 70, no. 8 (2010): 1171–75.

Henderson, Diedtra. "Drug Firms' Funding of Advocates Often Escapes Government Scrutiny." *Boston Globe*, March 18, 2007.

Herxheimer, Andrew. "Relationships Between the Pharmaceutical Industry and Patients' Organisations." *British Medical Journal* 326, no. 7400 (2003): 1208–10.

Hess, David J. "Antiangiogenesis Research and the Dynamics of Scientific Fields: Historical and Institutional Perspectives on the Sociology of Science." In *The New Political Sociology of Science*, edited by Scott Frickel and Kelly Moore, 122–47. Madison: University of Wisconsin Press, 2006.

Hess, David J. "Beyond Scientific Controversies: Scientific Counterpublics, Countervailing Industries, and Undone Science." In *The Public Shaping of Medical Research: Patient Associations, Health Movements and Biomedicine*, edited by Peter Wehling, Willy Viehover, and Sophia Koenen, 151–71. London: Routledge, 2015.

Hess, David J. "Medical Modernisation, Scientific Research Fields and the Epistemic Politics of Health Social Movements." *Sociology of Health and Illness* 26, no. 6 (2004): 695–709.

Hess, David, Steve Breyman, Nancy Campbell, and Brian Martin. "Science, Technology, and Social Movements." In *Handbook of Science and Technology Studies*, edited by E. J. Hackett, O. Amsterdamska, M. Lynch, and J. Wajcman, 473–97. Cambridge, MA: MIT Press, 2008.

Hilgartner, Stephen, and Charles L. Bosk. "The Rise and Fall of Social Problems: A Public Arenas Model." *American Journal of Sociology* 94, no. 1 (1988): 53–78.

Hiscock, Ira V. "Opportunities of Voluntary Health Agencies, with Special Reference to Social Hygiene." *Journal of Social Hygiene* 22, no. 2 (1936): 49–59.

Hobsbawm, Eric. "Identity Politics and the Left." *New Left Review* 217 (1996): 38–47.

Hoffman, Beatrix. *Health Care for Some: Rights and Rationing in the United States Since 1930*. Chicago and London: University of Chicago Press, 2012.

Hoffman, Beatrix. "Health Care Reform and Social Movements in the United States." *American Journal of Public Health* 93, no. 1 (2003): 75–85.

Hogg, Christine. *Patients, Power & Politics: From Patients to Citizens*. London and Thousand Oaks, CA: Sage Publications, 1999.

Hojnacki, Marie, David C. Kimball, Frank R. Baumgartner, Jeffrey M. Berry, and Beth L. Leech. "Studying Organizational Advocacy and Influence: Reexamining Interest Group Research." *Annual Review of Political Science* 15 (2012): 379–99.

hooks, bell. *Talking Back: Thinking Feminist, Thinking Black*. Boston: South End Press, 1989.

Hsu, Greta, Michael T. Hannan, and Özgecan Koçak. "Multiple Category Memberships in Markets: An Integrative Theory and Two Empirical Tests." *American Sociological Review* 74, no. 1 (2009): 150–69.

Huber, Evelyne, and John D. Stephens. *Development and Crisis of the Welfare State: Parties and Policies in Global Markets*. Chicago: University of Chicago Press, 2001.

Hughes, Gary, and Liz Minchin. "Drug Giants' Big-Money Pitch Exposed." *The Age*, December 13, 2003.

Huyard, Caroline. "How Did Uncommon Disorders Become 'Rare Diseases'? History of a Boundary Object." *Sociology of Health & Illness* 31, no. 4 (2009): 463–77.

Institute for Health Metrics and Evaluation. "Global Burden of Disease Study 2015 Data Input Sources Tool." Accessed February 1, 2017. http://ghdx.healthdata.org/gbd-2015/data-input-sources.

Insel, Thomas R., Nora Volkow, and Ting-Kai Li. "Research Funding: The View from NIH." *American Journal of Psychiatry* 163, no. 12 (2006): 2043–45.

Institute of Medicine. "For the Public's Health: Investing in a Healthier Future." Washington, DC: National Academies Press, 2012.

Institute of Medicine. *Scientific Opportunities and Public Needs: Improving Priority Setting and Public Input at the National Institutes of Health*. Washington, DC: National Academies Press, 1998.

Internal Revenue Service. "Exempt Organizations Annual Reporting Requirements." Accessed January 12, 2017. https://www.irs.gov/pub/irs-tege/faqs_annualreporting_overview.pdf.

Internal Revenue Service. "Lobbying." 2018. https://www.irs.gov/charities-non-profits/lobbying.

Istook, Ernest, Jr. "Research Funding on Major Diseases Is Not Proportionate to Taxpayers' Needs." *Journal of NIH Research* 9 (1997): 26–28.

Jain, S. Lochlann. "Be Prepared." In *Against Health: How Health Became the New Morality*, edited by Jonathan M. Metzl and Anna Kirkland, 170–82. New York: New York University Press, 2010.

Jenkins, Edward Corbin. *Philanthropy in America: An Introduction to the Practices and Prospects of Organizations Supported by Gifts and Endowments, 1924–1948.* New York: Association Press, 1950.

Jenkins, J. Craig. "Nonprofit Organizations and Political Advocacy." In *The Nonprofit Sector: A Research Handbook*, edited by Walter W. Powell and Richard Steinberg, 2nd ed., 307–32. New Haven, CT: Yale University Press, 2006.

Jenkins, J. Craig. "Radical Transformation of Organizational Goals." *Administrative Science Quarterly* 22, no. 4 (1977): 568–86.

Jenkins, J. Craig. "Resource Mobilization Theory and the Study of Social Movements." *Annual Review of Sociology* 9, no. 1 (1983): 527–53.

Jennings, Will, and Christopher Wlezien. "Distinguishing Between Most Important Problems and Issues." *Public Opinion Quarterly* 75, no. 3 (2011): 545–55.

Johnson, Erik W., and Scott Frickel. "Ecological Threat and the Founding of US National Environmental Movement Organizations, 1962–1998." *Social Problems* 58, no. 3 (2011): 305–29.

Johnson, Judith A. *AIDS and Other Diseases: Selected Federal Spending and Morbidity and Mortality Statistics.* Washington, DC: Congressional Research Service, 1994.

Johnson, Judith A. *Breast Cancer Research.* Washington, DC: Congressional Research Service, 1996.

Johnson, Judith A. *Disease Funding and NIH Priority Setting.* Washington, DC: Congressional Research Service, 1998.

Johnson, Michael P., and Karl Hufbauer. "Sudden Infant Death Syndrome as a Medical Research Problem Since 1945." *Social Problems* 30, no. 1 (1982): 65–81.

Jones, Bryan D., and Frank R. Baumgartner. *The Politics of Attention: How Government Prioritizes Problems.* Chicago: University of Chicago Press, 2005.

Jones, Kathryn. "In Whose Interest? Relationships Between Health Consumer Groups and the Pharmaceutical Industry in the UK." *Sociology of Health & Illness* 30, no. 6 (2008): 929–43.

Jørgensen, Karsten Juhl, and Peter C. Gøtzsche. "Presentation on Websites of Possible Benefits and Harms from Screening for Breast Cancer: Cross Sectional Study." *BMJ* 328, no. 7432 (2004): 148.

Jung, Wooseok, Brayden G. King, and Sarah A. Soule. "Issue Bricolage: Explaining the Configuration of the Social Movement Sector, 1960–1995." *American Journal of Sociology* 120, no. 1 (2014): 187–225.

Juvenile Diabetes Research Foundation. "JDRF Advocacy." Accessed December 22, 2016. http://www.jdrf.org/get-involved/advocacy/.

Kaiser Family Foundation. *Americans Distrust Government, but Want It to Do More.* 2000. https://kaiserfamilyfoundation.files.wordpress.com/2013/01/americans-trust-government-but-want-it-to-do-more.pdf.

Kaiser, Jocelyn. "A Bumpy Landing for Cancer Research." *Science* 303 (2004): 936–37.

Kaiser, Jocelyn. "Bid to Boost NIH Budget Fails in Senate." *Science* 301 (2003): 1647.

Kaiser, Jocelyn. "NIH Hopes Stimulus Isn't a Roller-Coaster Ride." *Science* 326 (2009): 1179–80.

Kaiser, Jocelyn. "NIH Set for Tiny Spending Hike in 2006." *Science* 310 (2005): 1256.

Kaiser, Jocelyn. "What Does a Disease Deserve?" *Science* 350 (2015): 900–902.

Kaiser, Jocelyn, David Malakoff, Erik Stokstad, Charles Siefe, Yudhijit Bhattacharjee, and Jeffrey Mervis. "2005 Budget Makes Flat a Virtue." *Science* 303 (2004): 748–50.

Kaitin, KI. "Deconstructing the Drug Development Process: The New Face of Innovation." *Clinical Pharmacology and Therapeutics* 87, no. 3 (2010): 356–61.

Kalberer, John T., and Michael D. Parkinson. "Workshop H: Involvement of Other PHS Agencies and Professional Societies in Prevention Research." *Preventive Medicine* 23, no. 5 (1994): 566–68.

Kamlet, Mark S., and David C. Mowery. "The Budgetary Base in Federal Resource Allocation." *American Journal of Political Science* 24, no. 4 (1980): 804–21.

Kamlet, Mark S., and David C. Mowery. "Influences on Executive and Congressional Budgetary Priorities, 1955–1981." *American Political Science Review* 81, no. 1 (1987): 155–78.

Kastor, John. *The National Institutes of Health: 1991–2008*. New York: Oxford University Press, 2010.

Katz, Alfred H. "Self-Help and Mutual Aid: An Emerging Social Movement?" *Annual Review of Sociology* 7 (1981): 129–55.

Katz, Alfred Hyman. *Self-Help in America: A Social Movement Perspective*. Woodbridge, CT: Twayne, 1993.

Kaufert, Patricia A. "Women, Resistance, and the Breast Cancer Movement." In *Pragmatic Women and Body Politics*, edited by Margaret Lock and Patricia A. Kaufert, 287–309. Cambridge: Cambridge University Press, 1998.

Kay Dickersin Papers. "August 15, 1991 meeting minutes (Federal Public Policy Task Force)." 1991a. Box 4, Folder 8. NBCC Working Board, Cambridge, MA.

Kay Dickersin Papers. "Board of Directors meeting, June 13, 1992." 1992. Box 4, Folder 10. NBCC Working Board, Cambridge, MA.

Kay Dickersin Papers. "History, Goals, Accomplishments." n.d. Box 13, Folder 10. NBCC History & General Info, Cambridge, MA.

Kay Dickersin Papers. "Memo to NBCC state coordinators from Fran Visco, March 24." 1994. Box 5, Folder 3. NBCC Working Board, Cambridge, MA.

Kay Dickersin Papers. "National Breast Cancer Coalition meeting, January 9." 1993. Box 5, Folder 3. NBCC Working Board, Cambridge, MA.

Kay Dickersin Papers. "Working Board meeting, Chicago, IL, July 25." 1991b. Box 4, Folder 8. NBCC Working Board, Cambridge, MA.

Kayal, Philip M. *Bearing Witness: Gay Men's Health Crisis and the Politics of AIDS*. Boulder, CO: Westview Press, 1993.

Kedrowski, Karen M., and Marilyn S. Sarow. *Cancer Activism: Gender, Media, and Public Policy*. Chicago: University of Illinois Press, 2007.

Keller, Ann C., and Laura Packel. "Going for the Cure: Patient Interest Groups and Health Advocacy in the United States." *Journal of Health Politics, Policy and Law* 39, no. 2 (2014): 331–67.

Kempner, Joanna. *Not Tonight: Migraine and the Politics of Gender and Health*. Chicago and London: University of Chicago Press, 2014.

King, Brayden G., Keith G. Bentele, and Sarah A. Soule. "Protest and Policymaking: Explaining Fluctuation in Congressional Attention to Rights Issues, 1960–1986." *Social Forces* 86, no. 1 (2007): 137–63.

King, Samantha. *Pink Ribbons, Inc.: Breast Cancer and the Politics of Philanthropy*. Minneapolis: University of Minnesota Press, 2006.

Kingdon, John W. *Agendas, Alternatives, and Public Policies*. New York: HarperCollins, 1984.

Kintisch, Eli. "Science Wins $21 Billion Boost as Stimulus Package Becomes Law." *Science* 323 (2009): 992–93.

Kintisch, Eli, and Jeffrey Mervis. "A Budget with Big Winners and Losers." *Science* 311 (2006): 762–64.

Klandermans, Bert. "The Social Construction of Protest and Multiorganizational Fields." In *Frontiers in Social Movement Theory*, edited by Aldon D. Morris and Carol McClurg Mueller, 77–103. New Haven, CT: Yale University Press, 1992.

Klawiter, Maren. *The Biopolitics of Breast Cancer: Changing Cultures of Disease and Activism*. Minneapolis: University of Minnesota Press, 2008.

Knopf, Sigard Adolphus. *A History of the National Tuberculosis Association: The Anti-Tuberculosis Movement in the United States*. New York: National Tuberculosis Association, 1922.

Koay, Pei P., and Richard R. Sharp. "The Role of Patient Advocacy Organizations in Shaping Genomic Science." *Annual Review of Genomics and Human Genetics* 14 (2013): 579–95.

Kolata, Gina. "Congress, NIH Open Coffers for AIDS." *Science* 221, no. 4609 (1983): 436–38.

Kolata, Gina. "Mammogram Debate Moving from Test's Merits to Its Cost." *New York Times*, December 27, 1993.

Kolker, Emily S. "Framing as a Cultural Resource in Health Social Movements: Funding Activism and the Breast Cancer Movement in the US 1990–1993." *Sociology of Health & Illness* 26, no. 6 (2004): 820–44.

Koopmans, Ruud, and Paul Statham. "Ethnic and Civic Conceptions of Nationhood and the Differential Success of the Extreme Right in Germany and Italy." In *How Social Movements Matter*, edited by Marco Giugni, Doug Mcadam, and Charles Tilly, 225–51. Minneapolis: University of Minnesota Press, 1999.

Kroll-Smith, J. Stephen, and H. Hugh Floyd. *Bodies in Protest: Environmental Illness and the Struggle over Medical Knowledge*. New York: New York University Press, 2000.

Kurtz, Russell H., ed. *Social Work Year Book 1939*. New York: Russell Sage Foundation, 1939.

Kushner, Howard I. "Competing Medical Cultures, Patient Support Groups, and the Construction of Tourette Syndrome." In *Emerging Illnesses and Society: Negotiating the Public Health Agenda*, edited by Randall M. Packard, Peter J. Brown, Ruth L. Berkelman, and Howard Frumkin, 39–70. Baltimore, MD: Johns Hopkins University Press, 2004.

Kushner, Rose. *Breast Cancer: A Personal History and an Investigative Report*. New York: Harcourt Brace Jovanovich, 1975.

Laffont, Kim. "Steady Progress." *University of Miami Medicine Magazine* 9, no. 2 (Summer 2007). http://www6.miami.edu/ummedicine-magazine/summer2007/featurestory3.html

Lake, David A., and Wendy H. Wong. "The Politics of Networks: Interests, Power, and Human Rights Norms." In *Networked Politics: Agency, Power, and Governance*, edited by Miles Kahler, 127–50. Ithaca, NY: Cornell University Press, 2009.

Lamont, Michèle. "Toward a Comparative Sociology of Valuation and Evaluation." *Annual Review of Sociology* 38, no. 1 (2012): 201–21.

Landzelius, Kyra. "Patient Organization Movements and New Metamorphoses in Patienthood." *Social Science & Medicine* 62, no. 3 (2006): 529–37.

Langstrup, Henriette. "Interpellating Patients as Future Users of Biomedical Technologies: The Case of Patient Associations and Stem Cell Research." In *The Public Shaping of Medical Research: Patient Associations, Health Movements and Biomedicine*, edited by Peter Wehling, Willy Viehover, and Sophia Koenen, 172–90. London: Routledge, 2015.

Larson, Jeff, and Sarah Soule. "Sector-Level Dynamics and Collective Action in the United States, 1965–1975." *Mobilization: An International Quarterly* 14, no. 3 (2009): 293–314.

Lauer, Mike. "NIH's Commitment to Basic Science." *Extramural Nexus* (blog), National Institutes of health, March 25, 2016. https://nexus.od.nih.gov/all/2016/03/25/nihs-commitment-to-basic-science/.

Lawler, Andrew. "Congress Targets Fusion, Favors NIH." *Science* 273 (1996a): 303–4.

Lawler, Andrew. "GOP Plans Would Reshuffle Science." *Science* 268 (1995): 964–67.

Lawler, Andrew. "Research Knows No Season as Budget Cycle Goes Awry." *Science* 271 (1996b): 589.

Lawler, Andrew. "Science Catches Clinton's Eye." *Science* 279 (1998a): 794–97.

Lawler, Andrew. "Senate Panel Backs Large NIH Increase." *Science* 279 (1998b): 2035.

Lawler, Andrew, and Jeffrey Mervis. "House Panel Homes in on NIH." *Science* 267 (1995): 1759.

Lawler, Andrew, Jeffrey Mervis, Charles Seife, Jocelyn Kaiser, Constance Holden, and Yudhijit Bhattacharjee. "Science Agencies Caught in Postelection Spending Squeeze." *Science* 306 (2004): 1662–63.

Layne, Linda L. "Pregnancy and Infant Loss Support: A New, Feminist, American, Patient Movement?" *Social Science & Medicine* 62, no. 3 (2006): 602–13.

Lear, John. "The Business of Giving." *Saturday Review*, December 2, 1961.

Lebel, Sophie, and Gerald M. Devins. "Stigma in Cancer Patients Whose Behavior May Have Contributed to Their Disease." *Future Oncology* 4, no. 5 (2008): 717–33.

Leech, Beth L. "Lobbying and Influence." In *The Oxford Handbook of American Political Parties and Interest Groups*, edited by L. Sandy Maisel and Jeffrey M. Berry, 534–51. New York: Oxford University Press, 2010.

Leichter, Howard M. "'Evil Habits' and 'Personal Choices': Assigning Responsibility for Health in the 20th Century." *Milbank Quarterly* 81, no. 4 (2003): 603–26.

Lenfant, Claude, Lawrence Friedman, and Thomas Thom. "Fifty Years of Death Certificates: The Framingham Heart Study." *Annals of Internal Medicine* 129, no. 12 (1998): 1066–67.

Leopold, Ellen. *A Darker Ribbon: Breast Cancer, Women, and Their Doctors in the Twentieth Century*. Boston: Beacon Press, 1999.

Lerner, Barron H. *The Breast Cancer Wars: Hope, Fear, and the Pursuit of a Cure in Twentieth-Century America*. New York: Oxford University Press, 2001.

Levitsky, Sandra R. *Caring for Our Own: Why There Is No Political Demand for New American Social Welfare Rights*. New York: Oxford University Press, 2014.

Levitsky, Sandra R. "Niche Activism: Constructing a Unified Movement Identity in a Heterogeneous Organizational Field." *Mobilization: An International Quarterly* 12, no. 3 (2007): 271–86.

Levitsky, Sandra R., and Jane Banaszak-Holl. "Introduction." In *Social Movements and the Transformation of American Health Care*, edited by Jane C. Banaszak-Holl, Sandra R. Levitsky, and Mayer N. Zald, 3–22. New York: Oxford University Press, 2010.

Ley, Barbara L. *From Pink to Green: Disease Prevention and the Environmental Breast Cancer Movement*. New Brunswick, NJ: Rutgers University Press, 2009.

Leyden, Kevin M. "Interest Group Resources and Testimony at Congressional Hearings." *Legislative Studies Quarterly* 20, no. 3 (1995): 431–39.

Li, Jie Jack. *Triumph of the Heart: The Story of Statins*. New York: Oxford University Press, 2009.

Lichtenberg, Frank R. "The Allocation of Publicly Funded Biomedical Research." In *Medical Care Output and Productivity*, edited by David M. Cutler and Ernst R. Berndt, 565–89. Chicago: University of Chicago Press, 2001.

Lichtenstiger, Dalrie S. "Philosophy and Significance of the Voluntary Health Agency Movement." In *The Voluntary Health Agency—Meeting Community Needs*, 3–8. San Francisco: American Public Health Association, 1961.

Lidz, Charles W., Paul S. Appelbaum, Thomas Grisso, and Michelle Renaud. "Therapeutic Misconception and the Appreciation of Risks in Clinical Trials." *Social Science & Medicine* 58, no. 9 (2004): 1689–97.

Lieberman, Evan S. *Boundaries of Contagion: How Ethnic Politics Have Shaped Government Responses to AIDS*. Princeton, NJ: Princeton University Press, 2009.

Link, Bruce G., and Jo Phelan. "Social Conditions as Fundamental Causes of Disease." Special issue, *Journal of Health and Social Behavior* (1995): 80–94.

Lipton, Eric, and Rachel Abrams. "EpiPen Maker Lobbies to Shift High Costs to Others." *New York Times*, September 16, 2016.

Little, Clarence C. *Civilization Against Cancer*. New York and Toronto: Farrar & Rinehart, 1939.

Lloyd-Jones, Donald M., David O. Martin, Martin G. Larson, and Daniel Levy. "Accuracy of Death Certificates for Coding Coronary Heart Disease as the Cause of Death." *Annals of Internal Medicine* 129, no. 12 (1998): 1020–26.

Lock, Margaret. "Biosociality and Susceptibility Genes: A Cautionary Tale." In *Biosocialities, Genetics and the Social Sciences: Making Biologies and Identities*, edited by Sahra Gibbon and Carlos Novas, 56–78. New York and London: Routledge, 2008.

Lofgren, Hans. "Pharmaceuticals and the Consumer Movement: The Ambivalences of 'Patient Power.'" *Australian Health Review* 28, no. 2 (2004): 228–37.

Lofland, John. "Consensus Movements: City Twinning and Derailed Dissent in the American Eighties." *Research in Social Movements, Conflict and Change* 11 (1989): 163–96.

Lofland, John. *Polite Protesters: The American Peace Movement of the 1980s*. Syracuse Studies on Peace and Conflict Resolution. Syracuse, NY: Syracuse University Press, 1993.

Lofland, John. *Social Movement Organizations: Guide to Research on Insurgent Realities*. New Brunswick, NJ: Transaction Publishers, 1996.

Lohmann, Raychelle Cassada. "2016 Awareness Calendar." *Psychology Today*, January 1, 2016. https://www.psychologytoday.com/blog/teen-angst/201601/2016-awareness-calendar.

Loomis, Burdett A., and Allan J. Cigler. "The Changing Nature of Interest Group Politics." In *Interest Group Politics*, edited by A. J. Cigler and Burdett A. Loomis, 4th ed., 1–31. Washington, DC: Congressional Quarterly Press, 1995.

Lorde, Audre. *The Cancer Journals*. San Francisco: Aunt Lute Books, 1980.

Lowi, Theodore J. "American Business, Public Policy, Case-Studies, and Political Theory." *World Politics* 16, no. 4 (1964): 677–715.

Lowrey, Annie. "Budget Battles Keep Agencies Guessing." *New York Times*, September 3, 2013.

Lupton, Deborah. *Medicine as Culture: Illness, Disease and the Body*. London: Sage, 1994.

Malakoff, David. "Biomedicine Gets Record Raise as Congress Sets 2002 Spending." *Science* 295 (2002): 24–25.

Malakoff, David. "Clinton's Science Legacy: Ending on a High Note." *Science* 290 (2000): 2234–36.

Malakoff, David. "NIH Gets $17.9 Billion in Another Record Year." *Science* 286 (1999): 1654.

Malakoff, David. "NIH Gets $2.5 Billion More as Congress Wraps up Budget." *Science* 290 (2000): 2226.

Malakoff, David. "NIH Prays for a Soft Landing After Its Doubling Ride Ends." *Science* 292 (2001): 1992–95.

Malakoff, David. "Science Lobbyists Aim for Better Balanced Budget." *Science* 291 (2001): 1882–84.

Malakoff, David, and Eliot Marshall. "NIH Wins Big as Congress Lumps Together Eight Bills." *Science* 282 (1998): 598–99.

Marks, Andrew R. "Rescuing the NIH Before It Is Too Late." *Journal of Clinical Investigation* 116, no. 4 (2006): 844.

Marshall, Eliot. "Last-Minute Deal Gives NIH 7.1% Raise." *Science* 278 (1997a): 1218.

Marshall, Eliot. "Lobbyists Seek to Reslice NIH's Pie." *Science* 276 (1997b): 344–46.

Marshall, Eliot. "OMB Stalks the 'Burgeoning Growth of Biomedicine.'" *Science* 237 (1987): 847–48.

Marshall, Eliot. "Plan to Reduce Number of New Grants Tempers Enthusiasm for NIH Budget Hike." *Science* 287 (2000): 953.

Marshall, Eliot. "Prevention Research: A New Growth Area for NIH?" *Science* 262 (1993): 1508–9.

Marshall, Eliot. "Research and the 'Flexible Freeze.'" *Science* 242 (1988): 1368–70.

Marshall, Eliot. "Science Funding: Up in Smoke?" *Science* 279 (1998): 974–75.

Marshall, Eliot. "Senate Restores NIH Funding Cut." *Science* 268 (1995): 1271–72.

Marshall, Eliot, and David P. Hamilton. "R&D Budget Collides with the Deficit." *Science* 258 (1992): 208–9.

Marshall, Eliot, and Andrew Lawler. "Congress: Biomedical Research Wins Big." *Science* 274 (1996): 27–28.

Marshall, Eliot, and Andrew Lawler. "R&D Budget Takes Shape in Congress, Piece by Piece." *Science* 269 (1995): 471–72.

Marshall, Eliot, and Andrew Lawler. "U.S. R&D Budget Becomes Political Football." *Science* 281 (1998): 16–17.

Marshall, Eliot, and Ellis Rubinstein. "NSF, NIH Under the Microscope." *Science* 255 (1992): 788–91.

Martin, Andrew W., Frank R. Baumgartner, and John D. McCarthy. "Measuring Association Populations Using the Encyclopedia of Associations: Evidence from the Field of Labor Unions." *Social Science Research* 35, no. 3 (2006): 771–78.

Martin, Jean. "Research in Biomedicine: Is Anyone Representing/Advocating the Public Interest?" *European Journal of Public Health* 11, no. 4 (2001): 458–59.

Marts, Arnaud C. *The Generosity of Americans*. Englewood Cliffs, NJ: Prentice Hall, 1966.

May, Peter J. "Reconsidering Policy Design: Policies and Publics." *Journal of Public Policy* 11, no. 2 (1991): 187–206.

McAdam, Doug. "'Initiator' and 'Spin-off' Movements: Diffusion Processes in Protest Cycles." In *Repertoires and Cycles of Collective Action*, edited by Mark Traugott, Charles Tilly, Marc W. Steinberg, Charles D. Brockett, and James W. White, 217–39. Durham, NC: Duke University Press, 1995.

McAdam, Doug. *Political Process and the Development of Black Insurgency, 1930–1970*. Chicago: University of Chicago Press, 1982.

McAdam, Doug, and W. Richard Scott. "Organizations and Movements." In *Social Movements and Organization Theory*, edited by Gerald F. Davis, Doug McAdam, W. Richard Scott, and Mayer N. Zald, 4–40. New York: Cambridge University Press, 2005.

McAdam, Doug, Sidney G. Tarrow, and Charles Tilly. *Dynamics of Contention*. New York: Cambridge University Press, 2001.

McCammon, Holly J., C. S. Muse, H. D. Newman, and T. M. Terrell. "Movement Framing and Discursive Opportunity Structures: The Political Successes of the US Women's Jury Movements." *American Sociological Review* 72, no. 5 (2007): 725–49.

McCarthy, John D., David W. Britt, and Mark Wolfson. "The Institutional Channeling of Social Movements by the State in the United States." *Research in Social Movements, Conflicts and Change* 13, no. 2 (1991): 45–76.

McCarthy, John D., and Mark Wolfson. "Consensus Movements, Conflict Movements, and the Cooptation of Civic and State Infrastructures." In *Frontiers in Social Movement Theory*, edited by Aldon D. Morris and Carol McClurg Mueller, 271–97. New Haven, CT: Yale University Press, 1992.

McCarthy, John D., and Mark Wolfson. "Resource Mobilization by Local Social Movement Organizations: Agency, Strategy, and Organization in the Movement Against Drinking and Driving." *American Sociological Review* 61, no. 6 (1996): 1070–88.

McCarthy, John D., and Mayer N. Zald. "Resource Mobilization and Social Movements: A Partial Theory." *American Journal of Sociology* 82, no. 6 (1977): 1212–41.

McCarthy, Kathleen D. "Women and Political Culture." In *Charity, Philanthropy, and Civility in American History*, edited by Lawrence J. Friedman and Mark D. McGarvie, 179–97. Cambridge: Cambridge University Press, 2003.

McCombs, Maxwell E. *Setting the Agenda: The Mass Media and Public Opinion*. Cambridge: Polity, 2004.

McCombs, Maxwell E., and Donald L. Shaw. "The Agenda-Setting Function of Mass Media." *Public Opinion Quarterly* 36, no. 2 (1972): 176–87.

McCombs, Maxwell, and Jian-Hua Zhu. "Capacity, Diversity, and Volatility of the Public Agenda: Trends from 1954 to 1994." *Public Opinion Quarterly* 59, no. 4 (1995): 495–525.

McCormick, Sabrina. *No Family History: The Environmental Links to Breast Cancer*. Lanham, MD: Rowman & Littlefield, 2009.

McCormick, Sabrina, Phil Brown, Stephen Zavestoski, and Alissa Cordner. "The Personal Is Scientific, the Scientific Is Political: The Public Paradigm of the Environmental Breast Cancer Movement." In *Contested Illnesses: Citizens, Science, and Health Social Movements*, edited by Phil Brown, Rachel Morello-Frosch, and Stephen Zavestoski, 147–68. Berkeley: University of California Press, 2011.

McDonnell, Terence E., Amy Jonason, and Kari Christoffersen. "Seeing Red and Wearing Pink: Trajectories of Cultural Power in the AIDS and Breast Cancer Ribbons." *Poetics* 60 (2017): 1–15.

McGinnis, J. Michael, Pamela Williams-Russo, and James R. Knickman. "The Case for More Active Policy Attention to Health Promotion." *Health Affairs* 21, no. 2 (2002): 78–93.

McManus, Rich. "Varmus Counsels Successor, Eyes Future in Final Remarks to Press." *NIH Record* 52, no. 2 (2000). https://nihrecord.nih.gov/newsletters/01_25_2000/story01.htm.

Mervis, Jeffrey. "Promising Year Ends Badly After Fiscal Showdown Squeezes Science." *Science* 319 (2008): 18–19.

Mervis, Jeffrey. "Science and the Stimulus." *Science* 326 (2009): 1176–77.

Mervis, Jeffrey. "Senate Bills Back Huge Increases." *Science* 275 (1997): 608.

Mervis, Jeffrey, Christopher Anderson, and Eliot Marshall. "Better for Science than Expected." *Science* 262 (1993): 836–38.

Mervis, Jeffrey, Yudhijit Bhattacharjee, Jocelyn Kaiser, and Andrew Lawler. "NIH Shrinks, NSF Crawls as Congress Finishes Spending Bills." *Science* 311 (2006): 28–29.

Mervis, Jeffrey, and Eliot Marshall. "When Federal Science Stopped." *Science* 271 (1996): 136–37.

Metzl, Jonathan, and Anna Kirkland, eds. *Against Health: How Health Became the New Morality.* New York: New York University Press, 2010.

Meyer, David S. "Protest and Political Opportunities." *Annual Review of Sociology* 30, no. 1 (2004): 125–45.

Meyer, David S., and Suzanne Staggenborg. "Movements, Countermovements, and the Structure of Political Opportunity." *American Journal of Sociology* 101, no. 6 (1996): 1628–60.

Meyer, David S., and Nancy Whittier. "Social Movement Spillover." *Social Problems* 41 (1994): 277.

Michels, Robert. *Political Parties: A Sociological Study of the Oligarchical Tendencies of Modern Democracy.* New York: Free Press, 1915.

Minkoff, Debra, Silke Aisenbrey, and Jon Agnone. "Organizational Diversity in the US Advocacy Sector." *Social Problems* 55, no. 4 (2008): 525–48.

Minkoff, Debra C. "Macro-Organizational Analysis." In *Methods of Social Movement Research*, edited by Bert Klandermans and Suzanne Staggenborg, 260–85. Minneapolis: University of Minnesota Press, 2002.

Minkoff, Debra C. *Organizing for Equality: The Evolution of Women's and Racial–Ethnic Organizations in America, 1955–1985.* New Brunswick, NJ: Rutgers University Press, 1995.

Minkoff, Debra C. "The Sequencing of Social Movements." *American Sociological Review* 62, no. 5 (1997): 779–99.

Mintzes, Barbara. "Should Patient Groups Accept Money from Drug Companies? No." *BMJ* 334, no. 7600 (2007): 935.

Mintzes, Barbara, and Catherine Hodgkin. "The Consumer Movement: From Single-Issue Campaigns to Long-Term Reform." In *Contested Ground: Public Purpose and Private Interest in the Regulation of Prescription Drugs*, edited by Peter Davis, 76–91. New York: Oxford University Press, 1996.

Modelmog, Dieter, Sibylle Rahlenbeck, and Dimitrios Trichopoulos. "Accuracy of Death Certificates: A Population-Based, Complete-Coverage, One-Year Autopsy Study in East Germany." *Cancer Causes & Control* 3, no. 6 (1992): 541–46.

Moffett, Jill. "Moving Beyond the Ribbon: An Examination of Breast Cancer Advocacy and Activism in the US and Canada." *Cultural Dynamics* 15 (2003): 287–306.

Mole, Beth. "Science Slowdown: Recent Federal Shutdown Just the Latest Shock in a Deepening Funding Crisis." *Science News* 184, no. 11 (2013): 14–16.

Montini, Theresa. "Resist and Redirect: Physicians Respond to Breast Cancer Informed Consent Legislation." *Women & Health* 26, no. 1 (1997): 85–105.

Morello, Lauren, Jessica Morrison, Sara Reardon, Jeff Tolleson, and Alexandra Witze. "Budget Offers Recovery Hope." *Nature* 505, no. 7484 (2014): 461–62.

Morganstern, Myrna. "The Rehabilitation and Continuing Care of the Cancer Patient." In *A History of Cancer Control in the United States, 1946–1971*, Book 1, 423–93. Washington, DC: US National Cancer Institute, 1979.

Morgen, Sandra. *Into Our Own Hands: The Women's Health Movement in the United States, 1969–1990*. New Brunswick, NJ: Rutgers University Press, 2002.

Morrow, Richard H., and John H. Bryant. "Health Policy Approaches to Measuring and Valuing Human Life: Conceptual and Ethical Issues." *American Journal of Public Health* 85, no. 10 (1995): 1356–60.

Moses, Hamilton III, E. Ray Dorsey, David H. M. Matheson, and Samuel O. Thier. "Financial Anatomy of Biomedical Research." *Journal of the American Medical Association* 294, no. 11 (2005): 1333–42.

Moynihan, Ray, and Alan Cassels. *Selling Sickness: How the World's Biggest Pharmaceutical Companies Are Turning Us All into Patients*. New York: Nation Books, 2005.

Mukherjee, Siddhartha. *The Emperor of All Maladies: A Biography of Cancer*. New York: Scribner, 2010.

Mukherjee, Siddhartha. "Fighting Chance." *New Republic* 226, no. 2 (2002): 16–19.

Mullin, Emily. "Congressional Budget Deal Would Ease NIH Sequester Cuts." In *FierceBioTechResearch*. Newton, MA: Questex Media Group, 2013.

Munguia, Hayley. "How Many People Really Showed Up to the People's Climate March?" *FiveThirtyEight* (blog), September 30, 2014. https://fivethirtyeight.com/features/peoples-climate-march-attendance/.

Murphy, Kevin M., and Robert H. Topel. *Measuring the Gains from Medical Research: An Economic Approach*. Chicago: University of Chicago Press, 2003.

Murphy, Kevin M., and Robert H. Topel. "Introduction." In *Measuring the Gains from Medical Research*, edited by Kevin M. Murphy and Robert H. Topel, 1–8. Chicago: University of Chicago Press, 2003.

Murphy, Michelle. *Sick Building Syndrome and the Problem of Uncertainty: Environmental Politics, Technoscience, and Women Workers*. Durham, NC: Duke University Press, 2006.

Murray, Christopher J. L., Theo Vos, Rafael Lozano, Mohsen Naghavi, Abraham D. Flaxman, Catherine Michaud, Majid Ezzati, et al. "Disability-Adjusted Life Years (DALYs) for 291 Diseases and Injuries in 21 Regions, 1990–2010: A Systematic Analysis for the Global Burden of Disease Study 2010." *Lancet* 380, no. 9859 (2012): 2197–2223.

Murray, Christopher J. L., and Arnab K. Acharya. "Understanding DALYs." *Journal of Health Economics* 16, no. 6 (1997): 703–30.

Muscular Dystrophy Association. "MDA—History." 2015. https://www.mda.org/about-mda/history.

Mushaben, Joyce Marie. "The Struggle Within: Conflict, Consensus, and Decision Making Among National Coordinators and Grass-Roots Organizers in the West German Peace Movement." *International Social Movement Research* 2 (1989): 267–98.

Mushkin, Selma J. *Biomedical Research: Costs and Benefits.* Cambridge, MA: Ballinger, 1979.

Myasthenia Gravis Foundation of America. "About MGFA." 2010. http://www.myasthenia.org/AboutMGFA.aspx.

Nathan, David G., and Alan N. Schechter. "NIH Support for Basic and Clinical Research: Biomedical Researcher Angst in 2006." *JAMA* 295, no. 22 (2006): 2656–58.

Nathanson, Constance A. *Disease Prevention as Social Change: The State, Society, and Public Health in the United States, France, Great Britain, and Canada.* New York: Russell Sage Foundation, 2007.

National Academy of Sciences. *Allocating Federal Funds for Science and Technology.* Washington, DC: National Academies Press, 1995.

National Breast Cancer Coalition. "Mammography for Breast Cancer Screening: Harm/Benefit Analysis." July 2011. http://www.breastcancerdeadline2020.org/searchresults.html?cx=014910871523269114435%3Ajyruobae2eu&cof=FORID%3A10&ie=UTF-8&q=mammography&x=0&y=0&siteurl=www.breastcancerdeadline2020.org%2F.

National Cancer Institute. "NCI Budget Fact Book Archive." 2016. https://www.cancer.gov/about-nci/budget/fact-book/archive.

National Center for Charitable Statistics. *Guide to Using NCCS Data.* Washington, DC: Urban Institute, 2006.

National Institute of Diabetes and Digestive and Kidney Diseases. "About the Special Diabetes Program." Accessed December 22, 2016. https://www.niddk.nih.gov/about-niddk/research-areas/diabetes/type-1-diabetes-special-statutory-funding-program/about-the-program/Pages/default.aspx.

National Institutes of Health. "August Crosswalk: Why the Categories are Different." *RCDC Fingerprint News*, September 2008, 5–7.

National Institutes of Health. "History of the Office of Disease Prevention." 2015. https://prevention.nih.gov/about/odp-history.

National Institutes of Health. "NIH Research Portfolio Online Reporting Tools (RePORT)—NIH Data Book." 2017. https://report.nih.gov/nihdatabook/.

National Institutes of Health. *Research in Prevention.* Washington, DC: US Department of Health and Human Services, 1984.

National Institutes of Health. *Setting Research Priorities at the National Institutes of Health.* Bethesda, MD: National Institutes of Health, 1997.

National Kidney Foundation. "History." 2016. https://www.kidney.org/about/history.

National Tay-Sachs and Allied Diseases Association. "Our History." 2016. https://ntsad.org/index.php/about-ntsad/our-history.

Nature. "NIH Budget Blues." *Nature* 497, no. 7449 (2013): 293.

Nature. "NIH Spared Budget Slash." *Nature* 473, no. 7345 (2011): 115.

Nature Medicine. "A Windfall for US Biomedical Science." *Nature Medicine* 22, no. 2 (2016): 115.

Nelson, Barbara J. *Making an Issue of Child Abuse: Political Agenda Setting for Social Problems.* Chicago: University of Chicago Press, 1984.

Neuman, W. Russell. "The Threshold of Public Attention." *Public Opinion Quarterly* 54, no. 2 (1990): 159.

New York Times. "AZT's Inhuman Cost." *New York Times,* August 28, 1989.

New York Times. "Mayor Is First Buyer of Christmas Seals." *New York Times,* November 30, 1923.

New York Times. "Medical Madness on Capitol Hill." *New York Times,* October 29, 1992.

Norman, Colin. "Congress Readies AIDS Funding Transfusion." *Science* 230 (1985): 418–19.

Norman, Colin. "Congress Votes NIH a Big Budget Boost." *Science* 226 (1984): 417–18.

Norman, Colin. "NIH Gets a Friendly Hearing on Capitol Hill." *Science* 231 (1986): 1364.

Norman, Colin. "Science Budget: Growth Amid Red Ink." *Science* 251 (1991): 616–18.

Norman, Colin. "Science Budget: More of the Same." *Science* 235 (1987): 151–53.

Norman, Colin. "Science Budget: Selective Growth." *Science* 255 (1992): 672–75.

Novas, Carlos. "The Political Economy of Hope: Patients' Organizations, Science and Biovalue." *BioSocieties* 1, no. 3 (2006): 289–305.

Nurse, Paul. "US Biomedical Research under Siege." *Cell* 124, no. 1 (2006): 9–12.

O'Connell, Brian. "What Voluntary Activity Can and Cannot Do for America." *Public Administration Review* 49, no. 5 (1989): 486–91.

O'Donovan, Orla. "Corporate Colonization of Health Activism? Irish Health Advocacy Organizations' Modes of Engagement with Pharmaceutical Corporations." *International Journal of Health Services* 37, no. 4 (2007): 711–33.

Okunade, Albert A., and Vasudeva N. R. Murthy. "Technology as a 'Major Driver' of Health Care Costs: A Cointegration Analysis of the Newhouse Conjecture." *Journal of Health Economics* 21, no. 1 (2002): 147–59.

Oliver, Pamela E., and Daniel J. Myers. "The Coevolution of Social Movements." *Mobilization: An International Quarterly* 8, no. 1 (2002): 1–24.

Oliver, Thomas R. "The Politics of Public Health Policy." *Annual Review of Public Health* 27, no. 1 (2006): 195–233.

Olson, Mancur. *The Logic of Collective Action: Public Goods and the Theory of Groups.* Cambridge, MA: Harvard University Press, 1965.

Olzak, Susan. "Analysis of Events in the Study of Collective Action." *Annual Review of Sociology* 15 (1989): 119–41.

Olzak, Susan. "The Effect of Category Spanning on the Lethality and Longevity of Terrorist Organizations." *Social Forces* 95, no. 2 (2016): 559–84.

Olzak, Susan, and Emily Ryo. "Organizational Diversity, Vitality and Outcomes in the Civil Rights Movement." *Social Forces* 85, no. 4 (2007): 1561–91.

O'Neill, Michael. *Third America: The Emergence of the Nonprofit Sector in the United States.* San Francisco: Jossey-Bass, 1989.

Orenstein, Peggy. "Our Feel-Good War on Breast Cancer." *New York Times,* April 25, 2013.

Orkin, Stuart H., and Arno G. Motulsky. *Report and Recommendations of the Panel to Assess the NIH Investment in Research on Gene Therapy.* Bethesda, MD: National Institutes of Health, 1995.

Orzag, Peter R. "Growth in Health Care Costs." Statement Before the Committee on the Budget, US Senate, January 31, 2008.

Oshinsky, David M. *Polio: An American Story.* New York: Oxford University Press, 2005.

Packard, Randall M., Peter J. Brown, Ruth L. Berkelman, and Howard Frumkin, eds. *Emerging Illnesses and Society: Negotiating the Public Health Agenda.* Baltimore, MD: Johns Hopkins University Press, 2004.

Padgett, John F. "Bounded Rationality in Budgetary Research." *American Political Science Review* 74, no. 2 (1980): 354–72.

Padgett, John F. "Hierarchy and Ecological Control in Federal Budgetary Decision Making." *American Journal of Sociology* 87, no. 1 (1981): 75–129.

Palca, Joseph. "Emphasizing the Health in NIH." *Science* 254 (1991): 23–24.

Palca, Joseph. "Hard Times at NIH." *Science* 246 (1989): 988–90.

Palca, Joseph. "NIH Grants: Better Late than Never?" *Science* 254, no. 5031 (1991): 513.

Pampel, Fred C., and John B. Williamson. "Welfare Spending in Advanced Industrial Democracies, 1950–1980." *American Journal of Sociology* 93, no. 6 (1988): 1424–56.

Panem, Sandra. "AIDS: Public Policy and Biomedical Research." *Hastings Center Report* 15, no. 4 (1985): 23–26.

Panofsky, Aaron. "Generating Sociability to Drive Science: Patient Advocacy Organizations and Genetics Research." *Social Studies of Science* 41, no. 1 (2011): 31–57.

Parker-Pope, Tara. "Plenty of Blame in a Health System 'Designed to Fail.'" *New York Times*, May 8, 2012.

Parkinson's Disease Foundation. "Parkinson's Disease Foundation 1957–2007: Fifty Years of Leadership and Commitment to the Parkinson's Disease Community." Accessed September 28, 2016. http://www.pdf.org/en/founder.

Parsons, Talcott. *The Social System*. London: Routledge, 1991.

Paschel, Tianna S. "The Right to Difference: Explaining Colombia's Shift from Color Blindness to the Law of Black Communities." *American Journal of Sociology* 116, no. 3 (2010): 729–69.

Patton, Cindy. *Inventing AIDS*. New York: Routledge, 1990.

Paulsen, Monte. "The Cancer Business: The Same Companies that Profit from Breast Cancer Treatments Also Manufacture Cancer-Causing Toxins." *Mother Jones* (May/ June 1994). https://www.motherjones.com/politics/1994/05/cancer-business/.

Payne, A. Abigail. "Earmarks and EPSCoR." In *Shaping Science and Technology Policy: The Next Generation of Research*, edited by David H. Guston and Daniel R. Sarewitz, 149–72. Madison: University of Wisconsin Press, 2006.

Pear, Robert. "Congress Rejects Trump Proposals to Cut Health Research Funds." *New York Times*, September 11, 2017.

Penner, Rudolph G., and C. Eugene Steuerle. "Budget Rules." *National Tax Journal* 57, no. 3 (2004): 547–57.

Perez-Pena, Richard. "Beyond 'I'm a Diabetic,' Little Common Ground." *New York Times*, May 17, 2006.

Pescosolido, Bernice A. "Professional Dominance and the Limits of Erosion." *Society* 43, no. 6 (2006): 21–29.

Pescosolido, Bernice A., and Jack K. Martin. "The Stigma Complex." *Annual Review of Sociology* 41 (2015): 87–116.

Pescosolido, Bernice A., Jack K. Martin, J. Scott Long, Tait R. Medina, Jo C. Phelan, and Bruce G. Link. "'A Disease Like Any Other'? A Decade of Change in Public Reactions to Schizophrenia, Depression, and Alcohol Dependence." *American Journal of Psychiatry* 167, no. 11 (2010): 1321–30.

Phelan, Jo C. "Geneticization of Deviant Behavior and Consequences for Stigma: The Case of Mental Illness." *Journal of Health and Social Behavior* 46, no. 4 (2005): 307–22.

Phelan, Jo C., Bruce G. Link, Ana Diez-Roux, Ichiro Kawachi, and Bruce Levin. "'Fundamental Causes' of Social Inequalities in Mortality: A Test of the Theory." *Journal of Health and Social Behavior* 45, no. 3 (2004): 265–85.

Phelan, Sean M., Joan M. Griffin, George L. Jackson, S. Yousuf Zafar, Wendy Hellerstedt, Mandy Stahre, David Nelson, Leah L. Zullig, Diana J. Burgess, and Michelle van Ryn. "Stigma, Perceived Blame, Self-Blame, and Depressive Symptoms in Men with Colorectal Cancer." *Psycho-Oncology* 22, no. 1 (2013): 65–73.

PhRMA. *Biopharmaceutical R&D: The Process Behind New Medicines.* Washington, DC: PhRMA, 2015.

Pichardo, Nelson A. "New Social Movements: A Critical Review." *Annual Review of Sociology* 23, no. 1 (1997): 411–30.

Pierson, Paul. "The Deficit and the Politics of Domestic Reform." In *The Social Divide: Political Parties and the Future of Activist Government*, edited by Margaret Weir, 126–78. Washington, DC, and New York: Brookings Institution Press and Russell Sage Foundation, 1998.

Pierson, Paul. "Not Just What, but When: Timing and Sequence in Political Processes." *Studies in American Political Development* 14, no. 1 (2000): 72–92.

Pinto, Deirdre, Dominique Martin, and Richard Chenhall. "Chasing Cures: Rewards and Risks for Rare Disease Patient Organisations Involved in Research." *BioSocieties* 13, no. 1 (2018): 123–47.

Pinto, Deirdre, Dominique Martin, and Richard Chenhall. "The Involvement of Patient Organisations in Rare Disease Research: A Mixed Methods Study in Australia." *Orphanet Journal of Rare Diseases* 11 (2016): 2.

Piore, Michael J. *Beyond Individualism.* Cambridge, MA: Harvard University Press, 1995.

Piven, Frances Fox. *Challenging Authority: How Ordinary People Change America.* Lanham, MD: Rowman & Littlefield, 2006.

Piven, Frances Fox, and Richard Cloward. *Poor People's Movements: Why They Succeed, How They Fail.* New York: Vintage, 1978.

Pollack, Harold, George A. Kaplan, James S. House, and Robert F. Schoeni. "Social and Economic Policies as Health Policy: Moving Toward a New Approach to Improving Health in America." In *Making Americans Healthier: Social and Economic Policy as Health Policy*, edited by Robert F. Schoeni, James S. House, George A. Kaplan, and Harold Pollack, 379–90. New York: Russell Sage Foundation, 2008.

Polletta, Francesca. "Mobilization Forum: Awkward Movements." *Mobilization: An International Quarterly* 11, no. 4 (2006): 475–500.

Polletta, Francesca. "Strategy and Identity in 1960s Black Protest." *Research in Social Movements, Conflict, and Change* 17 (1994): 85–114.

Polletta, Francesca, and James M. Jasper. "Collective Identity and Social Movements." *Annual Review of Sociology* 27, no. 1 (2001): 283–305.

Porter, Dorothy. *Health, Civilization, and the State: A History of Public Health from Ancient to Modern Times.* London and New York: Routledge, 1999.

Porter, Theodore M. *Trust in Numbers.* Princeton, NJ: Princeton University Press, 1995.

Poterba, James. "Federal Budget Policy in the 1980s." In *American Economic Policy in the 1980s*, edited by Martin Feldstein, 235–70. Chicago: University of Chicago Press, 1994.

Price, David E. "Policy Making in Congressional Committees: The Impact of 'Environmental' Factors." *American Political Science Review* 72, no. 2 (1978): 548–74.

Putnam, Robert D. *Bowling Alone: The Collapse and Revival of American Community.* New York: Touchstone Books, 2000.

Quadagno, Jill. *One Nation, Uninsured: Why the U.S. Has No National Health Insurance.* New York: Oxford University Press, 2005.

Quimby, Ernest, and Samuel R. Friedman. "Dynamics of Black Mobilization Against AIDS in New York City." *Social Problems* 36 (1989): 403–15.

Rabeharisoa, Vololona. "Experience, Knowledge and Empowerment: The Increasing Role of Patient Organizations in Staging, Weighting and Circulating Experience and Knowledge." In *The Dynamics of Patient Organizations in Europe*, edited by M. Akrich, Joao Nunes, Florence Paterson, and Vololona Rabeharisoa, 13–82. Collection Sciences Sociales. Paris: Presses de l'école des mines, 2008.

Rabeharisoa, Vololona. "The Struggle Against Neuromuscular Diseases in France and the Emergence of the 'Partnership Model' of Patient Organization." *Social Science and Medicine* 57 (2003): 2127–36.

Rabeharisoa, Vololona, and Michel Callon. "The Involvement of Patients' Associations in Research." *International Social Science Journal* 54, no. 171 (2002): 57–63.

Rabinow, Paul. "Artificiality and Enlightenment: From Sociobiology to Biosociality." In *Incorporations*, edited by Jonathan Crary and Sanford Kwinter, 234–52. New York: Zone Books, 1992.

Rabinow, Paul. "Concept Work." In *Biosocialities, Genetics and the Social Sciences: Making Biologies and Identities*, edited by Sahra Gibbon and Carlos Novas, 188–92. New York and London: Routledge, 2008.

Radcliff, Benjamin, and Martin Saiz. "Labor Organization and Public Policy in the American States." *Journal of Politics* 60, no. 1 (1998): 113–25.

Raffle, Angela E., and J. A. Muir Gray. *Screening: Evidence and Practice*. New York: Oxford University Press, 2007.

Raloff, Janet. "2012 Budget Offers Pain and Gain." *Science News* 179, no. 6 (2011): 15.

Ransohoff, David F., Mary McNaughton Collins, and Floyd J. Fowler. "Why Is Prostate Cancer Screening so Common When the Evidence Is so Uncertain? A System Without Negative Feedback." *American Journal of Medicine* 113, no. 8 (2002): 663–67.

Rehm, Philipp, Jacob S. Hacker, and Mark Schlesinger. "Insecure Alliances: Risk, Inequality, and Support for the Welfare State." *American Political Science Review* 106, no. 2 (2012): 386–406.

Reiser, Stanley Joel. *Medicine and the Reign of Technology*. Cambridge and New York: Cambridge University Press, 1978.

Reiser, Stanley Joel. "The Era of the Patient: Using the Experience of Illness in Shaping the Missions of Health Care." *JAMA* 269, no. 8 (1993): 1012–17.

Reiss, Tom. "Laugh Riots: The French Star Who Became a Demagogue." *New Yorker*, November 12, 2007. https://www.newyorker.com/magazine/2007/11/19/laugh-riots.

Resnik, David B. "Setting Biomedical Research Priorities: Justice, Science, and Public Participation." *Kennedy Institute of Ethics Journal* 11, no. 2 (2001): 181–204.

Rettig, Richard A. *Cancer Crusade: The Story of the National Cancer Act of 1971*. Lincoln, NE: Authors Choice Press, 2005.

Rigby, Elizabeth. "How the National Prevention Council Can Overcome Key Challenges and Improve Americans' Health." *Health Affairs* 30, no. 11 (2011): 2149–56.

Robbins, Kevin C. "The Nonprofit Sector in Historical Perspective: Traditions of Philanthropy in the West." In *The Nonprofit Sector: A Research Handbook*, edited by Walter W. Powell and Richard Steinberg, 2nd ed., 13–31. New Haven, CT: Yale University Press, 2006.

Rochefort, David A., and Roger W. Cobb. "Problem Definition: An Emerging Perspective." In *The Politics of Problem Definition: Shaping the Policy Agenda*, edited by David A. Rochefort and Roger W. Cobb, 1–31. Lawrence: University Press of Kansas, 1994.

Rochefort, David A., and Roger W. Cobb. "Problem Definition, Agenda Access, and Policy Choice." *Policy Studies Journal* 21, no. 1 (1993): 56–71.

Rodgers, Daniel T. "In Search of Progressivism." *Reviews in American History* 10, no. 4 (1982): 113–32.

Rodwin, Marc A. "Patient Accountability and Quality of Care: Lessons from Medical Consumerism and the Patients' Rights, Women's Health and Disability Rights Movements." *American Journal of Law & Medicine* 20 (1994): 147–67.

Rorty, Richard. *Achieving Our Country: Leftist Thought in Twentieth-Century America.* Cambridge, MA: Harvard University Press, 1999.

Rose, Nikolas. *The Politics of Life Itself: Biomedicine, Power, and Subjectivity in the Twenty-First Century.* Princeton, NJ: Princeton University Press, 2007.

Rose, Susannah L., Janelle Highland, Matthew T. Karafa, and Steven Joffe. "Patient Advocacy Organizations, Industry Funding, and Conflicts of Interest." *JAMA Internal Medicine* 177, no. 3 (2017): 344–50.

Rosenbaum, David E. "It's the Economy Again, as Democrats Attack the 'Contract with America.'" *New York Times*, November 1, 1994.

Rosenberg, Charles E. *Our Present Complaint: American Medicine, Then and Now.* Baltimore, MD: Johns Hopkins University Press, 2007.

Ross, Walter Sanford. *Crusade: The Official History of the American Cancer Society.* New York: Arbor House, 1987.

Rothman, Sheila M. *Living in the Shadow of Death: Tuberculosis and the Social Experience of Illness in America.* New York: Basic Books, 1994.

Rothman, Sheila M., Victoria H. Raveis, Anne Friedman, and David J. Rothman. "Health Advocacy Organizations and the Pharmaceutical Industry: An Analysis of Disclosure Practices." *American Journal of Public Health* 101, no. 4 (2011): 602–9.

Rowberg, Richard E. *Pharmaceutical Research and Development: A Description and Analysis of the Process.* Washington, DC: Congressional Research Service, Library of Congress, 2001.

Rubin, Irene. "Aaron Wildavsky and the Demise of Incrementalism." In *Public Budgeting: Policy, Process, and Politics*, edited by Irene Rubin, 171–85. Armonk, NY: M. E. Sharpe, 2008.

Rubin, Irene S. *The Politics of Public Budgeting: Getting and Spending, Borrowing and Balancing.* New York: Chatham House Publishers, 2000.

Rush, Ladonna L. "Affective Reactions to Multiple Social Stigmas." *Journal of Social Psychology* 138, no. 4 (1998): 421–30.

Russett, Bruce. "Defense Expenditures and National Well-Being." *American Political Science Review* 76, no. 4 (1982): 767–77.

Ruzek, Sheryl Burt. *The Women's Health Movement: Feminist Alternatives to Medical Control.* Santa Barbara, CA: Praeger, 1979.

Saad, Lydia. "Support for Active Government Up in U.S." Gallup, October 2, 2017. http://news.gallup.com/poll/220058/support-active-government.aspx.

Sack, Kevin. "Cancer Society Focuses Its Ads on the Uninsured." *New York Times*, August 31, 2007.

Saguy, Abigail C., and Kevin W. Riley. "Weighing Both Sides: Morality, Mortality, and Framing Contests over Obesity." *Journal of Health Politics, Policy and Law* 30, no. 5 (2005): 869–923.

Salamon, Lester M. *The Resilient Sector: The State of Nonprofit America.* Washington, DC: Brookings Institution Press, 2003.

Salamon, Lester M., and Alan J. Abramson. *The Federal Budget and the Nonprofit Sector.* Washington, DC: Urban Institute Press, 1982.

Sampat, Bhaven N. "Mission-Oriented Biomedical Research at the NIH." *Research Policy* 41, no. 10 (2012): 1729–41.

Sampat, Bhaven N. "The Dismal Science, the Crown Jewel and the Endless Frontier." In *The New Economics of Technology Policy*, edited by Dominique Foray, 148–62. Cheltenham, UK: Edward Elgar Publishing, 2009.

Sampat, Bhaven N., Kristin Buterbaugh, and Marcel Perl. "New Evidence on the Allocation of NIH Funds Across Diseases." *Milbank Quarterly* 91, no. 1 (2013): 163–85.

San Francisco Chronicle. "Tuberculosis Association Saves Lives: 80,000 Bottles of Milk Distributed Yearly to School Children." November 27, 1921.

Santoro, Wayne A., and Gail M. McGuire. "Social Movement Insiders: The Impact of Institutional Activists on Affirmative Action and Comparable Worth Policies." *Social Problems* 44 (1997): 503–19.

Sarewitz, Daniel. *Frontiers of Illusion: Science, Technology and the Politics of Progress.* Philadelphia: Temple University Press, 1996.

Schattschneider, E. E. *The Semi-Sovereign People: A Realist's View of Democracy in America.* Hinsdale, IL: Dryden Press, 1960.

Schlozman, Kay Lehman, Benjamin I. Page, Sidney Verba, and Morris P. Fiorina. "Inequalities of Political Voice." In *Inequality and American Democracy: What We Know and What We Need to Learn*, edited by Lawrence R. Jacobs and Theda Skocpol, 1st ed., 19–87. New York: Russell Sage Foundation, 2007.

Schlozman, Kay Lehman, and John T. Tierney. *Organized Interests and American Democracy.* New York: Harpercollins College, 1986.

Schneider, Anne, and Helen Ingram. "Social Construction of Target Populations: Implications for Politics and Policy." *American Political Science Review* 87, no. 2 (1993): 334–47.

Sczudlo, Lauren. "Positivity Is Bullshit When You Have Cancer." Gawker, November 23, 2013. http://gawker.com/positivity-is-bullshit-when-you-have-cancer-1469975747.

Sealander, Judith. "Curing Evils at Their Source: The Arrival of Scientific Giving." In *Charity, Philanthropy, and Civility in American History*, edited by Lawrence J. Friedman and Mark D. McGarvie, 217–39. New York and Cambridge: Cambridge University Press, 2003.

Serres, Chris. "Two Years Later, Ice Bucket Challenge Yields Huge Dose of Hope for Minnesotans with ALS." *Star Tribune*, July 30, 2016.

Shannon, James A. "The Advancement of Medical Research: A Twenty-Year View of the Role of the National Institutes of Health." *Journal of Medical Education* 42, no. 2 (1967): 97–108.

Shapiro, Joseph P. *No Pity: People with Disabilities Forging a New Civil Rights Movement.* New York: Times Books, 1993.

Shaw, Donald Lewis, and Maxwell E. McCombs. *The Emergence of American Political Issues: The Agenda-Setting Function of the Press.* St. Paul, MN: West Publishing, 1977.

Shiffman, Jeremy, David Berlan, and Tamara Hafner. "Has Aid for AIDS Raised All Health Funding Boats?" *JAIDS Journal of Acquired Immune Deficiency Syndromes* 52, no. S1 (2009): S45–48.

Shryock, Richard Harrison. *National Tuberculosis Association, 1904–1954: A Study of the Voluntary Health Movement in the United States.* New York: National Tuberculosis Association, 1957.

Silberman, Steve. *Neurotribes: The Legacy of Autism and the Future of Neurodiversity.* New York: Avery, 2015.

Sills, David L. *The Volunteers: Means and Ends in a National Organization.* Glencoe, IL: Free Press, 1957.

Silverstein, Ken. "Prozac.Org." *Mother Jones* 24, no. 6 (1999): 22–23.

Sinclair, Ward. "Disease Lobbies: Where, How, of NIH Spending." *Washington Post,* March 8, 1980.

Siplon, Patricia D. *AIDS and the Policy Struggle in the United States.* Washington, DC: Georgetown University Press, 2002.

Skocpol, Theda. *Boomerang: Health Care Reform and the Turn Against Government.* New York: W. W. Norton, 1997.

Skocpol, Theda. *Diminished Democracy: From Membership to Management in American Civic Life.* Norman: University of Oklahoma Press, 2003.

Skocpol, Theda. *Protecting Soldiers and Mothers: The Political Origins of Social Policy in United States.* Cambridge, MA: Harvard University Press, 1992.

Skrentny, John D. "Policy-Elite Perceptions and Social Movement Success: Understanding Variations in Group Inclusion in Affirmative Action." *American Journal of Sociology* 111, no. 6 (2006): 1762–1815.

Skrentny, John D. *The Ironies of Affirmative Action: Politics, Culture, and Justice in America.* Chicago: University of Chicago Press, 1996.

Skrentny, John D. *The Minority Rights Revolution.* Cambridge, MA: Harvard University Press, 2002.

Slonim, Amy B., Carol Callaghan, Lisa Daily, Barbara A. Leonard, Fran C. Wheeler, Charles W. Gollmar, and Walter F. Young. "Recommendations for Integration of Chronic Disease Programs: Are Your Programs Linked." *Preventing Chronic Disease* 4, no. 2 (2007): A34.

Smelser, Neil J. *Theory of Collective Behavior.* New York: Free Press, 1963.

Smith, Jeremy N. *Epic Measures: One Doctor. Seven Billion Patients.* New York: Harper Wave, 2015.

Smith, Katherine. "Institutional Filters: The Translation and Re-Circulation of Ideas About Health Inequalities Within Policy." *Policy & Politics* 41, no. 1 (2013): 81–100.

Smith, Mark F. "Washington Watch: Research Funding." *Academe* 84, no. 3 (1998): 79.

Smith, Philip M., and Michael McGeary. "Don't Look Back: Science Funding for the Future." *Issues in Science and Technology* 13, no. 3 (Spring 1997): 33–40.

Smith, Richard A. "Interest Group Influence in the U.S. Congress." *Legislative Studies Quarterly* 20, no. 1 (1995): 89–139.

Smith, Rogers M. "Identities, Interests, and the Future of Political Science." *Perspectives on Politics* 2, no. 2 (2004): 301–12.

Smith, Sheila, Joseph P. Newhouse, and Mark S. Freeland. "Income, Insurance, and Technology: Why Does Health Spending Outpace Economic Growth?" *Health Affairs* 28, no. 5 (2009): 1276–84.

Soule, Sarah A., and Brayden G. King. "Competition and Resource Partitioning in Three Social Movement Industries." *American Journal of Sociology* 113, no. 6 (2008): 1568–1610.

Spector, Malcolm, and John I. Kitsuse. *Constructing Social Problems.* Menlo Park, CA: Cummings Publishing, 1977.

Spingarn, Natalie Davis. *Heartbeat: The Politics of Health Research.* Washington, DC: Robert B. Luce, 1976.

Stabiner, Karen. *To Dance with the Devil: The New War on Breast Cancer; Politics, Power, People*. New York: Delta, 1997.

Staggenborg, Suzanne. "The Consequences of Professionalization and Formalization in the Pro-Choice Movement." *American Sociological Review* 53, no. 4 (1988): 585–605.

Stapleton, Stephanie. "Lobby for Labs: Biomed Research Campaigning for Funding Increase." *American Medical News* 41, no. 6 (February 1998).

Starr, Paul. *The Social Transformation of American Medicine: The Rise of a Sovereign Profession and the Making of a Vast Industry*. New York: Basic Books, 1982.

Starr, Paul. "The Sociology of Official Statistics." In *The Politics of Numbers: For the National Committee for Research on the 1980 Census*, edited by William Alonso and Paul Starr, 7–58. New York: Russell Sage Foundation, 1987.

Steel, Emily. "'Ice Bucket Challenge' Has Raised Millions for ALS Association." *New York Times*, August 17, 2014.

Steensland, Brian. "Cultural Categories and the American Welfare State: The Case of Guaranteed Income Policy." *American Journal of Sociology* 111, no. 5 (2006): 1273–1326.

Steensland, Brian. "Moral Classification and Social Policy." In *Handbook of the Sociology of Morality*, edited by S. Hitlin and S. Vaisey, 455–68. New York: Springer, 2010.

Steinberg, Daniel, and Antonio Gotto. "Preventing Coronary Artery Disease by Lowering Cholesterol Levels: Fifty Years from Bench to Bedside." *JAMA* 282, no. 21 (1999): 2043–50.

Steinberg, Marc W. "The Talk and Back Talk of Collective Action: A Dialogic Analysis of Repertoires of Discourse Among Nineteenth-Century English Cotton Spinners 1." *American Journal of Sociology* 105, no. 3 (1999): 736–80.

Stephan, Paula. *How Economics Shapes Science*. Cambridge, MA: Harvard University Press, 2012.

Stephan, Paula E., and Ronald G. Ehrenberg. "Introduction." In *Science and the University*, edited by Paula E. Stephan and Ronald G. Ehrenberg, 3–15. Science and Technology in Society. Madison: University of Wisconsin Press, 2007.

Stergiopoulos, Stella, and Kenneth A. Getz. "Mapping and Characterizing the Development Pathway from Non-Clinical Through Early Clinical Drug Development." *Pharmaceutical Medicine* 26, no. 5 (2012): 297–307.

Steuerle, C. Eugene. "Financing the American State at the Turn of the Century." In *Funding the Modern American State, 1941–1995: The Rise and Fall of the Era of Easy Finance*, edited by W. Elliot Brownlee, 409–44. New York: Cambridge University Press, 1996.

Stevenson, Richard W. "Surplus Dreams: A Debate over Dividing Tax Dollars Yet to Be Collected." *New York Times*, August 10, 1999.

Stewart, John David. *British Pressure Groups: Their Role in Relation to the House of Commons*. Oxford: Clarendon Press, 1958.

Stockdale, Alan. "Waiting for the Cure: Mapping the Social Relations of Human Gene Therapy Research." *Sociology of Health & Illness* 21, no. 5 (1999): 579–96.

Stolberg, Sheryl Gay. "Confronting Cancer: Advocates Strive to Defeat Cancer but Disagree on Methods." *New York Times*, April 9, 2002.

Stolberg, Sheryl Gay. "Patients Lobby for Cash for Research into Illness." *New York Times*, April 14, 1999.

Stone, Deborah. *Policy Paradox: The Art of Political Decision Making*. Rev. ed. New York: W. W. Norton, 2001.

Stone, Deborah A. "Causal Stories and the Formation of Policy Agendas." *Political Science Quarterly* 104, no. 2 (1989): 281–300.

Stoto, Michael A., David Blumenthal, Jane S. Durch, and Penny H. Feldman. "Federal Funding for AIDS Research: Decision Process and Results in Fiscal Year 1986." *Reviews of Infectious Diseases* 10, no. 2 (1988): 406–19.

Strach, Patricia. *Hiding Politics in Plain Sight: Cause Marketing, Corporate Influence, and Breast Cancer Policymaking.* New York: Oxford University Press, 2016.

Strang, David, and John W. Meyer. "Institutional Conditions for Diffusion." *Theory and Society* 22, no. 4 (1993): 487–511.

Strauss, Anselm L., and Barney Glaser. *Chronic Illness and the Quality of Life.* St. Louis, MO: Mosby, 1975.

Strickland, Stephen P. *Politics, Science, and Dread Disease: A Short History of United States Medical Research Policy.* Cambridge, MA: Harvard University Press, 1972.

Strickland, Stephen P. *The Story of the NIH Grants Programs.* Lanham, MD: University Press of America, 1988.

Strolovitch, Dara Z. *Affirmative Advocacy: Race, Class, and Gender in Interest Group Politics.* Chicago: University of Chicago Press, 2007.

Studer, Kenneth E., and Daryl E. Chubin. *The Cancer Mission: Social Contexts of Biomedical Research.* Beverly Hills, CA: Sage Publications, 1980.

Studwell, Karen. "NIH Launches New Research Project Tracking System." American Psychological Association, Psychological Science Agenda February 2009. http://www.apa.org/science/about/psa/2009/02/nih.aspx.

Suchman, Mark C. "Managing Legitimacy: Strategic and Institutional Approaches." *Academy of Management Review* 20 (1995): 571–610.

Sulik, Gayle A. *Pink Ribbon Blues: How Breast Cancer Culture Undermines Women's Health.* New York: Oxford University Press, 2011.

Susan G. Komen Breast Cancer Foundation. "Race for the Cure," 2018. http://ww5.komen.org/RaceForTheCure/.

Susan G. Komen for the Cure. *2010–2011 Annual Report.* Dallas, TX: Susan G. Komen for the Cure, 2011.

Taft Group. *Corporate Giving Directory.* Farmington Hills, MI: Taft Group, 1990.

Taft Group. *Corporate Giving Directory.* Farmington Hills, MI: Taft Group, 1995.

Taft Group. *Corporate Giving Directory.* Farmington Hills, MI: Taft Group, 2005.

Talley, Colin. "The Combined Efforts of Community and Science: American Culture, Patient Activism, and the Multiple Sclerosis Movement in the United States." In *Emerging Illnesses and Society: Negotiating the Public Health Agenda,* edited by Randall M. Packard, Peter J. Brown, Ruth L. Berkelman, and Howard Frumkin, 39–70. Baltimore, MD: Johns Hopkins University Press, 2004.

Tarrow, Sidney. "Foreword." In *How Social Movements Matter,* edited by Marco Giugni, Doug Mcadam, and Charles Tilly, vii–ix. Minneapolis: University of Minnesota Press, 1999.

Tarrow, Sidney G. *Power in Movement: Social Movements and Contentious Politics.* New York: Cambridge University Press, 1994.

Tarrow, Sidney G. *Struggle, Politics, and Reform: Collective Action, Social Movements and Cycles of Protest.* Ithaca, NY: Center for International Studies, Cornell University, 1991.

Taylor, Verta. *Rock-a-by Baby: Feminism, Self-Help and Postpartum Depression.* New York: Routledge, 1996.

Taylor, Verta. "Social Movement Continuity: The Women's Movement in Abeyance." *American Sociological Review* 54 (1989): 761–75.

Taylor, Verta, and Marieke Van Willigen. "Women's Self-Help and the Reconstruction of Gender: The Postpartum Support and Breast Cancer Movements." *Mobilization: An International Quarterly* 1, no. 2 (1996): 123–42.

Taylor, Verta, and Nancy Whittier. "Collective Identity in Social Movement Communities: Lesbian Feminist Mobilization." In *Frontiers in Social Movement Theory*, edited by Aldon D. Morris and Carol McClurg Mueller, 104–29. New Haven, CT: Yale University Press, 1992.

Taylor, Verta, and Mayer N. Zald. "The Shape of Collective Action in the U.S. Health Sector." In *Social Movements and the Transformation of American Health Care*, edited by Jane C. Banaszak-Holl, Sandra R. Levitsky, and Mayer N. Zald, 300–18. New York: Oxford University Press, 2010.

Teitelbaum, Michael S. *Falling Behind? Boom, Bust, and the Global Race for Scientific Talent*. Princeton, NJ: Princeton University Press, 2014.

Teitelbaum, Michael S. "Structural Disequilibria in Biomedical Research." *Science*, 321 (2008): 644–45.

Teller, Michael E. *The Tuberculosis Movement: A Public Health Campaign in the Progressive Era*. New York: Greenwood Press, 1988.

Thompson, Guy. "Community Chests and United Funds." In *Social Work Year Book 1957*, edited by Russell H. Kurtz, 175–78. New York: National Association of Social Workers, 1957.

Thurber, James A. "Congressional Budget Reform: Impact on the Appropriations Committees." *Public Budgeting & Finance* 17, no. 3 (1997): 62–73.

Thurber, James A. "Republican Roles in Congressional Budget Reform: Twenty-Five Years of Deficit and Conflict." In *New Majority or Old Minority? The Impact of Republicans on Congress*, edited by Nicol C. Rae and Colton C. Campbell, 135–52. Lanham, MD: Rowman & Littlefield, 1999.

Tichenor, Daniel J., and Richard A. Harris. "The Development of Interest Group Politics in America: Beyond the Conceits of Modern Times." *Annual Review of Political Science* 8 (2005): 251–70.

Tilly, Charles. "Contentious Repertoires in Great Britain, 1758–1834." *Social Science History* 17, no. 2 (1993): 253–80.

Time Magazine. "Cancer Army." *Time* 29, no. 12 (March 22, 1937): 59.

Timmermans, Stefan. *Postmortem: How Medical Examiners Explain Suspicious Deaths*. Chicago: University of Chicago Press, 2006.

Timmermans, Stefan. "Suicide Determination and the Professional Authority of Medical Examiners." *American Sociological Review* 70, no. 2 (2005): 311–33.

Timmermans, Stefan, and Steven Epstein. "A World of Standards but Not a Standard World: Toward a Sociology of Standards and Standardization." *Annual Review of Sociology* 36 (2010): 69–89.

Tobert, Jonathan A. "Lovastatin and Beyond: The History of the HMG-CoA Reductase Inhibitors." *Nature Reviews Drug Discovery* 2, no. 7 (2003): 517–26.

Tomes, Nancy. "Patients or Health-Care Consumers? Why the History of Contested Terms Matters." In *History and Health Policy in the United States: Putting the Past Back In*, edited by Rosemary Stevens, Charles E. Rosenberg, and Lawton R. Burns, 83–110. New Brunswick, NJ: Rutgers University Press, 2006.

Tomes, Nancy. *The Gospel of Germs: Men, Women, and the Microbe in American Life.* Cambridge, MA: Harvard University Press, 1998.

Tomes, Nancy. "The Patient as a Policy Factor: A Historical Case Study of the Consumer/ Survivor Movement in Mental Health." *Health Affairs* 25, no. 3 (2006): 720–29.

Tracy, George S., and Zachary Gussow. "Self-Help Health Groups: A Grass-Roots Response to a Need for Services." *Journal of Applied Behavioral Science* 12, no. 3 (1976): 381–96.

Truman, David B. *The Governmental Process.* New York: Alfred A. Knopf, 1951.

Turner, Ralph H., and Lewis M. Killian. *Collective Behavior.* Englewood Cliffs, NJ: Prentice Hall, 1972.

Turner, Sarah E., Thomas I. Nygren, and William G. Bowen. "The NTEE Classification System: Tests of Reliability/Validity in the Field of Higher Education." *Voluntas: International Journal of Voluntary and Nonprofit Organizations* 4, no. 1 (1993): 73–94.

Turner, Stephanie. "Intersex Identities: Locating New Intersections of Sex and Gender." *Gender & Society* 13, no. 4 (1999): 457–79.

US Commission on Chronic Illness. *Chronic Illness in the United States.* Vol. 1, *Prevention of Chronic Illness.* Cambridge, MA: Harvard University Press, 1957.

US House of Representatives. "Combating the Rising Influence of Breast Cancer." Washington, DC: US Government Printing Office, 1992.

US House of Representatives. "Departments of Labor and Health, Education, and Welfare Appropriations for 1960. Statements of Members of Congress, Interested Organizations, and Individuals." Washington, DC: US Government Printing Office, 1959.

US House of Representatives. "Departments of Labor and Health, Education, and Welfare Appropriations for 1961." Washington, DC: US Government Printing Office, 1960.

US House of Representatives. "Departments of Labor and Health, Education, and Welfare Appropriations for 1964, Part 3: National Institutes of Health." Washington, DC: US Government Printing Office, 1963.

US House of Representatives. "Departments of Labor and Health, Education, and Welfare Appropriations for 1970, Part 7: Testimony of Members of Congress and Other Interested Individuals and Organizations." Washington, DC: US Government Printing Office, 1969.

US House of Representatives. "Departments of Labor and Health, Education, and Welfare Appropriations for 1975, Part 4: National Institutes of Health." Washington, DC: US Government Printing Office, 1974.

US House of Representatives. "Departments of Labor and Health, Education, and Welfare Appropriations for 1975, Part 7: Testimony of Members of Congress and Other Interested Individuals and Organizations." Washington, DC: US Government Printing Office, 1974.

US House of Representatives. "Departments of Labor and Health, Education, and Welfare Appropriations for 1980, Part 4." Washington, DC: US Government Printing Office, 1979.

US House of Representatives. "Departments of Labor and Health, Education, and Welfare Appropriations for 1980, Part 8." Washington, DC: US Government Printing Office, 1979.

US House of Representatives. "Departments of Labor, Health and Human Services, Education, and Related Agencies Appropriations for 1985, Part 4a: National Institutes of Health." Washington, DC: US Government Printing Office, 1984.

US House of Representatives. "Departments of Labor, Health and Human Services, Education, and Related Agencies Appropriations for 1985, Part 10: Testimony of Members of Congress and Other Interested Individuals and Organizations." Washington, DC: US Government Printing Office, 1984.

US House of Representatives. "Departments of Labor, Health and Human Services, Education, and Related Agencies Appropriations for 1987, Part 9: Testimony of Members of Congress and Other Interested Individuals and Organizations." Washington, DC: US Government Printing Office, 1986.

US House of Representatives. "Departments of Labor, Health and Human Services, Education, and Related Agencies Appropriations for 1990, Part 8: Testimony of Members of Congress and Other Interested Individuals and Organizations." Washington, DC: US Government Printing Office, 1989.

US House of Representatives. "Departments of Labor, Health and Human Services, Education, and Related Agencies Appropriations for 1991, Part 8a: Testimony of Members of Congress and Other Interested Individuals and Organizations." Washington, DC: US Government Printing Office, 1990.

US House of Representatives. "Departments of Labor, Health and Human Services, Education, and Related Agencies Appropriations for 1993, Part 8a: Testimony of Members of Congress and Other Interested Individuals and Organizations." Washington, DC: US Government Printing Office, 1992.

US House of Representatives. "Departments of Labor, Health and Human Services, Education, and Related Agencies Appropriations for 1995, Part 4: National Institutes of Health." Washington, DC: US Government Printing Office, 1994.

US House of Representatives. "Departments of Labor, Health and Human Services, Education, and Related Agencies Appropriations for 1995, Part 7: Testimony of Members of Congress and Other Interested Individuals and Organizations." Washington, DC: US Government Printing Office, 1994.

US House of Representatives. "Departments of Labor, Health and Human Services, Education, and Related Agencies Appropriations for 1998, Part 4b: National Institutes of Health." Washington, DC: US Government Printing Office, 1997.

US House of Representatives. "Departments of Labor, Health and Human Services, Education, and Related Agencies Appropriations for 1998, Part 7a: Testimony of Members of Congress and Other Interested Individuals and Organizations." Washington, DC: US Government Printing Office, 1997.

US House of Representatives. "Departments of Labor, Health and Human Services, Education, and Related Agencies Appropriations for 2000, Part 4a: National Institutes of Health." Washington, DC: US Government Printing Office, 1999.

US House of Representatives. "Departments of Labor, Health and Human Services, Education, and Related Agencies Appropriations for 2000, Part 7a: Testimony of Members of Congress and Other Interested Individuals and Organizations." Washington, DC: US Government Printing Office, 1999.

US House of Representatives. "Departments of Labor, Health and Human Services, Education, and Related Agencies Appropriations for 2001, Part 7b: Testimony of Members of Congress and Other Interested Individuals and Organizations." Washington, DC: US Government Printing Office, 2000.

US House of Representatives. "Departments of Labor, Health and Human Services, Education, and Related Agencies Appropriations for 2009, Part 7: Statements of Members of Congress and Other Interested Individuals and Organizations." Washington, DC: US Government Printing Office, 2008.

US House of Representatives. "Lobbying Disclosure Act." 1995. http://lobbyingdisclosure. house.gov/lda.html.

US Senate. "Biomedical Research Priorities: Who Should Decide?" Washington, DC: US Government Printing Office, 1997.

US Senate. "Conquest of Cancer Act." Washington, DC: US Government Printing Office, 1971.

US Senate. "Lobbying Disclosure Act." 1995. http://www.senate.gov/legislative/ Lobbying/Lobby_Disclosure_Act/3_Definitions.htm.

US Senate. "Lobbying Disclosure Act Database." n.d. Accessed September 20, 2018. https://soprweb.senate.gov/index.cfm?event=selectfields.

Varmus, Harold. "Evaluating the Burden of Disease and Spending the Research Dollars of the National Institutes of Health." *New England Journal of Medicine* 349, no. 24 (1999): 1914–15.

Varmus, Harold E., and Marc W. Kirschner. "Don't Undermine Basic Research." *New York Times*, September 29, 1992.

Verba, Sidney, Kay Lehman Schlozman, and Henry E. Brady. *Voice and Equality: Civic Voluntarism in American Politics*. Cambridge, MA: Harvard University Press, 1995.

Voetsch, Karen, Sonia Sequeira, and Amy Holmes Chavez. "A Customizable Model for Chronic Disease Coordination: Lessons Learned from the Coordinated Chronic Disease Program." *Preventing Chronic Disease* 13 (2016): 150509.

Wachter, Robert M. "AIDS, Activism, and the Politics of Health." *New England Journal of Medicine* 326, no. 2 (1992): 128–33.

Walder, Andrew G. "Political Sociology and Social Movements." *Annual Review of Sociology* 35, no. 1 (2009): 393–412.

Walker, Edward T. *Grassroots for Hire: Public Affairs Consultants in American Democracy*. Cambridge and New York: Cambridge University Press, 2014.

Walker, Edward T., John D. McCarthy, and Frank Baumgartner. "Replacing Members with Managers? Mutualism Among Membership and Nonmembership Advocacy Organizations in the United States." *American Journal of Sociology* 116, no. 4 (2011): 1284–1337.

Walker, Edward T., and Lina Stepick. "Valuing the Cause: A Theory of Authenticity in Social Movements." *Mobilization*, forthcoming.

Walker, Jack L. *Mobilizing Interest Groups in America: Patrons, Professions, and Social Movements*. Ann Arbor: University of Michigan Press, 1991.

Walker, Jack L. "The Origins and Maintenance of Interest Groups in America." *American Political Science Review* 77, no. 2 (1983): 390–406.

Wang, Dan, Alessandro Piazza, and Sarah A. Soule. "Boundary-Spanning in Social Movements: Antecedents and Outcomes." *Annual Review of Sociology* 44, no. 1 (2018): 167–87.

Warner, John Harley. *The Therapeutic Perspective: Medical Practice, Knowledge, and Identity in America, 1820–1885*. Cambridge, MA: Harvard University Press, 1986.

Washington Post Editorial Board. "NIH Research Is Ailing from the Budget Squeeze." *Washington Post*, December 5, 2013.

Waters, Malcolm. "Succession in the Stratification System: A Contribution to the 'Death of Class' Debate." *International Sociology* 9, no. 3 (1994): 295–312.

Watkins-Hayes, Celeste. *Remaking a Life*. Berkeley: University of California Press, 2019.

Wayne, Alex. "GOP Budget Cuts Would Hurt Research, NIH Says." *Washington Post*, November 10, 2010.

Weakliem, David L. "Race versus Class? Racial Composition and Class Voting, 1936–1992." *Social Forces* 75, no. 3 (1997): 939–56.

Weber, Max. *General Economic History*. Mineola, NY: Dover Publications, 2003.

Wehling, Peter, Willy Viehover, and Sophia Koenen, eds. *The Public Shaping of Medical Research: Patient Associations, Health Movements and Biomedicine*. Routledge Studies in the Sociology of Health and Illness. London: Routledge, 2014.

Weiner, Bernard, Raymond P. Perry, and Jamie Magnusson. "An Attributional Analysis of Reactions to Stigmas." *Journal of Personality and Social Psychology* 55, no. 5 (1988): 738–48.

Weiner, Tim. "Congress Chafing at Spending Caps: Both Parties See Urgent Need to Evade '97 Budget Deal." *New York Times*. July 31, 1999.

Weiner, Tim. "Senate Approves Budget Package, Ending Deadlock." *New York Times*, November 20, 1999.

Weir, Margaret. "Ideas and the Politics of Bounded Innovation." In *Structuring Politics: Historical Institutionalism in Comparative Analysis*, edited by Sven Steinmo, Kathleen Ann Thelen, and Frank Longstreth, 188–216. Cambridge and New York: Cambridge University Press, 1992.

Weisman, Carol S. *Women's Health Care: Activist Traditions and Institutional Change*. Baltimore, MD: Johns Hopkins University Press, 1998.

Weiss, Rick. "War Between Sexes Rages over Research; Funds to Study Prostate, Breast Cancer at Issue." *Washington Post*, August 6, 1996.

Welch, H. Gilbert, Lisa M. Schwartz, and Steven Woloshin. *Overdiagnosed: Making People Sick in the Pursuit of Health*. Boston: Beacon Press, 2011.

Whetten, David A. "Albert and Whetten Revisited: Strengthening the Concept of Organizational Identity." *Journal of Management Inquiry* 15, no. 3 (2006): 219–34.

White, Joseph. "Budgeting and Health Policymaking." In *Intensive Care: How Congress Shapes Health Policy*, edited by Thomas E. Mann and Norman J. Ornstein, 53–78. Washington, DC: American Enterprise Institute and Brookings Institution, 1995.

Whittier, Nancy. "The Consequences of Social Movements for Each Other." In *The Blackwell Companion to Social Movements*, edited by David A. Snow, Sarah A. Soule, and Hanspeter Kriesi, 531–51. Oxford: Wiley-Blackwell, 2004.

Wiebe, Robert H. *The Search for Order, 1877–1920*. Making of America. New York: Hill and Wang, 1967.

Wildavsky, Aaron. *The New Politics of the Budgetary Process*. Glenview, IL: Scott, Foresman and Company, 1988.

Williams, Simon J., and Michael Calnan. "The 'Limits' of Medicalization? Modern Medicine and the Lay Populace in 'Late' Modernity." *Social Science & Medicine* 42, no. 12 (1996): 1609–20.

Wilson, James Q. *Political Organizations*. New York: Basic Books, 1973.

Wilson, James Q. *The Politics of Regulation*. New York: Basic Books, 1980.

Wilson, Scott. "Bruised by Stimulus Battle, Obama Changed His Approach to Washington." *Washington Post*, April 29, 2009.

Wolfe, Audra J. "Giving Philanthropy a New History." *Historical Studies in the Natural Sciences* 43, no. 5 (2013): 619–30.

Wolfson, Mark. *The Fight Against Big Tobacco: The Movement, the State, and the Public's Health*. New York: Aldine de Gruyter, 2001.

Women's Community Cancer Project Archives. "Report from Jean Powers, National Breast Cancer Coalition, December 12, 1994 Meeting, Washington, D.C." Box 1, Minutes. Cambridge, MA: Women's Community Cancer Project Archives, 1995.

Women's Community Cancer Project Archives. "Report from the March National Breast Cancer Coalition Board Meeting." Box 1, Minutes. Cambridge, MA: Women's Community Cancer Project Archives, 1995.

Wood, Bruce. *Patient Power? The Politics of Patients' Associations in Britain and America*. Philadelphia: Open University Press, 2000.

Wuthnow, Robert. *Sharing the Journey: Support Groups and America's New Quest for Community*. New York: Simon and Schuster, 1994.

Yeager, David Scott, Samuel B. Larson, Jon A. Krosnick, and Trevor Tompson. "Measuring Americans' Issue Priorities: A New Version of the Most Important Problem Question Reveals More Concern About Global Warming and the Environment." *Public Opinion Quarterly* 75, no. 1 (2011): 125–38.

Yetman, Michelle H., Robert J. Yetman, and Brad Badertscher. "Calibrating the Reliability of Publicly Available Nonprofit Taxable Activity Disclosures: Comparing IRS 990 and IRS 990-T Data." *Nonprofit and Voluntary Sector Quarterly* 38, no. 1 (2008): 95–116.

Zald, Mayer N., and Roberta Ash. "Social Movement Organizations: Growth, Decay and Change." *Social Forces* 44, no. 3 (1966): 327–41.

Zald, Mayer N., and John D. McCarthy. "Social Movement Industries: Competition and Cooperation Among Movement Organizations." *Research in Social Movements, Conflict, and Change* 3 (1980): 1–20.

Zavestoski, Stephen, Phil Brown, Meadow Linder, Sabrina McCormick, and Brian Mayer. "Science, Policy, Activism, and War: Defining the Health of Gulf War Veterans." *Science, Technology & Human Values* 27, no. 2 (2002): 171–205.

Zerhouni, Elias A. "NIH in the Post-Doubling Era: Realities and Strategies." *Science*, 314, no. 5802 (2006): 1088–90.

Zhu, Jian-Hua. "Issue Competition and Attention Distraction: A Zero-Sum Theory of Agenda-Setting." *Journalism Quarterly* 69, no. 4 (1992): 825–36.

Zones, Jane S. "Profits from Pain: The Political Economy of Breast Cancer." In *Breast Cancer: Society Shapes an Epidemic*, edited by Anne S. Kasper and Susan J. Ferguson, 119–52. New York: Palgrave Macmillan, 2002.

Zuckerman, Ezra W. "The Categorical Imperative: Securities Analysts and the Illegitimacy Discount." *American Journal of Sociology* 104, no. 5 (1999): 1398–1438.

Zunz, Olivier. *Philanthropy in America: A History*. Princeton, NJ: Princeton University Press, 2011.

Index